Healing
with Complementary
& Alternative Therapies

Healing
with Complementary
& Alternative Therapies

LYNN KEEGAN
RN, PhD, HNC, FAAN

DELMAR

™

THOMSON LEARNING

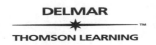

DELMAR

THOMSON LEARNING™

Healing with Complementary & Alternative Therapies
by Lynn Keegan RN, PhD, HNC, FAAN

Business Unit Director:
William Brottmiller

Product Development Manager:
Marion S. Waldman

Product Development Editor:
Jill Rembetski

Editorial Assistant:
Penelope Cartwright

Executive Marketing Manager:
Dawn Gerrain

Channel Manager:
Gretta Oliver

Executive Production Manager:
Karen Leet

Project Editor:
Mary Ellen Cox

Production Coordinator:
Nina Lontrato

Art/Design Coordinator:
Jay Purcell

Library of Congress Cataloging-in-Publication Data

Keegan, Lynn.
    Healing with complementary and alternative therapies / Lynn Keegan.
      p. cm.
    ISBN 0-7668-1890-X
    1. Alternative medicine. 2. Healing.
I. Title.
R733 .K44 2000
615.5—dc21

00-063858

NOTICE TO THE READER

Publisher does not warrant or guarantee any of the products described herein or perform any independent analysis in connection with any of the product information contained herein. Publisher does not assume, and expressly disclaims, any obligation to obtain and include information other than that provided to it by the manufacturer.

The reader is expressly warned to consider and adopt all safety precautions that might be indicated by the activities herein and to avoid all potential hazards. By following the instructions contained herein, the reader willingly assumes all risks in connection with such instructions.

The Publisher makes no representation or warranties of any kind, including but not limited to, the warranties of fitness for particular purpose or merchantability, nor are any such representations implied with respect to the material set forth herein, and the publisher takes no responsibility with respect to such material. The publisher shall not be liable for any special, consequential, or exemplary damages resulting, in whole or part, from the readers' use of, or reliance upon, this material.

CONTENTS

Preface   xv

PART I   THE JOURNEY

Chapter 1   CONCEPT OF HEALING   3

Introduction   3
Relationship of Healing to Alternative and
    Complementary Care   4
Healing Philosophies and Schools of Thought   4
    Allopathic (Western) Medicine   5
    Ayurvedic Medicine   6
    Chiropractic   6
    Environmental Medicine   7
    Herbalism   7
    Holistic Dentistry   8
    Homeopathy   8
    Midwifery   10
    Naturopathic Medicine   11
    Osteopathic Medicine   13
    Shamanism   13
    Traditional Chinese (Oriental) Medicine   14
Beliefs about Healing   15
    Faith Healing   15
    Mind Cures   15
    Metaphysical or Mental Healing   16
    Spiritualism   16
    Mesmerism   16
    Energy Medicine and Aura Fields   16
    Hypnotism   17
    Natural Healing   17
Resurgence of Natural Healing   17
Joining of Eastern and Western Philosophies   19
Healing versus Curing   21

Chapter 2   HISTORY AND FUTURE OF HEALING   24

Healing in Antiquity   24
    Primitive Cultures   24
    Eastern and Indian Cultures   25
    Ancient Greek and Roman Period   28
    The Enchanted World   29
The New Worldview   29
    Reawakening of Holistic Health Care   31
    Wellness Paradigm   31
    Modern Holistic Health Movement   33
Contemporary Times   33
    Changing Demographics   34
    Baby Boomers   34
    Multicultural Impact   35
Federal Government Initiatives   36
    What Is *Healthy People?*   36
    Healthy People 2010   37
Healing in the New Millennium   37
    Healing Centers   38

Chapter 3   DRIVING MARKET FORCES   41

Surge in Alternative Health Care   41
    Financial Factors   43
    Increase in Chronic Diseases   46
    Overreliance on Prescription Drugs   46
    Physician Referrals   47
State and Regional Differences   47
Education Changes   49
    Medical Schools   50
    Nursing Programs   50
Organizations   50
Societal Changes   51
    Change in Societal Self-Image   52
    Technology   52
Healing in the Arts   52
    Radio   52
Computer Influence   53
Healthy Partnerships: Hospitals Link Up
    with the Internet   54
Telemedicine   55
    In Education   55
    For Providers   55
    Consumer Use   56
Projections for the Future   57

PART II COMPLEMENTARY AND ALTERNATIVE APPROACHES TO HEALING

Chapter 4 ALTERNATIVE AND COMPLEMENTARY
THERAPIES   63

Nature of Alternative and Complementary
  Therapies   63
Office of Alternative Medicine   64
  History of the OAM   65
  Purpose of the OAM/NCCAM   66
  Mission of the OAM/NCCAM   66
  Budget of the OAM/NCCAM   66
  OAM Programs   66
  Sponsored Research   67
  Research Centers   68
  Research Database and Evaluation   68
Classification of CAM Practices   69
  Other Classification Systems   75
Strategies for Use and Practice   76
  Safety and Effectiveness of
    Alternative Therapies   76
  Practitioner's Expertise   77
  Service Delivery   78
  Costs   79
  Discussing All Issues with Your Client   79

Chapter 5 INTEGRATIVE MEDICINE   82

Introduction   82
Factors Influencing Development of
  Integrative Health Care Centers   82
Model Centers   83
  Wellness Centers   84
  Related Practices   84
Focus of Care   84
Healers Working in Wellness Centers   85
Continuing Education in Integrative Medicine   86
Existing Hospital Practice Implications   87
  Advantages to Hospital for Implementing
    a CAP Program   89
Business Aspects of Integrative Health Care
  Programs   89
  Budgetary Considerations   90
Projections for the Future   90

PART III   HEALING MODALITIES

Chapter 6   HERBAL MEDICINE, NUTRITION, AND
                  SUPPLEMENTS   100

                  Herbal Medicine   100
                       Overview   100
                       Practitioners   103
                       Training Requirements   104
                       Treatment   104
                       Advice to Patients   107
                       Research   107
                  Nutrition and Special Diet Therapies   109
                       Overview   110
                       Practitioners   114
                       Treatment   115
                       Advice to Patients   115
                       Research   117
                  Nutritional Supplements   119
                       Overview   119
                       Practitioners   121
                       Advice to Patients   121
                       Research   121

Chapter 7   HOMEOPATHY   130

                  Overview   130
                       History   132
                       Regulation   132
                  Practitioners   133
                       Training Requirements   134
                  Treatment   135
                  Advice to Patients   138
                  Research   139
                       Studies Supporting Use of Homeopathy   139
                       Studies Not Supporting Use of Homeopathy   139
                       Studies with Neutral Conclusions   141

Chapter 8   NATUROPATHY   147

                  Overview   147
                       History   147
                       Principles   148
                  Practitioners   149
                       Training Requirements   149
                       Licensure Requirements   151
                       Regulation   151

Treatment   151
Advice to Patients   153
Research   154

Chapter 9   MIND-BODY THERAPIES   158

Introduction   158
Psychotherapy   158
    Practitioners and Training Requirements   159
    Treatment   160
    Body-Oriented Psychotherapy   161
    Core Energetics   161
    Gestalt Therapy   162
    Pathwork   162
    Advice to Patients   162
    Research   163
Art Therapy   164
    Practitioners   165
    Treatment   166
    Research   168
Music (Sound) Therapies   168
    Overview   168
    Practitioners   170
    Treatment   170
    Research   170
Imagery   171
    Overview   171
    Practitioners   172
    Guided Imagery   172
    Treatment   173
    Rebirthing   175
Hypnosis   176
    Overview   176
    Practitioners   176
    Treatment   177
    Advice to Patients   178
    Research   179
Meditation   180
    History   181
    Practitioners   181
    Meditation Practice   181
    Mindfulness   182
    Focusing   182
    Relaxation Response   182
    Research   183

Chapter 10   POSTURE AND MOBILITY   189

Introduction   189
Movement Therapies   190
 Practitioners   191
 Alexander Technique   191
 Aston Patterning   192
 Body-Mind Centering   192
 Dance/Movement Therapies   192
 Feldenkrais Method   193
 Gyrotonics   194
 Pilates Method   194
 Rosen Method   195
 Advice to Patients   196
 Research   196
Tai Chi   196
 History   197
 Practitioners   198
 The Practice   198
 Qigong   199
 Advice to Patients   200
Yoga   203
 Practitioners   204
 Techniques of Yoga   205
 Phoenix Rising Yoga Therapy   205
 Kripalu Yoga   205
 Advice to Patients   206
 Research   206

Chapter 11   TOUCH THERAPIES AND BODYWORK   210

Introduction   210
The Modalities   211
Massage Therapy   212
 Overview   212
 Practitioners   214
 Treatment   214
 Infant Massage   217
 Bodywork   217
 Advice to Patients   222
Acupressure   224
 Overview   224
 Practitioners   224
 Treatment   225
 Advice to Patients   229

Chapter 12 CHIROPRACTIC   234
                Introduction   234
                    Overview   234
                    History   235
                Practitioners   236
                    Training Requirements   236
                    Licensure   237
                Treatment   238
                Advice to Patients   240
                    Cautions   241
                Research   242
                    U.S. Government Endorses Effectiveness   242
                    Cost-effectiveness: *The Manga Report, 1993*   243
                    Journal of Manipulative and Physiological
                        Therapeutics, 1993   243
                    Chiropractors Best Qualified to Perform
                        Manual Manipulation   243

Chapter 13 ENERGETIC THERAPIES   247
                Introduction   247
                    Overview   247
                    History   248
                Practitioners   248
                The Therapies   249
                    Barbara Brennan Healing Science   249
                    Bioenergetics   249
                    Biofeedback   250
                    Biological Terrain Assessment (BTA 1000)   250
                    Healing Touch   250
                    Magnet Therapy   252
                    Neurofeedback   256
                    Polarity Therapy   256
                    Reiki   257
                    Robert Jaffe Advanced Healing Energy   258
                    SHEN Therapy   258
                    Spiritual Healing   258
                    Therapeutic Touch   259
                Advice to Patients   261

Chapter 14 EASTERN THERAPIES   267
                Introduction   267
                Traditional Chinese Medicine   267
                Acupuncture   269
                    Overview   269
                    Practitioners   272

Treatment	273
Advice to Patients	275
Research	276
AMMA Therapy	278
Overview	278
Practitioners	279
Treatment	279
Advice to Patients	280

Chapter 15   MISCELLANEOUS THERAPIES   283

Introduction	283
Practitioners	284
Aquatherapy/Hydrotherapy	284
Aromatherapy	285
Astrology	285
Aura-Soma Color Therapy	287
Breathwork	287
Chanting	287
Chelation Therapy	288
Colon Therapy	288
Feng Shui	291
Holotrophic Breathwork	291
Iridology	291
Kinesiology	292
Applied Kinesiology	292
Educational Kinesiology	293
Health Kinesiology	293
Advice to Patients	293
Research	293
Light Therapy	295
Seasonal Affective Disorder (SAD)	296
Jaundice in Newborns	297
Pet Therapy	298
Rapid Eye Technology	298

PART IV   **HEALERS AND THE HEALED**

Chapter 16   THE PROCESS OF BECOMING A HEALER   303

Introduction	303
Developing Healing Traits	306
Living from a Place of Authenticity	306
Forgiveness	306
Love	309

| | Altruism | 313 |
| | Compassion | 313 |

Chapter 17 ATTITUDES AND BEHAVIORS OF HEALERS 318

Healing Attitudes	318
Joy and Empowerment through Service	318
Caring for Others as an Extension of the Self	321
A Sense of Purpose	322
Behaviors of Healers	325
Being Fully Present	325
Listening	327
Empathy	332
Attention to Detail	334

Chapter 18 HEALING OURSELVES AND OUR ENVIRONMENT 338

Introduction	338
Healing Yourself	338
Self-Care Begins with Assessment	339
Personal Options to Stay Fit	342
Chronic Disease and Self-Care	343
Basic Self-Care Approaches for Maintaining and Improving Your Health	343
Obesity in America	344
Start Good Eating Habits Early with Children	346
Healthy Digestion	348
Components of a Healthy Diet	348
Exercise	350
Relaxation Techniques	350
Massage	352
Healing Our Environment	354
Overview of Some Environmental Problems	355
Personal Space	357
Joint Space Work Environments	357

PART V   BODY-MIND-SPIRIT CONNECTION TO HEALTH AND ILLNESS

Chapter 19 CONSCIOUSNESS AND HEALING 365

History, Science, and a Shifting Paradigm	365
Awakening Consciousness	366
Mindful Living	366
Daily Ritual	367

Awareness in Healing 368
    Theories of Awareness 369
    Barriers to Awareness and Healing 371
    Creativity and Healing Awareness 372
Healing Meditation 374
    Meditation Process 374
    Modern Medicine and Ancient Therapeutics 374
    Elements of Meditation 375
    Behavioral Aspects of Meditation 375
    Meditation and Behavior Modification 376
Spirituality and Healing 378
    Forming a Spiritual Group 378

Chapter 20 STRESS AND ITS CONSEQUENCES 381
Introduction 381
What Is Stress and How Does It Occur? 382
    Factors That Contribute to Stress 383
    Determining Stress Levels 384
Fight-or-Flight Response 384
    How Stress Biochemistry Causes Illness 385
    Hans Selye 387
    Effect of Negative Stress 389
Types of Stressors 390
    Changes When the Body is under Stress 390
    Role of General Adaptation Syndrome 392
Stress and Illness 392
    Effects of Stress on the Body's Immune System 393
    Stress and Colds 394
    Stress and Skin Disease 394
    Stress and Heart Disease 395
Stress Management 396
    Learn to Change Anxiety to Concern 398
    Tolerance to Stress 398
    Coping Statements 399
    Behavioral Psychology 400
Stress and Exercise 401
    Using Tai Chi to Combat Stress 401
Coping with Stress 402
    Taking Care of Yourself 402

Chapter 21 BOLSTERING THE IMMUNE SYSTEM 406
Introduction 406
Our Immune Army 407
How the Immune System Works 407
    Organs of the Immune System 408
    Cells of the Immune System 408
    The Immune Response 410

Body-Mind Physiology and Neuropeptides   411
   Immunity and Stress   411
Learning and Memory   412
   Conditioned Response   412
   Psychedelic Drugs and the Immune System   413
Joy, Optimism, and Hope   414
Physical Exercise   415
   Beginning an Exercise Program   417
   Aerobic Fitness   418
   Recovery Phase   420
   Make It Fun   423
Healing Nutrition   423
   A Basic Plan   423
   Herbs as Immune Boosting Foods   425
   Herbs as Medicine   426
   Some Foods Harm   428
   Fuel for the Immune Cells   429
   Nutrition Cautions   430
   Imbalance in the Immune System   430
   Malnutrition and the Immune System   430
   Stress Reduction Is Essential to
      Immune Health   431

PART VI HEALING RESOURCES AND SUPPORT NETWORKS

Chapter 22 ALTERNATIVE AND COMPLEMENTARY
   HEALTH CARE RESOURCES   437
Introduction   437
Associations, Organizations, and Educational
   Institutions   437
On-Line Libraries and Journals   461
Conducting Internet Searches on Alternative
   Medicine Subjects   462
   Commercial Internet Sites   463
Conferences   465
Support Groups   465

Appendix 1 SUPPLEMENTARY RESEARCH DATA AND
   REPORTS   467

Appendix 2 INTEGRATIVE CARE CENTERS AND
   WELLNESS CENTERS   485

Glossary   489

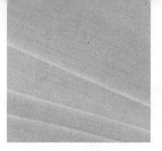

PREFACE

INTRODUCTION

The twenty-first century is upon us and health care providers have awakened to the paradigm shift that calls for the incorporation of alternative and complementary approaches into the traditional twentieth-century delivery system. Nurses, doctors, massage therapists, physical therapists, pharmacists, psychologists, insurance adjusters, and the whole field of allied health professionals are answering the call to use new methodologies to care for the ill and to augment the health levels of those who are well.

PURPOSE OF THIS BOOK

Why a new book on healing? Why now and why this book? *Healing with Complementary and Alternative Therapies* is a volume that has been in gestation for some time. It is the culmination of a long-term relationship between a leading edge publisher and an author who have worked on numerous projects together. In 1992, William Burgower, an editor at Delmar, asked me if I would like to author a book with the word *healer* in the title. Since at that time my work was directed solely toward nurses, it seemed natural to title the book *The Nurse as Healer*. Mr. Burgower had the vision to see the changes that were close at hand and wanted Delmar to lead the crest of the wave that was coming. This was the first professional nursing book to have the term *healer* in the title.

In 1994 *The Nurse as Healer* was published as one of the last books in Delmar's The Real Nursing Series. *The Nurse as Healer,* its message, and the concept were so well received that an entire new series bearing the same name as the first book was introduced in 1996. The titles in that series spread the concept of healing wide and far in the arena of nursing education, nursing practice, and allied health. After four years, those books are still so popular that new titles in the series are being added yearly.

The concept of the "nurse as healer" was not new; just as there is nothing new under the sun, simply new ways of looking at things, this concept has been around for awhile. Barbara Dossey first elucidated the idea in 1988 in the first edition of Aspen Publishers' coauthored text, *Holistic Nursing: A Handbook for Practice,* now available in the third edition. Since the 1980s, seminars, workshops, and keynote addresses have advanced the theory that nurses can also be healers.

Other professional and trade publishers soon followed the lead of the concepts introduced in the 1980s by including the term *healing* in the title of their publications. Shortly thereafter in the mid- to late 1990s, a plethora of books using the keywords healing, alternative health, and complementary therapies began appearing in the marketplace. These books were for physicians, nurses, and allied health professions, but most of all the books were directed to consumers of health care. A few reference books also appeared. Delmar Thomson Learning, who began the trend to offer healing-oriented books to professionals in the early 1990s, decided once again to lead by developing a definitive reference book for the new millennium. This time a new visionary editor, Marion Waldman, along with publisher William Brottmiller asked me if I was interested in the project. I agreed it would be a delight to develop a book about healing by blending and creating something new from the best of what is currently known and projecting all that is possible.

The staff at Delmar and I have worked closely together to bring you what we consider to be the most important elements of the state-of-the-art healing practices of today. This book and your own personal searching style will enable you to access the best of what is known to date and show you how to open the doors for your future.

ORGANIZATION OF THE TEXT

Healing with Complementary and Alternative Therapies is divided into six parts. Part I, Concept of Healing, has three chapters. The focus is on types of healing, the history and future of healing, and the driving market forces behind the surge in alternative health care. Part II, Complementary and Alternative Approaches to Healing, has two chapters, one that focuses on the nature and classification systems for the therapies and another that focuses on integrative health care. Part III, Healing Modalities, contains 10 chapters that discuss a wide range of selected healing modalities. Part IV, Healers and the Healed, has three chapters that relate to the process of becoming a healer, the attitudes and behaviors of healers, and a chapter about healing ourselves and our environment. Part V, Body-Mind-Spirit Connection to Health and Illness, contains three chapters that deal with consciousness and healing, stress and its consequences, and bolstering the immune system. Finally, Part VI covers alternative and complementary care resources and includes detailed information on organizations, Web sites, conferences, and support groups. The Appendices contain additional research reports and information about the modalities and philosophies described in the text as well as examples of an integrative care center. Finally there is a Glossary of terms.

FEATURES

Healing with Complementary and Alternative Therapies has several special features. Throughout the book, concepts are illustrated with healing stories that depict real-life anecdotes and experiences. These stories bring the concepts to life and deal with everyday occurrences that could be applicable to your setting. Another unique feature of this text is the use of research boxes. The shift to alternative and complementary care is toward an evidenced-based practice; that is, many traditional practitioners want to use therapies that have documented research findings to support and validate their effectiveness. Throughout the text, the most up-to-date research is cited to illustrate the concepts and give evidence of published scientific support. As new research becomes available in the coming years, you will find it on the Internet web site below. Also, many chapters include steps to implement the concepts and clinical implications.

ABOUT THE AUTHOR

Many of you may have heard me speak or may have read my work in previous journal or book publications as I have spoken at many conferences and published widely in journals for more than 20 years. My solo and co-authored book titles include:

Holistic Nursing: A Handbook for Practice, 3rd ed., Aspen Publishers, 2000

Healing Waters: The Miraculous Health Benefits of Earth's Most Essential Resource, Berkley/Putnam Publishers, 1998

Profiles of Nurse Healers, Delmar Publishers, 1997

The Art of Caring, Sounds True, 1997

Healing Nutrition, Delmar Publishers, 1996

The Nurse as Healer, Delmar Publishers, 1994

Self Care: A Program to Improve Your Life, Bodymind Systems, 1987

The Busy Person's Guide for Returning to School, Bodymind Systems, 1988

I earned my B.S. from Cornell University in New York, my M.S. from Loma Linda University in California, and my Ph.D. from The University of Texas at Austin. I have taught nursing at all levels at several major universities and colleges. These include Temple University in Philadelphia, Medical University of South Carolina, Texas Women's University, McLennan Community College in

Texas, and the University of Texas Health Science Center in San Antonio. In between teaching jobs I have held clinical positions, thus enabling me to continuously blend theory, research, and practice.

In 1997 I was inducted as a Fellow into The American Academy of Nursing (FAAN) and in 1998 became certified as a holistic nurse (HNC). Currently I work as an author and consultant in holistic health.

ACKNOWLEDGMENTS

The publisher, editors, and staff at Delmar Thomson Learning have been invaluable in bringing this book to fruition. Bill Brottmiller, Publisher, Marion Waldman, Project Development Manager, and Jill Rembetski, my Project Development Editor, were committed to the project from the onset and offered all the support any author could want. Mary Ellen Cox, Health Care Project Editor, was invaluable in fine tuning and bringing the project to closure.

I especially wish to thank all of the reviewers who took their time to read and comment on the manuscript. These professionals work hard behind the scenes to add important insights and suggestions prior to publication. Their names and affiliations are listed on the Reviewers Page.

AVENUE FOR FEEDBACK

Feedback is important to me and to Delmar Thomson Learning. Therefore, we have set up a mechanism for you to reach and dialogue with me. An Internet web page has been developed at: www.delmarnursing.com. Through this page you can ask questions, make comments, and read new material relating to alternative and complementary therapies. I encourage you to visit the site frequently and access as much material as you need about the exciting field of healing with alternative and complementary medicine.

Lynn Keegan, RN, PhD, HNC, FAAN

CONTRIBUTORS

Lennie Martin, RN, FNP, DPH
Sierra Family Medical Clinic
and Emeritus professor of nursing
Sonoma State University
Nevada City, CA
Co-author, Chapter 6

David Wells, DC, LAc
Medical Director
Landmark Healthcare
Sacramento, CA
Author, Chapter 12

REVIEWERS

Barry Bittman, MD
CEO
Mind-Body Wellness Center
Meadville, PA

Lea Gaydos, PhD, HNC, RN
Assistant Professor
Beth El College
Colorado Springs, CO

Karilee Halo Shames, RN, HNC, PhD
Assistant Professor
College of Nursing
Florida Atlantic University
Boca Raton, FL

Kathleen Palladino, BS, RN
Co-Director and Health Counselor
Angell Hill Wellness Center
Spencertown, NY

Kathleen Tanner
Health Care Consultant
Delmar, NY

Lizzie S. Teichler, RN-C, FNP, AHNC,
    PhD(C)
Assistant Professor
University of Colorado Health Science
    Center
School of Nursing
Denver, CO

Diane Wind Wardell, PhD, RNC, HNC,
    CHTP/I
Associate Professor
University of Texas Houston, Health
    Science Center
School of Nursing
Houston, TX

David Wells, DC, LAc
Medical Director
Landmark Healthcare
Sacramento, CA

The Journey

CHAPTER 1

Concept of Healing

Chapter Objectives

- Learn the range of and diversity between different healing philosophies.
- List types of healing and health care that are widely utilized.
- Learn about the resurgence of natural healing.
- Describe how patients may utilize different methods of healing.
- Understand how to implement alternative healing into caregiving.

INTRODUCTION

Healing is perhaps as mysterious and elusive as any term in our language. It is a word that conjures up thoughts of divinity in some and outright skepticism in others. It is a term that usually evokes an emotional reaction one way or the other. To those who have personally experienced healing episodes, it is a reality that the person feels strongly about and is often even eager to share. To others with minimal experience with disease and illness, the concept of healing may seem like an elusive phenomenon with no real relevance. Many view the healing phenomenon from their cultural background and philosophical viewpoint. Healing, therefore, is comprised of components of worldview, culture, and personal experience.

The *Webster's Collegiate American Dictionary, Tenth Edition*, defines *heal* as:

1. To make whole or sound; restore to health; free from ailment
2. To bring to an end or conclusion, as conflicts between two people, groups, etc., usually with the strong implication of restoring former amity; settle; reconcile
3. To free from evil; cleanse; purify; to heal the soul
4. To effect a cure
5. To become whole or sound; mend; get well

RELATIONSHIP OF HEALING TO ALTERNATIVE AND COMPLEMENTARY CARE

The concept of healing is as old as the history of people. *Alternative* and *complementary* care, although seemingly new terms, are likewise as old as the history of medicine. Accepted conventional medicine has undergone evolution solely because new and different methods of treatment, outside the mainstream, were tried. More times than not, these new methods were discarded when, because of trial and error, they were found ineffective or in some cases even dangerous. But in many instances the new alternative proved more effective than the accepted care. Thus the alternative became the conventional. In today's world, caregivers still seek to heal, while the controversy between conventional and alternative caregivers continues to evolve the practice.

HEALING PHILOSOPHIES AND SCHOOLS OF THOUGHT

Healing philosophies arise from a point of view, opinion, or method that has proven worthy over a period of time. Some of the philosophies cited in this chapter have their roots in antiquity, dating back many thousands of years, and represent many diverse cultures. Others began more recently, in the nineteenth and twentieth centuries, and have developed rapidly and have attracted many followers.

Individuals gravitate to a healing philosophy that mirrors their personality, culture, and/or worldview. Generally a philosophy offers broad principles and guidelines for practice.

The philosophies and schools of thought included in this chapter are not all inclusive but do contain those most commonly used. Many of the philosophies are derived from Western medicine but are different enough to stand alone. They are:

Allopathic or Western medicine

Ayurvedic medicine

Chiropractic

Environmental medicine

Herbal medicine

Holistic dentistry

Homeopathy

Midwifery

Natural medicine

Naturopathic medicine

Osteopathic medicine

Shamanism

Traditional Chinese medicine

Allopathic (Western) Medicine

Western medicine has its roots in Greek antiquity. Hippocrates, a Greek philosopher and physician, was the first to write about, catalog, and organize many of the disease conditions still recognized today. Although nursing nuns and nursing men worked alongside physicians throughout history, a nineteenth-century English nurse, Florence Nightingale, is recognized as the founder of modern, scientific nursing.

The term *allopathic* was originally coined by homeopathic physician Samuel Hahnemann in the nineteenth century, the term *allopathic medicine* is derived from Greek roots meaning "other than the disease." The term is used most often today to refer to conventional medical practice, as opposed to alternative practice philosophies such as homeopathy and herbal medicine. The thrust in allopathic medicine is to kill bacteria and to suppress symptoms such as fever, coughs, and diarrhea. The mechanism of action is to contradict and override the body's natural response to bacteria and viruses. Allopathic medicine is the most commonly practiced system of health care in America.

In the nineteenth and twentieth centuries, pathogenic organisms were discovered. Much of Western scientific medicine has developed because of this notion. Practitioners of germ theory believe that invading pathogenic organisms, that is, bacteria and viruses, cause most illness and disease. Many of these organisms can be prevented from entering the body with simple preventative techniques such as personal hygiene, public sanitation, and inoculations of vaccines. It is common for people to be immunized with tetanus, pertussis, diphtheria, polio, measles, and mumps vaccines. When one does become ill, scrupulous measures are then used to prevent the pathogenic organism from further multiplying. Sterile technique is employed to protect patients from further pathogen assault when the internal body undergoes surgery. Antibiotic and other pharmaceutical remedies are employed to combat the invading pathogens.

HOLISTIC HEALTH

Holistic health is a Western system of care directed toward integrating and balancing mind, body, and spirit. The word *holism* was first coined in South Africa in the mid-1920s and began its renaissance in North America in the 1970s. Holistic practitioners recognize that the causes of illness are complex. Disease is not seen as a purely external event, although environmental factors can be among the causative variables. In many instances, the mind and spirit, including thoughts, feelings, and emotions, are as important as the physical body's needs in maintaining health and recovering from illness. Holism embraces a philosophy that emphasizes personal responsibility and participation in one's own health care. It encompasses all safe modalities of diagnosis and treatment while emphasizing the whole person: physical, mental, emotional, and spiritual.

Holistic practitioners incorporate lifestyle patterning with other therapies that include the physical, mental, emotional, and spiritual aspects of intervention and support. In addition, these practitioners believe in the interrelationship of the body, mind, and spirit in an ever-changing environment. Many of the healing therapies are performed by an accomplished individual on her or his own behalf. It is more common, however, for another person serving as a conduit or channel to facilitate the process.

Ayurvedic Medicine

Practiced in India for more than 5000 years, the ayurvedic tradition views illness as a state of imbalance among the body's systems that can be detected through such diagnostic procedures as reading the pulse and examining the tongue. The term *ayurveda* is Sanskrit for "science of life," suggesting a holistic medicinal as well as spiritual orientation. Ayurveda maintains that illness is the result of falling out of balance with nature. Diagnosis is based on 3 metabolic body types called doshas: vata, pitta, and kapha. (There are an additional 10 subtypes based on these 3.) Treatment usually involves prescribing a diet, herbal remedies, breathwork, physical exercise, hatha yoga, meditation, and a rejuvenation or detoxification program. Nutrition counseling, massage, natural medications, meditation, and other healing modalities are used to address a broad spectrum of ailments, from allergies to acquired immunodeficiency syndrome (AIDS). Maharishi Ayur-Ved is a contemporary interpretation of ayurvedic medicine inspired by Maharishi Mahesh Yogi, the founder of transcendental meditation.

Chiropractic

The chiropractic system is based on the premise that the spine is literally the backbone of human health. Founded in 1895 by David Daniel Palmer of Iowa, chiropractic has a basic premise that is similar to osteopathic medicine in that it views the spinal column as central to one's entire well-being and instrumental in maintaining the health of the nervous system. Another basic belief is that if the body is functioning correctly, it will cure its own ills. Misalignments of the vertebrae caused by poor posture or trauma result in pressure on the spinal nerve roots, which may lead to diminished function and illness. The chiropractor seeks to analyze and correct these misalignments through spinal manipulation, abuse histories, eating disorders, and other concerns. Treatment involves the adjustment of the position of spinal vertebrae through manipulation and massage to restore the proper flow of nerve impulses to and from the spinal column. Various approaches are used by chiropractors. Some choose solely to free the spine from being misaligned, thereby allowing the body's "innate intelligence" to restore health. Others expand this process with diagnostic techniques, including X-rays, and may incorporate other modalities, such as Applied Kinesiology and nutritional counseling. Applied Kinesiology is a tradename and relates to the flow of nerve impulses from the brain through the spine to the whole body.

Environmental Medicine

Environmental medicine focuses on the relationship of environmental factors, such as allergens and chemical toxins, as a cause of chronic illness. Doctors of environmental medicine, whose focus is often primary or internal medicine, check for allergens in the environment and diet of the patient. Furnaces in the home or office building, for example, circulate dust as well as fuel fumes; household products, such as paints, synthetic fibers, and disinfectants that contain petrochemicals, can cause inorganic allergies; ammonia found in cleansers, fabric dyes, and fertilizers can cause allergic reactions—headaches, nausea, or panic attacks. Regarding diet, some individuals experience nausea, hives, or cold sores from the sulfites in wine or upset stomach and/or vomiting from dried fruit and nuts, which are often fumigated with methyl bromide. Homeopathy, nutritional supplements, diet, fasting, herbal remedies, and aromatherapy are some of the modalities used by doctors in environmental medicine to treat a multitude of allergic reactions that patients suffer as a consequence of environmental factors.

Herbalism

Herbalism is an ancient form of healing still widely used in much of the world. Herbalism uses plants or plant-based substances to treat illnesses and enhance the body's functioning. Though herbalism is not a licensed professional modality in the United States, herbs are "prescribed" by a range of practitioners from holistic doctors to acupuncturists to naturopathic physicians.

Records from ancient China, India, Rome, Egypt, and Persia reveal that herbs have been used throughout history as a basic practice in medicine. Today, virtually all naturopathic and homeopathic practitioners, and many holistic medical doctors, are trained in herbalism. The argument for using herbal medicines over pharmaceutical derivatives is that, when used in therapeutic doses, herbs are more natural, gentler, and less toxic for the body than synthetic drugs. Also, herbs can have multiple benefits, while drugs are often symptom specific. For instance, when used as prescribed, herbs can cleanse and purify the body without side effects, stimulate the body's immune system, and regulate and tone the lymphatic system.

Herbalists believe that the activity and therapeutic effects of a plant result from the combined action of the many constituents working together. This is reflected in holistic thought—"the whole is greater than the sum of the parts." Another tenent of herbal medicine is that some constituents in the whole plant may "buffer" some otherwise harmful side effects.

CLASSIFICATION OF HERBS

Because herbs have multiple constituents, most have a broad spectrum of uses. However, most can be classified according to the body systems over which they have the most influence (see Table 1-1).

TABLE 1-1	Classification of Herbs
NERVINES: USED TO TREAT DISORDERS OF THE NERVOUS SYSTEM St. John's wort Valerian Vervain Skullcap	**CIRCULATORY STIMULANTS** Hawthorn Rosemary Gingko Capsicum Ginger Bog myrtle

Holistic Dentistry

Holistic dentists are licensed dentists who practice an interdisciplinary approach, often working with other alternative treatment modalities. They often incorporate such methods as homeopathy, nutrition, and acupuncture into their treatment plans. Most holistic dentists emphasize wellness and preventive care, focusing on the interrelation of mouth to body. A holistic dentist will treat the teeth after first collecting information about the person's past and present health issues, because work done on the mouth can affect the patient's overall well-being. No silver filling material is used (silver alloy contains mercury, which is toxic to human tissues), and many holistic dentists will recommend removal of mercury amalgam fillings and instead use fillings that do not contain mercury. Patients are tested to see if gold is a compatible metal before it is used in the mouth.

Homeopathy

Homeopathy is a medical system that uses infinitesimal doses of natural substances, called remedies, to stimulate a person's immune and defense system. A remedy is individually chosen for a sick person based on its capacity to cause, if given in overdose, physical and psychological symptoms similar to those a patient is experiencing. Homeopathy addresses such common conditions as infant and childhood diseases, infections, fatigue, allergies, and chronic illnesses, including arthritis and asthma.

Homoios means "similar" and *pathos* means "disease." Homeopathy operates on the principle that, upon introduction of a substance that is similar to the disease the patient is suffering from, the body will respond by mobilizing its natural defenses against the disease agent. Therefore, homeopathy primarily works with remedies that are solutions containing infinitesimal doses of plant, mineral, and

RESEARCH BOX: Clinical Effects of Homeopathy

Homeopathy seems scientifically implausible but has widespread use. In this study, scientists assessed whether the clinical effect reported in randomized controlled trials of homeopathic remedies is equivalent to that reported for placebo. The methods they used were made from studies of computerized bibliographies and contracts with researchers, institutions, manufacturers, individual collectors, homeopathic conference proceedings, and books. Double-blind and/or randomized placebo-controlled trials of clinical conditions were considered. A review of 185 trials identified 119 that met the inclusion criteria. Eighty-nine had adequate data for meta-analysis, and two sets of trials were used to assess reproducibility. Two reviewers assessed study quality with two scales and extracted data for information on clinical condition, homeopathy type, dilution, "remedy," population, and outcomes. The combined odds ratio for the 89 studies entered into the main meta-analysis was 2.45 (95% CI 2.05, 2.93) in favor of homeopathy. The odds ratio for the 26 good-quality studies was 1.66 (1.33, 2.08), and that corrected for publication bias was 1.78 (1.03, 3.10). Four studies on the effects of a single remedy on seasonal allergies had a pooled odds ratio for ocular symptoms at 4 weeks of 2.03 (1.51, 2.74). Five studies on postoperative ileus had a pooled mean effect size difference of -0.22 standard deviations (SD; 95% CI -0.36, -0.09) for flatus and -0.18 SD (-0.33, -0.03) for stool (both $p < 0.05$). The results of the meta-analysis are not compatible with the hypothesis that the clinical effects of homeopathy are completely due to placebo.

Source: Linde, K., Clausius, N., Ramirez, G., Melchart, D., Eitel, F., Hedges, L. V., & Jonas, W. B. (1998). Are the clinical effects of homeopathy placebo effects? A meta-analysis of placebo-controlled trials. *Lancet, 350*(9081), 834–843.

animal matter that, when administered in prescribed doses, gently affect the desired healing response in the body. Homeopaths interview their patients in great detail to discover all physical and psychological symptoms they may be experiencing.

FLOWER ESSENCES

Flower essence therapy was first developed in England in the 1930s by Edward Bach, a physician. Flower essences fall under the umbrella of homeopathic remedies, although they differ slightly in content, theory, and approach from other types of homeopathic remedies. Bach believed that many illnesses were the result of an imbalance of negative emotions and that the "essence" of certain flowers helped balance these emotions. Flower essences are intended to alleviate negative emotional states that may contribute to illness or hinder personal growth. Once balanced, the body could then mobilize naturally against such a disease state and restore itself to health. Bach created 38 remedies derived from flowers and divided them into seven groups to cover all known negative emotional states; the most famous is an all-purpose remedy called the "rescue remedy," to be taken during an emotional crisis. Flower essences are usually found in the form of a tincture of flower essence and alcoholic extract; drops are administered either under the tongue or by rubbing them in on pulse points. The practitioner helps the client choose appropriate essences, focusing on the client's emotional state rather than on a particular physical condition.

Flower essences are subtle liquid extracts that are used to address profound issues of emotional well-being. They are generally prepared from a sun infusion (tincture) of wildflowers or garden blossoms in a bowl of distilled or purified water, then diluted, potentized, and preserved in a combined solution of brandy and, in some cases, spring water.

Like homeopathic remedies, flower essences are believed to be vibrational in nature and work through the various human energy fields, which in turn influence emotional and physical well-being. Flower essence therapy is thought to be a way to nurture and sustain health with the beneficent forces of nature.

Midwifery

Midwifery is the age-old practice of assisting and overseeing the birth of children. Midwives provide education and support during pregnancy, assist mothers during labor and delivery, and provide follow-up care. With the growing interest in natural childbirth, midwifery has become an increasingly popular alternative to typical hospital birthing care. Today, midwives assist in both hospital and home births, as many nurses are now trained midwives. In some hospitals, instead of a physician, the nurse-midwife provides care for women with uncomplicated pregnancies and supervises the birth. Midwives are trained to provide support during pregnancy and labor and following birth.

Practitioners of childbirth support teams include childbirth educators, childbirth assistants, and *doulas* (women labor coaches). Doulas provide labor support for the birthing woman and her partner and some postpartum home assistance. In some states, midwives can attend home births or practice in birthing clinics in hospitals. Some midwives are also licensed to provide "well-woman" gynecological care, including screening tests and birth control.

Naturopathic Medicine

Naturopathic medicine is a primary health care system with philosophical roots dating back to Hippocrates. Naturopathic medicine is founded on a belief in the innate wisdom of nature and in the body's ability to heal itself. It uses many natural therapies to help restore health and balance in the body: nutrition, herbal medicine, hydrotherapy, acupuncture, homeopathy, therapeutic massage, and Oriental medicine. Naturopathic medicine emphasizes the curative power of nature and treats acute and chronic illnesses in all age groups.

A licensed naturopathic physician attends a four-year graduate-level naturopathic medical school and is educated in all of the same basic sciences as a medical doctor, but also studies holistic and nontoxic approaches to therapy with a strong emphasis on disease prevention and optimizing wellness. In addition to a standard medical curriculum, the naturopathic physician is required to complete four years of training in clinical nutrition, acupuncture, homeopathic medicine, botanical medicine, psychology, and counseling (to encourage people to make lifestyle changes in support of their personal health). A naturopathic physician takes rigorous professional board exams so that he or she may be licensed by a state or jurisdiction as a primary care general practice physician.

In the United States, there is only one accrediting agency recognized by the American Association of Naturopathic Physicians to accredit naturopathic programs and colleges. That agency is the Council on Naturopathic Medical Education (CNME). The CNME issues a bulletin twice a year giving the accrediting status of each of the institutions with which it is engaged. At this time, there are three accredited institutions:

1. National College of Naturopathic Medicine, Portland, Oregon
2. Bastyr University, Seattle, Washington
3. Southwest College of Naturopathic Medicine, Tempe, Arizona

There is also one institution that is a candidate for accreditation status:

4. Canadian College of Naturopathic Medicine, Toronto, Canada

RESEARCH BOX: Naturopathic Practitioners' Different Worldviews

This study describes naturopathic practitioners with two different world-views—holistic and scientific—and explores the relationship of practitioners' socialization experiences and practice patterns with these two worldviews. Data were gathered by a variety of methods, including (1) a 14-page questionnaire mailed to all 296 naturopathic practitioners licensed in Canada, (2) a participant observation study at the Canadian College of Naturopathic Medicine (CCNM), and (3) open-ended interviews with 16 students attending CCNM and 41 naturopathic practitioners, which were audiotaped and transcribed verbatim. Individuals with both holistic and scientific worldviews entered naturopathic training, and none of the practitioners who were interviewed reported a change in worldview while at naturopathic college. However, practitioners reported a newfound appreciation of the "other" worldview on completion of their training, indicating the occurrence of a socialization effect. Many decisions involved in setting up a practice and seeing patients were affected by the practitioners' worldviews. For example, there were distinct differences in the way the practitioners with different worldviews who were interviewed chose treatment modalities. Practitioners with scientific worldviews reported choosing treatments based on the available "scientific evidence," while practitioners with holistic worldviews included a careful exploration of the patient's spirituality and their own intuition in their treatment decisions. In addition, practitioners with holistic worldviews reported significantly longer patient visits than practitioners with scientific worldviews. The data presented here suggest that one's worldview influences one's perceptions of socialization experiences and social situations and modulates the effects of both on practice patterns.

Source: Boon H. (1998). Canadian naturopathic practitioners: Holistic and scientific worldviews. *Social Science and Medicine*, 46(9), 1213–1225.

Naturopathic physicians use similar diagnostic and testing procedures as do medical doctors, although a naturopathic doctor will often address a broader range of lifestyle factors that may affect a patient's health than an allopath might. A naturopath may spend an hour gathering information on health history and pertinent lifestyle data. Naturopaths recommend appropriate lifestyle and dietary changes as well as encourage patients to play an active role in their own healing process and in disease prevention.

Osteopathic Medicine

Osteopathic medicine is a form of medical care founded on the philosophy that all body systems are interrelated and dependent upon each other for good health. This philosophy originated in 1874 with Andrew Taylor Still, a Missouri physician and surgeon, who championed the concept of "wellness" and established The American School of Osteopathy. This system is concerned with establishing and maintaining the normal structural integrity of the body.

Osteopathic physicians, like their medical counterparts, must pass a national or state medical board examination in order to obtain a license to practice. There are approximately 37,000 osteopathic physicians practicing in the United States. Like medical doctors, osteopathic physicians provide comprehensive medical care, including preventive medicine, diagnosis, surgery, prescription medications, and hospital referrals. In diagnosis and treatment, they pay particular attention to the joints, bones, muscles, and nerves. One aspect of treatment is through manipulation of the body's joints and tissues in order to restore them to their normal positions and mobility, thereby releasing tension in muscles and ligaments. They are specially trained in osteopathic manipulative treatment, using their hands to diagnose, treat, and prevent illness.

Traditionally the work of osteopaths focuses on the spinal column, since it houses the spinal cord, through which the autonomic nervous system exercises its authority. However, today, most osteopathic physicians practice very much like medical doctors. Though often compared to chiropractors, osteopathic physicians go through a training and licensure process similar to that of medical doctors; osteopaths prescribe medications, practice surgery, and provide comprehensive medical care.

Shamanism

The word *shaman* comes from the Tungusic language of Russia. The word has come into usage by anthropologists, historians of religion, and others in contemporary society to designate the experience and practices of the shaman. Its usage has grown to include similar experiences and practices in cultures outside of the original Siberian cultures from which the term shaman originated.

Shamanism is classified by anthropologists as an archaic magico-religious phenomenon in which the shaman is the great master of ecstasy. A shaman may exhibit a particular magical specialty (such as control over fire, wind, or magical flight). When a specialization is present, the most common is as a healer. The distinguishing characteristic of shamanism is its focus on an ecstatic trance state in which the soul of the shaman is believed to leave the body and ascend to the sky (heavens) or descend into the earth (underworld). The shaman makes use of spirit helpers, with whom he or she communicates, all the while retaining control over his or her own consciousness. It is also important to note that while most shamans in traditional societies are men, both women and men may and have become shamans.

Traditional shamans developed techniques for lucid dreaming and what is today called the out-of-body experience (OOBE). These methods for exploring the inner landscape are being investigated. These techniques and the near-death experience (NDE) have played a significant role in shamanic practice.

The ability to consciously move beyond the physical body is the particular specialty of the traditional shaman. These journeys of the soul may take the shaman to the nether realms, higher levels of existence, or parallel physical worlds or other regions of this world. Shamanic flight is in most instances an experience, not of an inner imaginary landscape, but of flight beyond the limitations of the physical body.

For many the call to shamanize is often directly related to an NDE by the prospective shaman. Among the traditional examples are being struck by lightning, a fall from a height, a serious life-threatening illness, or a lucid dream experience in which the person dies and is reborn. Survival of these initial inner and outer brushes with death provides the shaman with personal experiences, which strengthen his or her ability to work effectively with others. Having experienced something, a shaman is more likely to understand what must be done to help others correct a condition or situation.

Traditional Chinese (Oriental) Medicine

Traditional Chinese medicine (TCM) is a comprehensive system of diagnosis and treatment. It is one of the world's oldest practiced medicines, with one-quarter of the world's population using one or another TCM therapy. Diagnosis in TCM is based on patient history, observation of the body (especially the tongue), palpation, and pulse diagnosis. Treatment usually consists of a combination of therapies: acupuncture, acupressure, herbal remedies, massage, dietary changes, and internal energy exercises such as tai chi, breathing, and meditation. Conditions commonly treated include fertility problems, asthma, arthritis, skin disorders, and pain control. Traditional Chinese medicine is based on the philosophy of Taoism, wherein everything in the world is related to the balance of yin and yang, the two dynamic forces of the universe, along with the five elements of nature (see Figure 1-1). Man as an integral part of the universe must also be kept in balance; harmony in one's life is reflected by the state of one's health.

The yin and yang are fundamentally female and male energies, with many attributes accorded to each. When the flow of yin and yang is blocked, illness occurs. One of the treatments for illness is insertion of acupuncture needles in one or more of the hundreds of points along the meridians for the purpose of stimulation and restoring the flow of the ch'i energy. In the tai chi symbol, which illustrates yin and yang thought, the white dot on the black portion and the black dot on the white section are reminders that each quality contains some of its opposite.

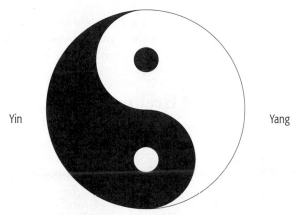

Figure 1-1 The yin and yang symbol

BELIEFS ABOUT HEALING

The dictionary definition of healing offers a standard, generic meaning that, although comprehensive, certainly does not encompass the broad range of how many people view the concept. Healing can occur in a variety of ways. Some believe it is primarily spiritual, while others reject the notion of spirituality, believing physiological or physical cures are the only healing possible. The actual mechanism of healing is still unknown. Health care professionals and the general public may think of the concept very differently, and that is why we should explore healing from a variety of perspectives and belief systems. Several categories of these phenomena are described here, depicting a variety of theories. Belief systems arise from one's culture, philosophy, and worldview.

Faith Healing

Based on prayer and religious faith, healing within this domain occurs because the faith of the supplicant has been answered by the mysterious power of the divine. Cures such as the ones at Lourdes and other holy shrines fall within this category. The method of prayer is common to evangelical practitioners, charismatics, and some one-on-one relationship counselors.

Mind Cures

Healing in this domain relates to the supposition that the diseased states of the body are caused by an aberrant or confused condition of the mind. Adherents to this method attempt to change the state of the mental processes of the client or patient—hence the development of the term "mental therapies." Many contemporary practitioners and groups engage in mind cures. To some extent, psychiatric nurses and holistic practitioners subscribe to this belief system. Approaches such as scientology, concept therapy, humanities, Silva mind control, and others use some portion of this thesis in their healing work.

Metaphysical or Mental Healing

Healers following Christian Science and related systems believe in the nonreality of matter. They assume that our bodies are not real and that, consequently, there is no such thing as disease. They feel that the manifestation of illness and disease is solely an aberration of the mind. Other esoteric and metaphysical groups also subscribe to this conceptual belief.

Spiritualism

Historically this system was derived from the belief that spirits of the dead could operate directly, or indirectly through a medium, to heal a patient. In recent years spiritualism has evolved the belief that the source of healing is directly from the Holy Spirit or some greater source flowing into and through the physical form. Opinions vary whether the healing occurs from the realignment of the molecular structure or from an infusion of light into the cellular substance.

Mesmerism

This system was founded on the supposition that in each person there exists a vital fluid, the free circulation of which results in a state of health and the blocking of the effects of disease. It was believed that this vital fluid could be transmitted to another at will if the recipient was willing to receive it and that the movement of the fluid in the recipient provided therapeutic action.

Energy Medicine and Aura Fields

This theory has grown in popularity during the past decade, deriving part of its origin from mesmerism and the esoteric practices that were popular during the 1800s. This practice has also been augmented and intertwined with the belief in Oriental meridian theories and the Indian science of chakras. Energy and aura theory is based on the belief that energy fields surround the physical body. A practitioner moving the energy through the aural field can alter these fields that surround the patient's body. The purpose of the practice is to open blocked channels and, thereby, realign the unbalanced energy system. An entire school of practice has developed based on this theory. Therapeutic touch, healing touch, aura healing, chakra opening or closing, and electromagnetic healings all fall within this domain.

Hypnotism

In this method it is believed that persons in the hypnotic condition can be guided by the power of suggestion. Suggestion is used by hypnotists to control pain, alter body functions, and change lifestyle habits. This is a popular method for smoking cessation and behavior modification. Subliminal tapes use this technique to subtly direct listeners to change their behaviors.

Natural Healing

"Natural healing" has its roots in the remedies used by tribes, settlers, and rural dwellers and occurs in the folklore of our ancestors. Natural healing recognizes that the body is superbly designed to resist disease and heal injuries. However, when disease or injury occurs, the first course in natural healing is to see what can be done to strengthen the body's natural resistance and healing powers so it can act against the disease or injury process. Since natural healing takes a slower, more organic approach, results are not expected with the immediacy that some people expect with conventional medicine. The flip side of this approach is that cures often occur without the potentially deleterious side effects so common with conventional therapy. A natural healing orientation means that when you have a symptom, instead of reaching for the first available analgesic or rushing to the doctor to ask for treatment, you try the use of naturally occurring remedies and approaches first.

RESURGENCE OF NATURAL HEALING

Toward the end of the twentieth century it became evident that the marvels of modern, conventional medicine did not have the answers for all our ills. In many cases it was discovered that the treatment even caused disease. A case in point, the overuse of antibiotics caused two untoward consequences. First, resistance to the drugs became widespread and, second, other conditions developed in many who took antibiotics. *Candida* infections, yeast problems, even canker sores are but a few of the problems that can develop in those who overuse antibiotics.

People became savvy to the secondary problems of contemporary medicine and began to look elsewhere for other ways of healing. However, some parts of the country seem to be more open to the emergence of natural healing than others. On the Pacific coast, for instance, schools of naturopathic medicine, Oriental medicine, and a host of alternative schools have developed. It was from this movement, away from the sometimes hazardous, overzealous reliance on conventional medicine, that the appeal to alternative medicine originated.

Natural healing methods have been practiced since the beginning of human history. It was during the middle of the twentieth century that the natural healing approach fell out of favor. During the surge and forward thrust of the scientific revolution, modern medicine became all-powerful. When penicillin was

HEALING STORY: Natural Healing for Headache

Matt has a headache. He has been working at the computer in his home office for several consecutive hours. Before he learned about natural healing, he would simply reach for the handy bottle of aspirin, pop three, and return to his job. Since Matt joined a health care interest group at his local church, he has learned some new approaches and uses one for this headache. His group leader, a parish nurse, explained that aspirin can irritate the stomach lining in some people; with others it may cause tinnitis. Additionally the analgesic only treats the symptom by blocking the perception of pain and by blocking the pain; it often numbs the sufferer of trying to understand the cause of the problem. Now Matt knows better. He closes down the program he is working on and heads to the couch. On the way he goes to the freezer and pulls out an ice pack. He lies back on the couch, places the flannel-wrapped pack in the area of pain, and closes his eyes. Within 5 minutes he is asleep and in 15 more he awakens, refreshed, without pain. The throbbing, dilated vessels along the scalp had been constricted and now the stress that originated it has been curtailed. He lies there another few minutes, analyzing why this happened and concludes that, in addition to too much eye strain, he has done no exercise and has been hunched over his desk too long. Matt decides to go for a walk before continuing his work.

Observations and Insights

In this story, the individual decided not to opt for a conventional pharmaceutical usage or to seek the services of a physician, but first try a more conservative approach. This individual was able to successfully bypass medication. In essence, the natural healing approach is conservative. Natural, noninvasive methods are tried first before resorting to more complicated approaches. In general, these natural healing techniques are simpler, safer, and cheaper.

discovered in 1939, everyone thought that miraculous cures were here to stay. Antibiotics and their derivatives became so effective that both professionals and consumers were willing to put aside the old remedies in favor of the new scientific methods. Thus people flocked to physicians and clinics seeking the new therapies. During this period many Americans joined the fast track and became part of the technological revolution. Televisions and computers were developed and society learned new ways of communicating. We changed our lifestyle, moving from an agrarian, industrial people to increasingly technology-dependent citizens.

The practice of natural healing became less well-known and rarely practiced during the mid-twentieth-century years; reliance for health care was on the scientifically trained health care professional. As we neared the close of the twentieth century, it became evident that many of the great scientific breakthroughs and discoveries also had some downsides. As mentioned above, we began developing resistance to antibiotics. Newer and stronger drugs proliferated to keep pace with the increased strength necessary to combat newer, more virulent bacteria. Chronic diseases developed in number and range never before experienced, and the new scientific advances have proven to be of little effect in many of them.

JOINING OF EASTERN AND WESTERN PHILOSOPHIES

Many of the newly developed modalities now practiced in the West have come from Eastern philosophy and healing tradition. For centuries, techniques such as tai chi, acupuncture, and shiatsu were commonplace in the Orient while relatively unheard of in the West. During the last quarter of the twentieth century practitioners of myriad techniques, modalities, and philosophies made their way across the Pacific Ocean and expanded the knowledge base of American healers. Today Eastern therapies and approaches have become integrated with Western techniques with a resultant benefit to all peoples.

HEALING STORY: Use of Tai Chi for Healing in Hypertension

Tina buckled with the news—hypertension? No, not me, she thought. Yet here she was, 55 years old, facing a diagnosis that required attention. She was aware of the possible consequences: stroke, kidney disease, and a host of other not-so-pleasant possibilities. Her doctor had told her to cut back on salty and fat foods, but she was already doing that, and frankly she really did not need to lose weight. What her doctor had not asked was her stress level.

Tina was an overachiever, disciplined, and upwardly mobile. At 40, she had made it to middle management and now at 55 she had broken through the glass ceiling to the top ranks as a vice president in her company. Tina, however, was accustomed to overcoming obstacles and she took on her new medical diagnosis the same way she addressed projects

(Continued on next page)

at work. She learned all she could about the condition and all the treatment options. She agreed to take the antihypertensive medications since she realized the risks if she did not. But, other than diet and exercise, she knew there must be more. Eventually her explorations led her to some of the Eastern healing approaches.

She discovered a class in tai chi (see Chapter 10) at the local Cultural Activities Center and enrolled. She committed to spending every Tuesday and Friday in a one-hour session with the Master and six other long-time pupils. Becoming a student at the back of the class was a feat in itself. It required Tina to relinquish control and humble herself to the instructor and all the other students that seemed so advanced to her. From this group Tina learned about meditation (see Chapter 10). She got some books and audiocassette tapes on the subject and set up a personal space to practice the system at home. During the months she was honing the art of tai chi and meditation, she gradually released some of her other activities that she had done for years. Her meditation experience helped her to understand the need for the release of old ways to make room for the new. She tried to apply the slow, methodical movements of tai chi to a new way of addressing the tasks of everyday life.

While embracing these new Eastern modalities, Tina continued on her antihypertensive prescription. On her six-month follow-up visit, Tina's blood pressure was stable and low. She told the practitioner she had modified her lifestyle, and together they agreed upon a plan to wean Tina off her medication. By Tina's 56th birthday, she so effectively altered her lifestyle and changed her behavior that she reversed the potentially lethal condition of hypertension and developed new patterns for healthful living.

Observations and Insights

Learning how to cut stress in her life not only helped Tina improve her hypertensive disorder, but also helped her to learn how to more effectively manage her everyday life. In what ways can you cut down the chances of high blood pressure, hypertension, or another disorder by changing your lifestyle?

Tai chi promotes calming meditation and teaches physical control. Do you currently participate in any activites that help you physically or mentally? If you don't, why not?

In this story, Tina made it her cause to learn as much as possible about her disorder. Do you encourage others and yourself to understand medical problems? Do you think that individuals should learn more about their disorders? Why or why not?

HEALING VERSUS CURING

There is a vast difference between healing and curing. Curing relates to the reversal of symptoms related to "dis-ease," illness, and/or sorrow. It is the absence of illness and disease. According to *Dorlands' Medical Dictionary*, cure means the course of treatment of any disease or wound, a system of treating diseases, or a medicine effective in treating a disease. An analysis of *Dorland's* definition clearly shows that the term disease is inherent in the definition.

Healing, as referred to previously, has to do with moving from a place of pain, discomfort, disease, and/or sorrow into a dimension of acceptance, understanding, and/or transformation. This occurrence may include recognition of facts and perceptions through an epiphany or spiritual experience. Healing is a condition of life or a way of living. A person can actually be dying yet be in a state of healing characterized by integration, balance, and satisfaction deep within. Healing involves expanding our inner potentials, and therefore, death is not seen as a failure but as a natural consequence of life (Bar, 1998). Table 1-2 details some of the differences between curing and healing.

TABLE 1-2	Differences between Curing and Healing	
CURING	**HEALING**	
Focus on disease pathophysiology	Focus on origin of symptoms and the total body-mind-spirit connection	
Medicating to stop or prevent the perception of pain	Medicating to stop the perception of pain plus searching to discover the complex origin of the symptom(s)	
Patient taking passive role with the practitioner as the authority	A joint partnership between the practitioner and the patient	
Focus of care to combat illness or disease	Focus of care is to restore balance and harmony within the patient	
First-line treatments are medications, surgery, radiation, and chemotherapy for cancer	As soon as symptoms are controlled, treatments focus on lifestyle behaviors, including diet, exercise, stress management, and alternative/complementary therapies Referral to a conventional practitioner for acute or serious pathology	
Death seen as failure	Death perceived as part of the whole life process and the practitioner attempts to aid the patient to harmonize and balance the process	

HEALING STORY: The Difference between Healing and Curing

Senator Johnson was rushed to the emergency room with a gastric bleed. He was transfused and then admitted to the medical floor for observation. He was in the terminal phase of cirrhosis. This time he swore he would never take another drink. Nevertheless, he complained to the staff and made demands of his wife. By and large his behavior was the same as ever. The first week of Senator Johnson's hospitalization drifted into the second and then to the third. One medical and surgical intervention after another was performed on him. However, nothing seemed to halt his deteriorating condition.

It is rare for a patient to be hospitalized so long, but in this case the medical team was determined to reverse his demise and give him more time to live; thus Senator Johnson remained in the hospital. The longer he stayed, the more his physical condition deteriorated. Eventually a total parenteral nutrition (TPN) feeding line was inserted so he could receive nourishment. The medical and surgical teams continued to do morning and afternoon rounds on him, but nothing they did halted his steady physical decline.

What was significant was the change in Senator Johnson's behavior. The staff noticed that his attitude softened. Demands gradually shifted to requests, and increasingly expressions of thanks were given despite the fact that he became progressively sicker. He also requested that a priest come regularly. They were most impressed when they heard laughter during his wife's visits whereas during the first month there was only silence. During the last few days, Senator Johnson's face relaxed and for the first time in years he was at peace with himself, his wife, and those in his environment. When he took his last breath, those around him declared he had experienced a genuine healing.

Observations and Insights

For many individuals with terminal diseases finding mental and emotional healing is a very important part of their life. How did Senator Johnson discover healing? How did the medical staff affect this process? How do you think the healing process is different from that of curing the disease? Do you practice both healing and curing in the care you render?

SUMMARY

Many philosophies of healing coexist in the contemporary health care system. Most have their roots in antiquity while others are relatively recent. Still others are on the frontier of tomorrow. Knowledge of alternative philosophies, concepts, beliefs, and types of healing will aid the caregiver in numerous ways. They offer the provider an insight into clients' perspectives. Alternative philosophies and therapies range from herbal remedies to the belief in energy or aura fields.

ASK YOURSELF

1. Which of the philosophies best fits with your view of healing?
2. Name at least two different cultural groups that evolved healing philosophies.
3. Why do you think belief systems vary so broadly?
4. How does one's culture and worldview relate to healing?
5. What is the difference between healing and curing?

SUGGESTED READINGS

Bradford, N. (Ed.). (1997). *Alternative health care.* Holt, MI: Thunder Bay Press.

Bratman, S. (1999). *The alternative medicine sourcebook: A realistic evaluation of alternative healing methods.* Lowell House.

Cassileth, B. R. (1999). *The alternative medicine handbook: The complete reference guide to alternative and complementary therapies.* W. W. Norton.

Dossey, B., Keegan, L., & Guzzetta, C. (2000). *Holistic nursing: A handbook for practice.* Gaithersburg, MD: Aspen.

Fugh-Berman, A. (1997). *Alternative medicine: What works.* Baltimore, MD: Lippincott Williams & Wilkins Healthcare.

Jacobs, J. (Ed.). (1996). *The encyclopedia of alternative medicine.* Boston, MA: Journey Editions.

Jager, M., & Buchman, D. (1999). *Alternative healing secrets: An A-to-Z guide to alternative therapies.* Grammercy.

Kastner, M., & Burroughs, H. (1996). *Alternative healing: The complete A–Z guide to more than 150 alternative therapies.* Owlet.

Keegan, L. (1994). *The nurse as healing.* Albany, NY: Delmar.

Thomas, R., & Shealy, C. N. (Eds). (1996). *The complete family guide to alternative medicine: An illustrated encyclopedia of natural healing.* Element Books.

History and Future of Healing

Chapter Objectives

- Discover how history impacts the future of health care.
- Analyze how medicine in antiquity relates to medicine today.
- Identify how changing demographics and multiculturalism affect the delivery of health care.
- Explore the wellness paradigm and learn how it affects us.
- Identify some ways healing will change during the twenty-first century.

The American health care system is in the midst of a major shift in the way care is delivered. Both professionals and clients alike are searching for ways to actively participate in maximizing their own health and treating illness and disease. Therapies that support and enhance the innate healing potential of individuals are gaining acceptance with both practitioners and consumers. For example, someone receiving a medication to lower blood pressure might also be advised to get a series of massages and have some biofeedback training. Today's renaissance has its roots in antiquity—much of what is new today is an extension of what began centuries ago.

HEALING IN ANTIQUITY

From the dawn of humankind healing has fascinated people. The healing arts have always attracted the most creative and intellectually curious among us. And from the very earliest times, healers have used their creative force to explore and utilize the tools, resources, and theories that their time and culture afforded them to augment the still mysterious healing process

Primitive Cultures

Primitive cultures were closely tied to nature, thus having an affinity to the animal and plant kingdoms. In the United States, these people were the Native

Americans; in other countries, such as India, China, and Africa, some primitive cultures still exist today. Because of this intimacy with nature, primitive (aboriginal) peoples ascribed human qualities to all life forms. They believed that natural objects—rocks, rivers, trees, wind, and animals—were alive and possessed a spirit or soul. This belief in *animism*—any of various beliefs that natural phenomena and things animate and inanimate possess an innate soul—profoundly affected the development of the practices related to the treatment of maladies.

Because the cause of illness might be due to spiritual woes, many cures were attempted through spiritual intervention. Consequently, a great body of tribal lore developed that included incantations, rites, rituals, and spells. The primary goal was to manipulate the body in such a fashion as to make it an unpleasant place for evil spirits, thereby ridding the body of the cause of the illness.

As this magical lore accumulated, it became too complex to be easily understood by tribes people, so individuals with special insight were selected to devote their time to mastering and interpreting the spiritual realms to the others. The possession of life-giving powers granted these "medicine men and women," or "shamans," a place of prestige and set them above the ordinary person. Thus, the esoteric position of the healer and his or her devotion to the pursuit of the alleviation of pain and suffering began.

Eastern and Indian Cultures

Healing in Far Eastern cultures, both in ancient times and the present, focuses upon the movement of life energy, which is called ch'i, along a system of unseen but recognized meridians. It is these meridians that contain the acupuncture and acupressure points (see Figure 2-1).

Ch'i is affected by how the opposing energies, called yin and yang, are ordered. The yin and yang are fundamentally female and male, complementary opposing energies with many attributes accorded to each. When the flow between yin and yang is blocked or out of balance, illness occurs. A treatment for illness is the insertion of acupuncture needles in one or more of the hundreds of points along the meridians for the purpose of stimulating and restoring the flow of the ch'i energy.

CHINESE MEDICINE

The sciences of organic anatomy, histology, and biochemistry were not developed in the Chinese medical system because they did not fit into their theoretical framework of healing. The Chinese treated illness according to how the patient's energy flowed in relation to the energy of the universe. In spite of their knowledge of anatomy and physiology, they chose to adopt belief in this energy system as they did dissections and studied anatomy over 2000 years ago.

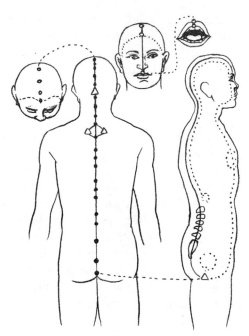

Figure 2-1 Human meridian lines

The development of medicine in China was based on the following applied sciences:

- Orbisiconography (functional relationships within the body)
- Sinarteriology (the natural channeling of ch'i energy through meridians of the body)
- Pharmaceutical agents, change in climatic environment, and immunology

Chinese traditional medicine is a complex system of thought and is further detailed in other sections of this book.

AYURVEDA: INDIAN MEDICINE

Ayurveda, the Indian Hindu system of healing, was developed more than 2000 years ago and is concerned with eight branches of medicine: pediatrics, gynecology, obstetrics, ophthalmology, geriatrics, otolaryngology, general medicine, and surgery. Each ailment is addressed according to theories of the five elements (ether, air, fire, water, and earth), the body humors, the body tissues, the body excretions, and the trinity of life: body, mind, and spiritual awareness. To understand healing from this perspective, one must realize that it is primarily the inward search and quest for soul growth that is important. The theory of reincarnation affects every aspect of life, including the treatment of illness and the acceptance of death.

One of the primary approaches utilized in the Vedic (also called Ayurveda) system is Yoga. Yoga is the science of union with the Divine and with truth. Its purpose is to help the individual achieve longevity, rejuvenation, and self-realization. Yoga deals with the unfoldment, or opening, of human consciousness with the goal of reaching total enlightenment. Yoga, which can be practiced in a variety of ways, is done to speed up the natural evolution of the individual. It is believed that when an individual is left on his or her own without the discipline of Yoga, they will evolve more slowly through the inevitable suffering that is a condition of earthly life.

It was through the Indian healing system that Western culture gained knowledge of chakras. Chakras are unseen energy fields consisting of vortices of energy that can be activated by concentration or meditation. The chakras, like the Oriental meridians, can become stagnant or blocked, giving rise to illness. There are seven major chakras located along the anterior human body from the top of the head to the base of the spinal column (see Figure 2-2). In contrast to Western healers, who tended to do something to someone else to alleviate sickness, the Vedic Indians learned to activate the chakra energy centers for self-healing. However, they, too, had knowledge of herbs and roots and had rudimentary understanding of anatomy and physiology.

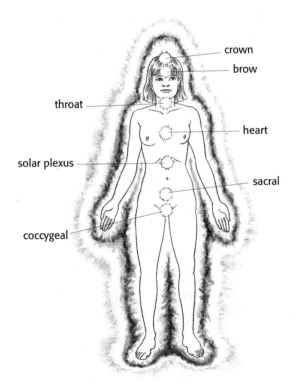

Figure 2-2 Seven major chakras

Ancient Greek and Roman Period

In ancient Greece, institutions dedicated to healing arose. There were as many as 200 temples, called Asclepions, after Asclepius, the god of healing. These centers, which existed for approximately a thousand years, from 700 B.C. to A.D. 300, had complete systems of mythology, symbolism, and priest healers and a method of healing that incorporated all the knowledge of the era. When an ill person sought healing, total immersion in a physical, mental, and spiritual healing environment followed. Dreams, drama, music, art, laughter, massage, bathing, and rest were used, along with herbs and the basic surgical treatments available during that period. By 500 B.C. Hippocrates had catalogued many methods of scientific treatment. The 57 surviving volumes of his writings were divided into many of the subspecialty categories that we use today. For example, medicine, surgery, obstetrics, and pediatrics are a few categories. The method of inquiry and scientific practice was at its height during the Grecian era, before the Western world began its long dark descent through the Middle Ages. In a way, Hippocrates represented a revolution against Egyptian medicine (similar to allopathic) in that his medicine was holistic and focused on overall lifestyle changes (a regimen). Hippocrates also focused on the person, not the disease, using the "humours" or "Hippocratic types" similar to the Chinese and Vedic systems.

From the time of Christ well into the 1600s, healers were imbued with a mystical aspect. From the third to the twelfth century, the Catholic Church served as the authority in health care as well as doctrinal concerns. Christian healers derived this orientation from the New Testament, which not only suggests the presence of God in all matters but also encourages seeing the image of Christ in all humans. For example, consider the Christian verse, "It is no longer I who live, but Christ that lives in me" (Gal. 2: 19–20).

Whatever you do for the least of my people you do for me

Feed the hungry

Give drink to the thirsty

Clothe the naked

Visit the imprisoned

Shelter the homeless

Visit the sick

Bury the dead

Figure 2-3 Corporal works of mercy

The origins of the healing professions in the West were based on these early Christian concepts. For a thousand years following the birth of Christ, monastic orders, made up of both men and women, made a virtue of what were called the corporal works of mercy. These healers based their caring on the concept of Christian charity and its imagery of the presence of the spirit in the body of humans. These works of mercy nourished the spirit through the care of the body. Figure 2-3 illustrates this concept.

The orientation of healers during this 1000-year period was holistic; it incorporated into every healing process an interlinking of body, mind, and spirit, to the point of considering some diseases as caused by the presence of evil spirits and treating these maladies by exorcism. From our modern view we can see both the error in this thought process as well as its inherent symbolic wisdom.

The Enchanted World

The view of nature that predominated before the dawn of the Scientific Revolution (early 1600s) was that of an enchanted world. Everything was seen as wondrous and alive. The cosmos was a place of belonging. As a member of this cosmos, one was not an alienated observer, but rather a direct participant in its drama. One's personal destiny was bound up with nature's destiny, and this known relationship gave meaning to life. This participating consciousness involved merging with one's surroundings and being part of a psychic wholeness. For example, when the Native Americans killed and ate an animal, they considered that the animal's soul or spirit mingled with theirs. Another example is that people existed in harmony with the weather. When it was cold and dreary, they stayed indoors and were quiet. When it was sunny and warm, they gathered, hunted, cleaned, washed, and stored, thus aligning their activities with the weather. In stark contrast, in contemporary society, no attention is given to the weather. People get up and go to work despite the darkness and bad weather. Thus, the ancient's sense of participating wholeness has for the most part been lost with the emergence of the modern scientific era. It is this concept of psychic wholeness that holistic healers are now reconstructing.

THE NEW WORLDVIEW

By the nineteenth century the Western scientific approach was well integrated into the healing arts of North America. Both physicians and nurses followed scientific curricula and worked diligently to serve the sick using their best atomistic or allopathic approaches. *Atomistic* or *allopathic* has to do with the approach of contemporary medicine based on treatments using remedies producing effects opposite from those produced by the disease being treated. For example, an antibiotic is designed to kill the invading bacteria.

The religious communities, which educated many nurses, continued to embody a spiritual approach in their practices. However, holistic health care in the early years of American history suffered a serious setback. The evolution of an agrarian to an industrialized society coupled with the cities' burgeoning immigrant population left little time for holistic health concerns. Early American practitioners waged battles with sanitation, basic hygiene, and immunization to combat the serious physical health problems of the era. Again, with the exception of hospitals run by religious orders, less and less attention was given to the mental and spiritual aspects of healing.

In the late nineteenth and first half of the twentieth centuries, increased diversification of doctors and nurses and increased specialization within the medical field pushed the concept of whole-body healing farther and farther into the recesses of the past. The more specialized and technical delivery systems became, the less attention was given to the spiritual aspect of care. Except for the work of a few healers, by the 1960s the pendulum had swung away from holistic health care. The holistic approaches remained alive and well in chiropractic, naturopathy, homeopathy, clinical nutritionists, etc., during this time. For the most part, however, illness was perceived as a strictly pathophysiological event, with the cure being completely allopathic (pertaining to the treatment of disease by creating conditions that are opposite or hostile to the conditions resulting from the disease itself, i.e., using antibiotics for bacterial infection).

The work of the isolated few in the technological West, however, kept the concept of wholeness alive. South African Prime Minister Jan Smuts introduced the term holistic health in 1926. He theorized that nature tends to bring things together to form whole organisms and that the determining factors in nature and evolution are wholes and not their constituent parts.

The first scientifically trained nurse recognized for her holistic orientation was Florence Nightingale. In her now classic book, *Notes on Nursing* originally published in1859, she shared the essence of her knowledge and wisdom. Some of her deceptively simple ideas are implemented in current-day practices. She called attention to the natural antidotes to disease: fresh air, the reparative importance of quiet in the hospital, good lighting, and a properly managed environment. She is remembered not only for the theory she generated but also for her political activism and the pursuit of a cause greater than herself. She was truly concerned with the body, mind, and spirit of the sick. Nightingale, an upper class British women, opted out of a life of leisure in her quest for helping and healing. Her actions and behavior startled those about her. She dared to move beyond the accepted customs of her day, thereby leading her peers, not always with their approval, to higher levels of thinking and performance. Nightingale scholar Barbara Dossey (2000) concludes that "Florence Nightingale's life embodied social action and a profound spiritual calling and purpose, which our world sorely needs."

During the middle of the twentieth century, when scientific curricula were gaining ascendancy, the gradual decline and ultimate dissolution of the feminine influence on medicine occurred. As the scientific content of health care curricula increased, the feminine qualities of nurturance, intuition, and empathy decreased. These qualities were seen as threats and impediments to the progression of the new scientific order.

Reawakening of Holistic Health Care

The reawakening of whole-person thought related to health and illness probably began in New York in the 1940s. It was here that Flanders Dunbar, a psychiatrist at Columbia Presbyterian Medical Center, did pioneer work in psychosomatic medicine. In her clinical studies she analyzed the relationships among personality type, stress, and physical illness in over 1600 patients over a period of 12 years (Dunbar, 1945). These patients suffered from cardiovascular disease, diabetes, fractures, allergies, and gastrointestinal disease. In each type of malady, Dunbar found certain personality characteristics typical of the majority of patients suffering from that particular disorder. Case histories revealed that the stressful emotional situations that patients experienced shortly before the onset of illness included moving to a new home, neighborhood, or town; death of a close friend or relative; a recent marriage; marital problems and poor sexual adjustment; problems with in-laws; increased family size; and problems with a job, job change, or job loss. It was information gleaned in the early psychosomatic studies that led another pioneer to the exploration of the related phenomenon of the psychophysiology of stress. Hans Selye (1956) developed the theory of stress based upon what he termed the general adaptation syndrome (GAS).

Although Flanders Dunbar's work in the 1940s was sometimes criticized as speculative and nonscientific, two researchers expanded on it in the 1960s. Building on Dunbar's stressful emotional situation categories, in 1967 Holmes and Rahe developed a 43-item questionnaire that elicited information on the occurrence of significant life events during the previous year. Each item was given a point value. The researchers predicted that when the point value reached a certain level, there was an increased likelihood that a physical illness would soon occur. This questionnaire has been used in many studies to document the relationship between the occurrence of the stresses of significant life events and the onset of illness or disease. Findings generated by a revised version of the tool revealed that the more change individuals underwent, the more likely they were to become sick. Thus, a correlation between lifestyle and the onset of illness was established.

Wellness Paradigm

In the early 1960s the concept of wellness was first addressed by Halpert Dunn, who is known as the founder of the wellness movement in the twentieth century. His now-classic definition of "high-level wellness" was an integrated method of functioning, which is oriented toward maximizing the potential of which the individual is capable within the environment where he is functioning. Wellness is an ongoing process toward higher potential, not a static goal, and high-level wellness is a feeling of being alive to the tips of the fingers, with energy to burn, tingling with vitality (Dunn, 1961). Health professionals tend to focus on disease, rather than wellness or prevention, because it is easier to fight against sickness than to fight for a condition of greater wellness.

The Canadian government made the first public and political statement about whole health. In 1974, the Canadian Ministry of Health and Welfare released a publication entitled A *New Perspective on the Health of Canadians* (LaLonde, 1974). This important document presented epidemiological evidence for the significance of lifestyle and environmental factors on health and illness. The report called for a host of health promotion strategies and presented evidence that health status would improve only when people began to assume more responsibility for their own health. When circulated in the United States, this document became the impetus for American political action.

In 1977, the U.S. Senate Select Committee released a landmark report on nutrition and human needs. *Dietary Goals for the United States* revealed the link between diet and disease and called for sweeping changes in American food consumption patterns. This was the first time foods with high-fat content were linked to heart disease. This report paved the way for changes in the ways Americans eat.

The number and scope of holistic practitioners began to increase in the late 1970s. These practitioner-nurses, physicians, allied health care professionals, and nontraditionally prepared practitioners began to integrate a wellness lifestyle as a major factor in the health process. New techniques were tried and new ways explored. Major emphasis was placed on four dimensions: nutrition, physical awareness, stress reduction, and self-responsibility. Out of this new practice, literature and research emerged that helped influence the way Americans conceptualized health and healing.

Ferguson (1980), in her now-classic book *The Aquarian Conspiracy,* sparked the interest of health care professionals when she wrote that a tremendous social transformation was taking place. This transformation embodied a new sense of spirituality and a mind evolution that encompassed consciousness raising. She postulated that individuals were developing an increased interpersonal awareness of their own body-mind-spirit connection as well as their interrelationships with others. She wrote that when individuals develop a new awareness of the body-mind-spirit connection, they focus their attention on a search for patterns and causes of their symptoms. They develop a new body-mind perspective and seek additional ways to prevent the occurrence of illness. Individuals take more responsibility for developing and maintaining a state of wellness.

As new theory and practice literature emerged, scientific studies were undertaken to document some of the suppositions underlying holistic concepts. The findings of one of the most extensive scientific investigations were published in

1982 as the Multiple Risk Factor Intervention Trial (MRFIT). This study was an outgrowth of a recommendation to do this research from the National Heart and Lung Institute. It was a randomized primary prevention trial to test the effect of a multifactor intervention program on mortality from coronary heart disease (CHD) in 12,866 men aged 35–57 years who were at high risk for CHD. The findings, from a seven-year follow-up period, were that men in special intervention programs consisting of counseling for cigarette smoking, stepped-care treatment for hypertension, and dietary advice for lowering blood cholesterol levels had a lower mortality rate than their control group counterparts. This major, broad-based study awakened the scientific community to the importance of education and prevention and opened the doors for numerous ongoing scientific investigations.

Modern Holistic Health Movement

Modern holistic practitioners assume more responsibility for total health care by combining new knowledge with skills organized around the basic life processes of self-responsibility, caring, stress management, lifestyle, communication, and change. Nursing research and publications were part of taking more responsibility. Nurses began developing literature in the holistic arena at the same time as physicians and lay counterparts in the late 1970s and early 1980s.

As practitioners continue to develop holistic approaches, they should take into account both their experience and those ineffable, immeasurable, nonmaterial, and spiritual values that have motivated our predecessors in their search for truth. Let us acknowledge that we are the sons and daughters of the earth and have access to its tools (Dossey, 1984). The world of empiricism has yielded valuable insight that should continue to be used, but our efforts must be blended with an understanding of the higher level of spirit. Our objective now is to learn from the past to help restore a balance, for true science combines the philosophical sciences with the natural sciences. In this way, we may return to our ancient roots in which all healing professions are based. We must search for ends and goals and become truly *teleologic,* that is, believe that the natural processes are determined not by mechanism but rather by their utility in an overall natural design. When using this approach to truth and value, we ultimately discover that they are the same reality.

Today, we are functioning at the end of one paradigm and the beginning of a new one. Our present health care delivery system copes well with trauma and technology but has made little progress with many crippling chronic conditions. In contrast, the new paradigm sees humankind as embedded in nature. It promotes and supports the autonomous individual in a decentralized society. We are at the threshold of awakening as stewards of all our resources, both inner and outer. As this paradigm shift advances, emphasis for both the individual and society will be placed on achieving maximum wellness.

CONTEMPORARY TIMES

Much has happened to change things in the past thousand years, yet surprisingly much remains the same. Human nature for the most part has not changed, but one thing that has is the number of us that share the planet.

Changing Demographics

There are more than 6 billion human beings on Earth. According to population estimates from the United Nations, the 6 billion mark was reached on October 12, 1999. Every second 5 people are born and 2 people die, a net gain of 3 persons. At this rate, the world population is doubling every 40 years and could be:

- 12 billion in 40 years (2040)
- 24 billion in 80 years (2080)
- 48 billion in 120 years (2120)

Without planetary birth control or natural catastrophe that reduces the population, the world will continue to evolve into a teeming mass of people who will live longer and have more health needs.

Baby Boomers

A rapidly growing subset of the U.S. population are the baby boomers. Baby boomers are those Americans born between 1946 and 1964. Every 7 seconds, a baby boomer turns 50. These 77 million aging people will transform health care with their nontraditional expectations and their willingness to move in new directions with their discretionary dollars, as are the subsequent generations—"echo generation," "generation Y," and "generation X." In fact, because these younger segments fly below (not being noticed by) the conventional health care radar, they may hold far more promise for utilizing the upcoming changes in the health care system. With the increasing popularity of alternative medicine and the trend toward direct commerce between consumers and providers, health care will become unlike anything seen before (Bartlett, 1999).

Baby boomers will reshape health care in the twenty-first century just as they sculpted education in the 1960s, housing in the 1970s, the workplace in the 1980s, and the stock market in the 1990s. By dint of their numbers, their affluence, and their sophisticated consumption, baby boomers will leave no stone unturned in the health care world.

Because of these boomers, during the coming years the highest health care–consuming segment of the population will increase by 135% between 2011 and 2029; in contrast, the U.S. population as a whole will grow by only 50%. During this same period, the baby boomer generation will expand the over-65 population by 77 million persons. By comparison, in 1990 there were only 30 million people over the age of 65.

Baby boomers spend freely, too. According to an estimate by the U.S. Department of Health and Human Services, people in this age bracket spent $203 billion out-of-pocket on health care in 1995 (Levit et al., 1994), which constituted 18% of overall U.S. health care spending and outpaced both Medicare (17% of total expenditures) and Medicaid (13% of expenditures) (Bartlett, 1999).

Multicultural Impact

One of the major influences of change is that the complexion of America is changing. In addition to the new age differences, there are racial and ethnic demographic changes. According to projections by the U.S. Census Bureau, non-Hispanic whites will comprise 62.4% of the U.S. population by the year 2025, down from 72.5% in 1998.

Amish	Buddhist	Catholic	Christian	Hindu	Islam
Jehovah's Witness	Judaism	Mormon	Quaker	Seventh Day Adventist	

Figure 2-4 Predominant American Religious Groups

Along with acculturation of new peoples comes new ways of looking at things and inclusion of new ideas. The United States is made up of a variety of religious and ethnic groups, each of which makes a contribution to our new multiculturalism. Figure 2-4 presents the predominant religious groups; Figure 2-5 lists the primary ethnic groups. As we plan ways to deliver complementary and alternative therapies, we will want to realize who we are.

African Americans	Alaskans, natives	Asian and Pacific Islanders	Caucasians	Chinese
Cambodian	Hispanic	Hmong	Indian	Japanese
Korean	Native Americans	Thai	Tibetan	Vietnamese

Figure 2-5 Predominant Ethnic Groups in the United States

Because of our diversity in religion, race, and special populations such as children, the elderly, and homosexuals, we are a cultural blend. Culture involves individuals functioning with a complex set of relationships. On the one side, the individual determines the culture; on the other, the individual is determined by culture. By contributing to the culture around him, the individual is part of the cultural change. Various concepts are often displayed as the basic differentiation of cultures. Table 2-1 lists the most common concepts that constitute a culture.

TABLE 2-4	Characteristics That Constitute a Culture			
National character/ basic personality	Language	Nonverbal communication	Behavior: norms, rules, manners	Social groupings and relationships
Thinking	Time concept	Space concept	Perception	Values

As health care providers move to deliver more complementary and alternative therapies, it is helpful to know more about the people who interrelate to both provide and receive the services.

FEDERAL GOVERNMENT INITIATIVES

In January 2000, the President's Initiative on Race was the cornerstone of the Department of Health and Human Services new program of health prevention and delivery. A goal was set for the year 2010: Eliminate the disparities in six areas of health status experienced by racial and ethnic minority populations while continuing the progress we have made in improving the overall health of the American people. This goal parallels the focus of *Healthy People 2010,* which contains the nation's health objectives for the twenty-first century and is designed to focus on six areas: infant mortality, cancer screening and management, cardiovascular disease, diabetes, human immunodeficiency virus (HIV)/acquired immunodeficiency syndrome (AIDS), and immunizations.

What Is *Healthy People?*

Healthy People is the health prevention agenda for the United States. It is a statement of national opportunities, a tool that identifies the most significant preventable threats to health and focuses public and private sector efforts to address those threats. *Healthy People* offers a simple but powerful idea: Provide the information and knowledge about how to improve health in a format that enables diverse groups to combine their efforts and work as a team. It is a road map to better health for all that can be used by many different people, states and communities, businesses, professional organizations, groups whose concern is a particular threat to health, or a particular population group. *Healthy People* is based on scientific knowledge and is used for decision making and for action.

BACKGROUND

The first set of national health targets was published in 1979 in *Healthy People: The Surgeon General's Report on Health Promotion and Disease Prevention.* This set of five challenging goals, to reduce mortality among four age groups—infants, children, adolescents and young adults, and adults—and increase independence among older adults, was supported by objectives with 1990 targets. The second document, *Healthy People 2000*, was released in 1990. It was a comprehensive agenda organized into 22 priority areas, with 319 supporting objectives. According to the Office of Disease Prevention and Health Promotion, U.S. Department of Health and Human Services in Washington, D.C., three overarching goals were to increase years of healthy life, reduce disparities in health among different population groups, and achieve access to preventive health services.

Healthy People 2010

The new *Healthy People 2010* goals and objectives were launched by U.S. Department of Health and Human Services Secretary Donna E. Shalala and U.S. Surgeon General David Satcher at the Partnerships for Health in the New Millennium Conference, January 2000, in Washington, D.C. *Healthy People 2010* is designed to achieve two overarching goals: increase quality and years of healthy life and eliminate health disparities.

FOCUS AREAS AND OBJECTIVES

The nation's progress in achieving the two overarching goals of *Healthy People 2010* will be monitored through 467 objectives in 28 focus areas. Many objectives focus on interventions designed to reduce or eliminate illness, disability, and premature death among individuals and communities. Others focus on broader issues, such as improving access to quality health care, strengthening public health services, and improving the availability and dissemination of health-related information. Each objective has a target for specific improvements to be achieved by the year 2010.

HEALING IN THE NEW MILLENNIUM

Healing in the new millennium will focus on health prevention, meeting the needs of a diverse society, and exploring new delivery systems. One thing we can be sure of is that complementary and alternative care will be matched by alternative delivery systems.

It is paradoxical, but at this time in our evolution we, as a society, are simultaneously functioning in three distinct health delivery paradigms. Health futurist Larry Dossey (1989, 1999) describes three eras of medicine operant in the West. Era I is technological and based on the pathophysiological system of cause and effect. In many institutional settings this is the mode of current conceptualization and concurrent medical practice. It is true that era I has led to miraculous breakthroughs in diagnosis and treatment, but at a cost. For one thing, it is wildly expensive. In addition, it has made little advance against catastrophic illness while at the same time it has become increasingly impersonal and intrusive. Some, like Dossey, forecast that the health care delivery system, as we know it in era I, is at the end of its time.

Era II medicine, operant in some contemporary settings, utilizes the mind-body connection and takes into account psychological principles and the effect of emotions on psychophysiology and pathophysiology. Bodywork, biofeedback laboratories, and settings that utilize music, aesthetics, and laughter are all part of the emerging era II domain. Dossey predicts era III medicine to be the norm in the new millennium. Era III is based on the metaphysical concept of the development of changes in consciousness occurring prior to changes in matter and energy.

We are in the midst of paradigm shifts. Eras I, II, and III are in flux and the best of all three will likely result in era IV. We are at the threshold of awakening as stewards of all our resources, both inner and outer. We are at the place where science, medicine, and spirituality will be embraced by those with healing attitudes to create new possibilities for all people. As this shift advances, emphasis for both the individual and society will be on achieving maximum wellness.

Many of the oncoming changes will evolve from societal changes. These include demographic, economic, science, and technology. There will be, for example, increasing numbers of elderly and intensifying diversity from continuing immigration. The economy and science will support new health care options. Technology will continue to advance as we move into the twenty-first century

As we advance, society will see itself in the image of a complex organism and, as such, will begin to design health care communities as living organic wholes. We can expect the emergence of renewal centers dedicated to healing; these centers will be reminiscent of the Greek Asclepions. Hundreds of Asclepion sites existed throughout the Greek world. Patrons went to an Asclepion when they needed healing or when they needed to make a transition to a higher level of well-being. These centers offered medical diagnosis and treatments. The therapies included rest and restoration using all the modalities of the period: aquatherapy, massage, dream work, journaling, herbs, nutrition, dance, drama, exercise, and sleep as well as the most current pharmaceutical and surgical interventions.

Today many who seek medical attention do not have organic disease. They have symptoms and seek therapy, but there is no pathology. There are already some sites where these people can go for nontraditional treatment, and healing centers that would benefit these people are being developed. These centers would address the problems of symptoms without pathology or disease and the prevention of disease emergence.

Healing Centers

Many healers are in the process of conceptualizing the kind of therapy centers needed. Future health centers will contain all the finest elements of antiquity but will house and utilize the most modern technology. There will be, for example, flotation tanks, quadraphonic-sound relaxation units, light and color therapy, and biofeedback devices, just to name a few. These units will be planned in ecological settings and utilize both professional and lay people.

Healing will evolve from the unifocused sterile, technological mode of the modern hospital into high-technology, high-touch care with a multidimensional focus on body, mind, and spirit. There will be new modes of therapy that include a variety of new practices. Health care delivery will include such practices as music, imagery, energy movement, humor, food, and friendship. In the new millennium a new definition of healing will emerge that includes caring alongside curing (Keegan, 1994).

HEALTH CARE PRACTITIONERS

Health care providers are moving into the forefront of consciousness and the arena of a transcendent practice. Many already direct their practice from this vantage point. Thousands of others are poised on the threshold waiting to follow the lead and move into a new perception of a new dimension of healing in the twenty-first century. Healing attitudes and behaviors, as well as interconnectedness and wholeness, are being applied to the earth as a living organism. The concept of healing as making whole is rapidly emerging as a force in world politics. Visionary healers are leading the way in helping to redefine what it means to heal and to make whole.

SUMMARY

Healing has evolved through many eras and cultures into the current intertwining of the best of Western empiricism and Eastern mysticism. The future of healing holds promise for disease prevention by modeling and teaching healthy lifestyles, the avoidance of unnecessary drugs and chemical manipulation, and maximizing potentials by learning new skills. Health care practitioners will teach the exploration of inner environments and offer new and alternative treatments to those who desire them. This will be done when we ultimately recognize that many diseases arise in response to a disturbed physical, mental, or spiritual environment.

ASK YOURSELF

1. How has the past influenced the American health care system?
2. What government reports relate to the way health care will be delivered in the future?
3. How do demographics and culture impact on health care?
4. Describe an ideal health care setting.

REFERENCES

Bartlett, D. F. (1999). The new health consumer. *Health Care Finance,* 25(3), 44–51.

Dossey, B. (2000). *Florence Nightingale: Mystic, visionary, healer.* Springhouse, PA: Springhouse.

Dossey, L. (1984). *Beyond illness.* Boston, MA: New Science Library.

Dossey, L. (1989). *Recovering the soul.* New York: Bantam Books.

Dossey, L. (1999). *Reinventing medicine: Beyond mind-body to a new era of healing.* New York: HarperCollins.

Dunbar, F. (1945). *Psychosomatic diagnosis.* New York: Paul B. Haeber.

Dunn, H. (1961). *High level wellness.* Arlington, VA: R.W. Beatty.

Ferguson, M. (1980). *The Aquarian conspiracy.* Los Angeles: J. P. Tarcher.

Holmes, T. H., & Rahe, R. (1967). The social readjustment rating scale. *Journal of Psychosomatic Research, 11,* 213–218.

Keegan, L. (1994) *The nurse as healer.* Albany, NY: Delmar.

LaLonde, M. (1974). *A new perspective on the health of Canadians.* Ottawa: Government of Canada.

Levit, K. R., Lazenby, H. C., Braden, B. R., Cowan, C. A., McDonnell, P. A., Sivarajan, L., Stiller, J. M., Won, D. K., Donham, C. S., Long, A. M., Stewart, M. W. (1996). National Health Expenditures, 1995. *Healthcare Financing Review,* 18(1), 175–214.

Nightingale, F. (1969). *Notes on nursing: What it is, & what it is not.* New York: Dover.

Selye, H. (1956). *The stress of life.* New York: McGraw-Hill.

U. S. Senate Select Committee on Nutrition and Human Needs. (1977). *Dietary goals for the United States.* Washington, D. C.: U. S. Government Printing Office.

CHAPTER 3

Driving Market Forces

Chapter Objectives

- Identify trends in health care that affect alternative and complementary therapies.
- Learn about the increase in chronic diseases and how this affects health care.
- Discuss the effects of technology on patient awareness of available health care options.
- Discuss projections for the future in alternative health care.

SURGE IN ALTERNATIVE HEALTH CARE

Alternative medicine has had a major presence and persuasive attraction in the industrialized Western world. The extent to which these practices have clinical efficacy according to biomedical criteria is a matter of ongoing research and debate. It may be that independent of any such efficacy, the attraction of alternative medicine is related to the power of its underlying shared beliefs and cultural assumptions. The fundamental premises are an advocacy of nature (becoming attuned to the environment), vitalism (feeling energetic and vital), science (validating theories with research and technology), and spirituality (being connected to or with a higher source). These themes offer people a participatory experience of empowerment, authenticity, and enlarged self-identity when illness threatens their sense of intactness and connection to the world. A discussion of these themes may enable conventionally trained clinicians to better understand their patients' attraction to and acceptance of alternative medical therapies (Kaptchuk & Eisenberg, 1998).

The results of a nationwide survey of 1539 adults published in the *New England Journal of Medicine* indicated that one in three Americans use therapies considered to be unconventional (Eisenberg et al., 1993). This was the landmark study that opened the floodgates to exploring and understanding these new therapies and how they worked. The most frequently used therapies identified in the survey were relaxation techniques, chiropractic, massage therapy, imagery, spiritual healing, lifestyle diets, herbal medicine, megavitamin therapy, self-help groups, energy healing, biofeedback, hypnosis, homeopathy, acupuncture, folk remedies, exercise, and prayer. However, some of these therapies are no longer "unconventional" since some of them have recently found their way into mainstream medicine. Medical schools are teaching them, hospitals and health maintenance organizations are offering them, and laws in some states require health plans to cover them. Even major pharmaceutical companies are participating in the rapidly growing industry of herbs and supplements (Johnson, 1999).

A follow-up national survey led by the same Eisenberg team as the 1993 research was done to document trends in alternative medicine use in the United States between 1990 and 1997. The investigators conducted random household telephone surveys. Among other issues, respondents were asked about their use of 16 alternative therapies, including relaxation techniques, herbal medicine, megavitamins, massage, chiropractic, diet, hypnosis, biofeedback, and acupuncture. A total of 1539 adults participated in 1991 and 2055 in 1997. Results found use of at least 1 of 16 alternative therapies during the previous year increased from 33.8% in 1990 to 42.1% in 1997. Overall, use of alternative therapies increased by 25%, total visits to alternative medicine practitioners increased by 47%, and expenditures for alternative goods and services increased by 45% (exclusive of inflation). Results from the follow-up study also showed that ailing individuals most often seek nonmainstream treatments for chronic conditions, such as back problems, anxiety, depression, and headaches. In 1990, an estimated 3 in 10 Americans used at least one alternative therapy; in 1997, the rate was 4 in 10. Of additional interest is the fact that the increased use does not appear to be linked to any particular sociodemographic group (Eisenberg et al., 1998). When extrapolating results to the entire U.S. adult population, the results suggest that Americans made 629 million visits to alternative medicine practitioners in 1997, thus exceeding total visits to all U.S. primary care physicians (Editor, 1999a).

The 1993 published survey estimated that 34% of the U.S. adult population (60 million persons) used at least one alternative therapy in the 12 months prior to study participation. For 1998, that proportion increased significantly to 42% (80 million). The 1998 results showed, for instance, that study respondents sought expertise for five therapies: massage, chiropractic, hypnosis, biofeedback, and acupuncture. Use of most therapies occurred without the supervision of a physician or conventional practitioner. In another study, Astin (1998) found that the majority of alternative medicine users were more educated and reported poorer health status. They used the alternative therapies not so much as a result of being dissatisfied with conventional medicine, but largely because they found these health care alternatives to be more congruent with their own values, beliefs, and philosophical orientations toward health and life.

Between survey years, the average number of visits per person to an alternative therapy practitioner remained consistent, but the total number of visits increased 47%. Relaxation therapy, massage, chiropractic, self-help, and energy healing were among the therapies that increased in patient use (see Figure 3-1). Chiropractors and massage therapists accounted for nearly one-half of all 1997 alternative therapy visits. Among respondents who reported using energy healing,

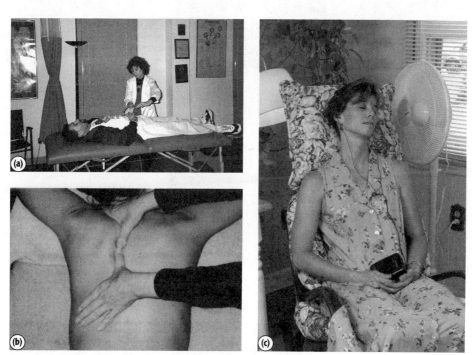

Figure 3-1 Examples of alternative therapies: (a) therapeutic touch, (b) Shiatsu massage, and (c) relaxation

"magnet therapy" was the most frequently cited technique. Therapies gaining the most popularity between 1990 and 1997 were herbal medicine, massage, megavitamins, self-help groups, folk remedies, energy healing, and homeopathy.

Health maintenance organizations (HMOs) are increasingly covering complementary or alternative medical care, according to a national survey of 449 HMOs by Landmark Healthcare, Sacramento, California. The survey found that 67% of HMOs offer at least one form of alternative care. The most common offerings are chiropractic (65%) and acupuncture (31%). Factors that influenced HMOs to make these benefits available were member and employer demand (38%) and mandates or legal requirements (38%). The types of care HMOs currently offer to their participants are detailed in Figure 3-3.

Financial Factors

The United States has one of the finest health care systems in the world. However, it is expensive and flawed, a situation that threatens to worsen as our population ages. By 2030, the United States will have 1.2 million people over 100. This is a figure we need to consider as we plan for the future. Some believe we are currently squandering our national resources, even as we fail to control our epidemic of chronic diseases, including heart disease and cancer.

Types of alternative care currently offered by HMOs

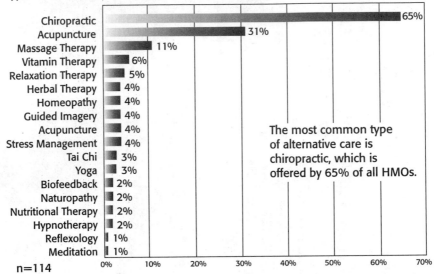

n=114

Figure 3-2 U.S. trends in annual visits to practitioners of alternative therapies versus visits to primary care physicians: 1990, 1997 (*Source*: Landmark Healthcare, 1998)

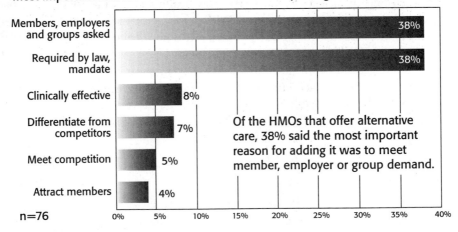

n=76

Figure 3-3 Types of alternative care offered by HMOs (*Source*: Landmark Healthcare, 1998)

RESEARCH BOX: Use of Alternative Therapies by Individuals with Physical Disabilities

A telephone survey of a cross-sectional convenience sample of 401 working-age people with disabilities was done to investigate the use of alternative therapies by individuals with physical disabilities. The results found that, compared to a randomized, national sample of the general population, more individuals with physical disabilities used alternative therapies (57.1% vs. 34% in the general population) and saw providers of those therapies (22% vs. 10%). Among individuals in the current sample, significant positive relationships between use of alternative therapies and higher education and income levels were discovered. The use of alternative therapies by this sample, however, was not associated with racial identity, gender, or age. Compared with the general population, this study's respondents reported a higher proportion of chronic pain (14% vs. 8%) and depression (14% vs. 8%) and a lower proportion of severe headache (9.2% vs. 13%). Alternative therapies were chosen more often than conventional therapies by those with physical disabilities for pain (51.8% vs. 33.9%), depression (33.9% vs. 25%), anxiety (42.1% vs. 13.1%), insomnia (32.3% vs. 16.1%), and headaches (51.4% vs. 18.9%). The conclusion one can draw is that physically disabled individuals are more likely to (1) use alternative therapies than the general population and to see providers for them, (2) have their use recommended by their physicians, and (3) be reimbursed by their health insurance.

Source: Krauss, H. H., Godfrey, C., Kirk, J., & Eisenberg, D. M. (1998) Alternative health care: Its use by individuals with physical disabilities. *Archives of Physical Medicine and Rehabilitation, 79*(11): 1440–1447.

In the 1990s we learned that the population was willing to go outside the system to try something new. The field of alternative and complementary health care is estimated to represent more than $13–$14 billion in spending, most of it out of pocket. The 1993 Eisenberg et al. study found that one-third of respondents utilized alternative modalities. Americans spent $137 billion on 425 million visits to alternative practitioners while spending $12.8 billion on 385 million visits to primary care allopathic (conventional) physicians (Eisenberg et al., 1993). Other estimates are that $27 billion was spent on such treatments in 1997.

Increase in Chronic Diseases

One reason people give when they turn to alternative medicine is that the mainstream medical system does not meet their needs. As our average age increases, so does the rate of inadequately treated chronic illness. Sixty million Americans have hypertension, 40 million suffer from arthritis, and 23 million have migraine headaches. A million Americans each year are being diagnosed with cancer, and close to 40% of us will, at one point or another, have this disease. The prevalence of asthma, multiple sclerosis, chronic fatigue, immune deficiency syndrome, HIV, and a host of other debilitating conditions is increasing. Conventional biomedicine, while successful in treating overwhelming infections, surgical and medical emergencies, and congenital defects, has been unable to stem the tide of these conditions (Carper, 1997).

Over-reliance on Prescription Drugs

The search for more natural benign medicines has occurred because of the alternative complementary care movement. Seeking more intrinsic remedies is triggered by growing concern over the hazards of our current pharmaceutical climate where physicians dispense so many drugs for numerous disorders and their side effects. Unquestionably, the U.S. drug industry manufactures countless products that can greatly benefit patients. However, many drugs are over-promoted in a way that overstates their benefits and understates their risks. The $10 billion per year of often dangerously misleading drug promotional expenditures coincides with inadequate education of doctors about drugs and, together, place people at risk of serious adverse drug reactions. According to Carper (1997), each year, for example, more than 1 million Americans have to be hospitalized because of adverse drug reactions, 61,000 people get drug-induced parkinsonism, 16,000 people have injurious auto accidents caused by prescription drugs, 163,000 people have drug-induced or drug-worsened memory loss, and 32,000 people have hip fractures caused by drug-induced falls. Most—at least two-thirds—of these are preventable.

The excessive, often indiscriminate, dispensing of prescription drugs has also made us a nation of unwitting drug dependents. Although we spend millions to stamp out illegal drugs that destroy human beings, our major addiction problem stems, not from heroin or cocaine or other illegal drugs, but from legal prescription drugs, many given out by doctors without thought of addiction. A number of studies address prescription drug abuse (Boulton, 1998; Chabal et al., 1997; Parran, 1997; Simoni-Wastila, 2000). More than 6 million Americans abused prescription drugs, such as widely used antianxiety drugs. This is far more than abuses of heroin and cocaine together. The consequences of such legal accidental addiction can be devastating, destroying the lives of people who were crying for help to treat a legitimate problem such as panic attacks and ended up either hopelessly addicted or in detoxification programs.

Physician Referrals

Studies suggest that between 30% and 50% of the adult population in industrialized nations use some form of complementary and/or alternative medicine (CAM) to prevent or treat a variety of health-related problems. A comprehensive literature search identified 25 surveys conducted between 1982 and 1995 that examined the practices and beliefs of conventional physicians with regard to five of the more prominent CAM therapies: acupuncture, chiropractic, homeopathy, herbal medicine, and massage. Six studies were excluded owing to their methodological limitations. Survey results showed that acupuncture had the highest rate of physician referral (43%) among the five CAM therapies, followed by chiropractic (40%) and massage (21%). Rates of CAM practice by conventional physicians varied from a low of 9% for homeopathy to a high of 19% for chiropractic and massage therapy. Approximately half of the surveyed physicians believed in the efficacy of acupuncture (51%), chiropractic (53%), and massage (48%), while fewer believed in the value of homeopathy (26%) and herbal approaches (13%). This suggests that large numbers of physicians are either referring to or practicing some of the more prominent and well-known forms of CAM and that many physicians believe that these therapies are useful or efficacious (Astin et al., 1998).

STATE AND REGIONAL DIFFERENCES

Ten years ago, the idea of getting acupuncture or herbal therapy at a traditional hospital would have seemed ridiculous, and expecting medical insurance to pay for such care was out of the question. However, within just one decade such prestigious institutions as New York's Columbia Presbyterian Medical Center, the University of California at Los Angeles Medical Center, and Ravenswood Hospital in Chicago as well as some major insurance companies have finally realized that alternative therapies can be less expensive and more effective than traditional treatments (Plank, 1999). In some states, provision of access to complementary medicine by managed-care organizations (MCOs) is mandated. The scope of complementary or alternative medicine ranges from the more familiar forms of chiropractic medicine and biofeedback to herbal medicine and macrobiotics.

In 1996, Washington State residents won the right to insurance-paid benefits for a number of alternative therapies. This right was challenged in 1999, but the U.S. Supreme Court refused to hear a case challenging Washington State's three-year-old law requiring health insurers to give enrollees access to all state-licensed health care providers, including chiropractors, naturopaths, acupuncturists, and massage therapists. In doing so, the Supreme Court allowed the ruling by the Ninth Circuit Court of Appeals to stand. It determined that the mandate falls within the state's jurisdiction. The Supreme Court's action paves the way for Washington's insurance commissioner to draft compliance regulations. It also positions the state law to become a national model (Gemignani, 1999).

To keep up with the growing demand of alternative and complementary therapies (and maintain profit margins), there are now more than 100 hospital-affiliated alternative care centers in the United States. They treat everything from depression to cancer, with treatments ranging from massage to acupuncture to herbal therapy.

These alternatives to traditional health care are emerging as an important element in the mix of services offered by managed-care plans. Integrating these non-traditional services, such as chiropractic, presents special challenges for plan managers. ChiroNet, an Oregon-based chiropractic specialty preferred provider organization (PPO), has formed partnerships with a variety of managed-care plans, bringing managed chiropractic services to the new PPO environments. Practical experience with benefit design, access protocols, utilization management, quality assurance, provider credentialing, and administrative integration has been developed over the period of the network's cooperation with its managed-care partners. Successful integration of these nontraditional provider groups depends on alignment of goals and incentives among all players in the system, including providers, their network, the patients, and the managed-care plan (Simpson, 1996).

In the mid-1990s, the utilization of chiropractic services was assessed in the continuously enrolled, non-Medicaid membership of the Group Health Cooperative of South Central Wisconsin. A random sample of 500 members using chiropractic services in the last quarter of 1994 was surveyed about satisfaction with the services. A total of 5.1% and 5.3% of members used the services in 1993 and 1994, respectively. Highest utilization occurred among women aged 35–49, with rates of 9.5% and 9.9%. Satisfaction levels were high in all areas; 95.8% indicated overall satisfaction with chiropractic care and services (Hansen & Futch, 1997).

Most hospitals set up programs because of patient demand. As more hospitals come to accept and offer alternative therapies, large health insurance companies like Blue Shield of California and Mutual of Omaha, who once scoffed at these treatments, are being forced to rethink their positions. Many offer supplemental coverage that pays for a broader range of nontraditional care; some even include these options as part of their basic plans. Other companies, such as Regence Blue Shield of Washington State, permit members to choose naturopaths as their primary care physician. Interestingly, these steps are being urged by the carrier's own medical advisers. All these health plans and hospitals have physicians on staff who are respected in their own fields and have become interested in complementary medicine.

Such acceptance is long overdue. According to the World Health Organization, 65%–80% of standard health care services overseas is what Americans would call "alternative." Germany has long offered massage and other complementary treatments in its hospitals, and in China, acupuncture is often used as an anesthesia during surgery. These therapies become complementary, alternative, or unconventional only when used in Western countries (Plank, 1999). We can learn something about the human complexities and traditions involved in healing, not only from Asian healers, but also from scientifically minded Western physicians in Germany and France. In these countries natural remedies are treated as legitimate mainstream medicines, not as aberrations of an unenlightened populace.

EDUCATION CHANGES

In 1996, a panel convened by the Office of Alternative Medicine recommended all medical and nursing students be exposed to alternative theories and techniques. Since then curriculum committees all over the country have been busy making revisions to include these approaches. Unfortunately there has been a haphazard approach, with schools designing their own courses, which range from an integrated curriculum to a brown-bag luncheon series.

RESEARCH BOX: Courses Involving Complementary and Alternative Medicine at U.S. Medical Schools

A study conducted in 1997–1998 was done to document the prevalence, scope, and diversity of medical school education in complementary and alternative therapy topics and to obtain information about the organizational and academic features of these courses. A mail survey and follow-up letter was sent to academic or curriculum deans and faculty at each of the 125 U.S. medical schools. Replies were received from 117 (94%) of the 125 U.S. medical schools. Of schools that replied, 75 (64%) reported offering elective courses in complementary or alternative medicine or including these topics in required courses. Of the 123 courses reported, 84 (68%) were stand-alone electives, 38 (31%) were part of required courses, and 1 (1%) was part of an elective. Thirty-eight courses (31%) were offered by departments of family practice and 14 (11%) by departments of medicine or internal medicine. Educational formats included lectures, practitioner lecture and/or demonstration, and patient presentations. Common topics included chiropractic, acupuncture, homeopathy, herbal therapies, and mind-body techniques. The conclusion is that there is tremendous heterogeneity and diversity in content, format, and requirements among courses in complementary and alternative medicine at U.S. medical schools.

Source: Wetzel, M. S., Eisenberg, D. M., Kaptchuk, T. J. (1998). Courses involving complementary and alternative medicine at US medical schools. *Journal of the American Medical Association, 280* (9), 784–787.

Medical Schools

With the public's increasing use of complementary and alternative medicine, medical schools are answering the challenge of educating physicians about these therapies.

A major indication that alternative medicine is being integrated into the mainstream is that a number of nonconventional approaches are being taught in at least 50 U.S. medical schools. That number represents a 29% increase over just three years ago. And even many seasoned doctors are acknowledging that alternative treatments are a way to improve a patient's quality of life. For example, one general practitioner in practice for over 30 years initially scoffed at the idea of alternative medicine, but then he saw a patient who had been using narcotics to manage chronic pain for seven years. He followed through by prescribing acupuncture and massage and eventually weaned the patient off the drugs. Since that episode he has prescribed similar therapies for patients suffering from a host of disorders, including high blood sugar and cancer (Plank, 1999).

Nursing Programs

Certification programs have been developed in a number of holistic programs and modalities. Holistic nursing, healing touch, imagery, and aromatherapy are but a few examples, with others being planned. Because of this, the third edition of Snyder and Lindquist's (1998) book on independent nursing interventions had a name change, to *Complementary and Alternative Therapies in Nursing*, claiming that there is a greater demand by individuals and health professionals for this kind of information. It is indeed time for nursing education to include complementary/alternative therapies in every nursing student's experience.

ORGANIZATIONS

Does alternative medicine have a place in the world of managed care? According to a nationwide study of 114 surveyed HMO executives, 85% believe that the relationship between traditional and alternative medical care is growing stronger, 47% perceive the two as being complementary, and 67% work for an HMO that offers at least one form of alternative care. A full 100% believe that consumer demand for alternative care will continue (Landmark Healthcare Report, 1998).

Under pressure from consumers, a growing number of health plans are offering a variety of nontraditional treatments, such as acupuncture and Chinese herbal medications (Rauber, 1998). In one study random samples of adult primary care physicians, obstetrics-gynecology physicians and nurse practitioners, and adult members of a large northern California group practice model HMO were surveyed by mail to assess the use of alternative therapies and the extent of interest in having them incorporated into HMO-delivered care. Two-thirds of adult primary care physicians and three-fourths of obstetrics-gynecology clinicians were at least moderately interested in using alternative therapies with patients, and nearly 70% of young and middle-aged adult and half of senior adult members were interested in having alternative therapies incorporated into their health care. Adult primary care physicians and members were more interested in having the HMO cover manipulative and behavioral medicine therapies than homeopathic or herbal medicines (Gordon et al., 1998). Some managed-care organizations now offer these therapies as an "expanded benefit." Managed-care members are seeking relief from a wide variety of maladies, from low back pain and asthma to depression and cancer

Among HMOs that offer alternative care benefits, 47% of their members are covered. In addition, half the HMOs contract with outside providers for alternative care services. Forty-seven percent of all respondents expect the relationship between traditional and alternative medical care to grow closer (Editor, 1999b).

According to the American Chiropractic Association, 46% of the nation's PPOs and 47% of its HMOs include chiropractors in their networks. Dozens of the country's largest health care organizations currently offer alternative medicine benefits to group purchasers.

We are moving in the direction of HMOs, the government, and other payers of health care coverage having a larger voice in the delivery of health care. Active, knowledgeable practitioners can help these organizations be aware of the value of these therapies to the consumer.

Manifestations of this vision can be seen in the growth of professional, holistically oriented organizations since the 1980s. In the 1980s there were only a few; today there are hundreds. There are as many organizations now as there are kinds of individual practitioners and modalities. See Chapter 22 for more information and specific details.

SOCIETAL CHANGES

No matter where you look, society has changed. Whether you are 20 and remembering 10 years ago or you are 50 reflecting 40 years back, you see change. Changes have occurred in the way we dress, eat, engage in recreation, and most certainly in the way we partake in health care. Even nomenclature has changed. What used to be called a general practitioner is now called the family practitioner. In addition, we now also have the nurse practitioner, a nurse with a specialized advanced practice degree. The overall umbrella term "health care industry" has been added to our descriptive vocabulary resulting in a new way of conceptualizing what used to be a simpler system.

Change in Societal Self-Image

The model of society as a complex organism will gain strength, leading to the design of health care communities as living, organic, integrated wholes. New types of healing centers are now being created. For example, Walt Disney Company is developing a "hospital" called Celebration as a prototype care center in a Florida community. Celebration is a hospital without beds, a place where doctors and patients will be called by their first names.

Because of the emerging orientation to combine the sacred and the secular, many of these centers will have the potential to become the new holy places of our society. Imagine new healing centers filled with ideals from the myths of the past, such as the Greek Asclepions, the best of the projections of the future, all combined with the latest in medical technology.

Technology

The vast increase in the sophistication and complexity of technology will continue as we move into the twenty-first century. The development of telematics (i.e., cardiac telemetry units) and biotechnology (i.e., human fertility implementation) will also continue. To realize the speed with which changes will occur, consider that, as recently as 1970, computer chips did not even exist. Today, there are more of them than people on the face of the earth.

HEALING IN THE ARTS

Art includes more than paintings, photography, theatre, and dance. Television, radio, and journalism are other forms of art that allow a medium for expression of who we are. And in these three areas there has been a proliferation of exposition about health and wellness. Countless televised "investigative reports," news stories, and dramas that focus on health appear weekly. Another art medium with daily coverage of health news is the radio.

Radio

More Americans listen to the radio than ever before. Talk programs can be heard on one station or another 24 hours a day. There are early morning programs, daytime shows, and late-night call-in programs for night owls and insomniacs. Interspersed between the politically focused programs, sports, and news shows are an ever-increasing number of health-oriented programs.

Programs dealing with personal relationships led this increasingly popular trend. Joy Brown and Laura Scleshinger, both registered clinical psychologists, are

TABLE 3-1	Radio Health Programs
SHOW TITLE	**DESCRIPTION**
The Doctor Dean Edell Show	Callers ask the full range of medical questions and Dr. Edell answers and gives commentary.
HealthStyles Radio	In this program Doctor Bob and Nurse Judy explore the frontiers of mind, body, and spirit on the Healthradio Network.
American Health and Herbs	A nondenominational group of Christian natural health professionals committed to helping people to better health through God, healing, education, and manufacturing the highest quality tried and proven herbal and natural products.
Doctors Online Radio Network	This program is designed for Canadian Family Physicians.
Johns Hopkins Gazette	Mike Field distributes 60-second stories about Hopkins medicine to radio stations around the country.
Jukebox Radio	Provides a forum for area physicians and health care professionals to discuss and answer questions about their practice, families, and expertise, as well as a wide array of medical health care issues of concern to area residents.
Healthwise	Jefferson Health Systems offers Philadelphia listeners the opportunity to have a radio doctor in their house.
National Public Radio (NPR)	Dr. Barry Bittman interviews health care professionals on BodyMind Matters.

examples of radio personalities who assist callers to sort out mental and emotional health problems manifested in relationship crises.

In the early 1990s, Dean Edell, a medical doctor, led the way to more physical health-oriented programs by hosting a still popular call-in radio talk show on all aspects of health. Many programs followed so that now there are syndicated programs on most local stations. A few of the more popular are depicted in Table 3-1. What the stations have discovered is that the general public is keenly interested in their health and want the interactive medium that talk radio supports.

COMPUTER INFLUENCE

You may ask yourself why innovate? Perhaps an appropriate answer is that health care is a fast-changing business. In the world of the Internet, many consumers believe they can become as knowledgeable as their health care provider. The old proverb "a little knowledge is a dangerous thing" is probably true. Practitioners sometimes get frustrated dealing with more sophisticated patients who come to them armed with Internet printouts and ideas for treatment. But the practitioner's information base is not always better; in some cases it's worse.

In any case, a good deal of the interaction that could have been spent productively dealing with the patient's problems is instead spent sorting through an assorted set of unscientific sources. Yet no matter how tiring to the health care provider, more and more consumers are doing this because the health care system is not meeting all their needs and they want more input (Morrison, 1999).

HEALTHY PARTNERSHIPS:
HOSPITALS LINK UP WITH THE INTERNET

Hospitals are beginning to develop their own Web sites and some even link with national sites. For example, in central Texas a new Internet partnership was launched between Scott & White Hospital and C. Everett Koop, former U.S. Surgeon General. The partnership includes interactive chat rooms, medical links, and resources so that patients can find accurate, dependable health and wellness information at their fingertips.

The Internet partnership means that viewers can access the extensive health care content and tools available through the virtual address sw.drkoop.com with the click of a mouse. Scott & White is the first Texas health care organization to become a drkoop.com community partner. Koop describes the partnership as "sitting down with your doctor in your kitchen and talking." There's no prescription more valuable than knowledge. Describing patients and physicians linking through the Internet, the former Surgeon General compared it to making a house call.

The Internet has given health care providers an unprecedented vehicle to provide timely and valuable information. A hospital can now make more informed decisions regarding health issues. Some hospitals provide links with current Internet sites and patients. Visitors to the site can gain access to searchable health resources, drug information, interactive chats, and forums assisting consumers in taking charge of their health.

Some Web sites offer world-class reference sources for consumers with dedicated channels focused on such topics as children, women, men, and healthy aging. Someone using the computer can find hundreds of health and wellness topics with in-depth content from a variety of distinguished health care sources. For example, the drkoop.com site, launched in July 1998, was the most visited health care site on the Internet in its first 100 days. It has more than 110 interactive communities, has received more than 4.5 million visitors, and has more than 100,000 registered users. It and other similar sites have thousands of pages on the Internet.

TELEMEDICINE

Telemedicine makes use of various electronic communications techniques to link practitioners to patients, educators to students, and consumers to services. Health care e-commerce, which includes the subset telemedicine, is poised to jump from $6.4 billion spending in 1999 to $370 billion in 2004. That equates to a projected growth of nearly 5800% in five years (Barrett, 2000). Health care providers will increasingly use the Internet to improve the flow of information, gain transaction efficiencies, and buy and sell medical supplies (Chin, 2000).

Because this technology is so new, there are novel problems to consider. For example, telemedicine involves a number of interstate issues that will create new procedures and methodologies, such as cross-state licensing.

In Education

Some states have large telemedicine programs. Texas, for example, is a leader in telemedicine and has extensive programs at the University of Texas Medical Branch at Galveston (UTMB), the Health Science Centers in San Antonio and Lubbock, and another at M.D. Anderson Cancer Center in Houston. The Texas Medical Association reports more than 3200 interactive consultations at four remote sites at UTMB during the first two years of the program. Recently, UTMB began a two-year program linking five hospitals serving remote areas to provide care for elderly patients. The program at the Health Science Center in Lubbock, HealthNet, serves rural communities in 108 counties, connecting specialists hundreds of miles away with local physicians and nurse practitioners' examining rooms using live, interactive connections. In certain conditions, such as soft tissue injury, it may be hard to know when and how much progress the patient is making. However, if magnetic resonance imaging (MRI) is performed and the first practitioner concludes there is nothing there, a second opinion can be obtained in a few days by providing a videotape to a second practitioner instead of waiting months for a second MRI. Patients in remote areas can have their records and tests sent to the regional center for evaluation without making the long-distance trip.

For Providers

Telemedicine allows providers to diagnose and treat patients without being with them. An example of one new on-line program is VidiMedix. The technology in this program uses Internet software to transmit live audio and video images between the provider and the distant patient in a remote site. The provider and patient can visually see one another via two-way screens while the provider uses controls to magnify, rotate, crop, color, and size high-resolution images: X-rays, computerized tomography (CT) scans, and MRIs. The provider can zoom in to look at an incision or to note the color and texture of a patient's skin and then proceed to pan and tilt the screen to talk to another provider in the same room as the patient (Foltz-Gray, 2000).

This technology will evolve into "virtual clinics," that is, compact telemedicine stations within many workplace environments. For example, if an employee had an ear ache while at work, he or she would report to the "clinic" and be supervised by a technician. The technician would put the otoscope into the person's ear and attach the other end to the computer. A digital image of the ear goes through cyberspace to the provider's screen, who diagnoses an inflamed membrane. The provider then writes the prescription on-line and the employee can pick it up from the pharmacy on the way home. Instead of taking half a day off, the employee and employer save time by having the "virtual office" in-house.

Consumer Use

Universities and hospitals are not the only groups surging into network computer and satellite links. The Internet is opening up avenues for the savvy consumer (Winters, 2000). Multiple new on-line services help users track personal health histories, manage medical bills and claim forms, and communicate with providers about prescriptions and other issues. Generally these services are free to consumers. The provider get its revenues by charging employers and insurance companies for the services. Examples of the sites are WellMed.com, IntelliHealth.com, and AllHealth.com.

With each service there is a registration and setup process where the person opening the account provides information about emergency contacts, allergies, blood type, and primary care provider. The service then assigns a log-in name and password and organizes the data into a record. Doctors, other providers, insurance companies, laboratories, and family members can have access to the health record when the account holder grants permission on the account options setup page. The person is then issued an information card to carry in their wallet, which prompts medical personnel to contact the Internet server.

Another type of site allows doctors to write prescriptions electronically that can be filled at participating on-line pharmacies. The doctor is then able to log on and learn when the patient filled the prescription and confirm what drug was given. These sites also help patients with instructions. For example, a patient with an asthma inhaler can go on-line and get instructions from a pharmacist. The doctor can see a log of these entries as well. An example of this site is eMD.com.

For consumers that are overwhelmed by a plethora of medical bills, Internet sites such as eHealthclaim.com are rushing to their aid. These Internet providers will help consumers manage their bills, benefits, and claims. These services are designed to help consumers better navigate the often confusing, frustrating world of health care. As telemedicine advances, both provider and consumer alike will find new ways to access and utilize information.

TELEMEDICINE CAUTIONS

The new on-line services are a great convenience, but patients should use caution before giving out personal information:

1. *Find out the site's privacy policy.* The health information, along with the person's name, may be sold to other companies for marketing or research. Patients should ask what the site plans to do with the data, and whether it is possible to keep the disclosed information private.

2. *Look for experts.* The site should have a medical advisory board with recognizable individuals or institutions represented.

3. *Test the site before signing up.* Suggest that your patient first test a prescription site with a question for the pharmacy to see how quick and correct the response is.

4. *Scrutinize the source.* Any sponsorship, advertising, or attempt to sell a product should be clearly marked and separated from the editorial content. If it is hard to tell what is an ad from what is not, the patient should be wary.

5. *Be selective about spam.* Many sites will offer personalized health news and information via e-mail. If the patient does not want messages arriving in their mail box that could possibly refer to their specific health problem, tell them to be sure to opt in the setup process not to receive these e-mails.

PROJECTIONS FOR THE FUTURE

Try to imagine a better future for health care. Today we have the ability to combine the power of new information technology, the needs and wants of sophisticated consumers, and a broader definition of what creates health to imagine a better future.

Twenty years ago no one would have predicted the rapid emergence of technologies such as the Internet, fax machines, and cellular telephones. The tacit suggestion is that similar biological advances are waiting right around the turn of the century. At NextMed2, a conference to envision the future of medicine, scientists and physicians shared findings, theories, and philosophies that hinted at turning cancer into a manageable disease like diabetes, eliminating cardiovascular disease as a leading cause of mortality, expanding the human lifespan to 150 years, and even reversing the aging process (Mitka, 1999).

The growth of alternative therapies and of patients communicating through the Internet may have an even greater impact on physicians' control of medicine. The Internet brings the capability for people globally to talk to one another about their medical care in ways they haven't done before. One of the interesting possibilities is that the conventional medical system might lose control of the system to groups of patients—groups of people who are ill talking to one another and convincing themselves that the alternatives lie elsewhere than in the clinical system (Mitka, 1999).

Futurist Morrison (1999) suggests that physicians consider the following new delivery methods. Other practitioners may want to modify them for their practices.

- *Microfee-for-service.* Many sophisticated consumers want a quick answer from their doctor. Nurse advice lines are great, but sometimes patients want an answer from their physician. Maybe we might consider microtransactions. For example, doctors could get paid a microfee by patients who hit on the "frequently asked questions" section of their physician's Web site. Practitioners could get paid a microfee for answering e-mails and voicemails from patients. Lastly, practitioners could make electronic housecalls and charge a microfee for service.

- *Group and community visits.* Many patients have chronic conditions; they need a lot of teaching and dialogue about their disease and the consequences for daily living. Sometimes the office visit is not the best model for imparting this information. Why are there not more group and community teaching and serving opportunities such as diabetic day clinics where internal medicine specialists, nephrologists, nurses, and dietitians give 15 or 30 patients at a time a group health experience? Similarly, perhaps a provider can be paid for being a "sysop": a host in a chatroom where he or she tends a chronically ill flock electronically. We need compensation schemes to make these types of encounters a reality.

- *Personal health coach.* Many consumers want their health providers to take a holistic view of health. Practitioners could be coaching and advising more than diagnosing and treating. We need reimbursement schemes and health plans that offer the opportunity for longer coaching interactions.

SUMMARY

As alternative health care and remedies continue to become a growing part of medicine, health care providers need to become knowledgeable of the trends to better understand their patients. Furthermore, as we understand more about the long-term effects of prescription drugs, the increase in chronic disease, and state and regional differences in health care problems, we will all gain a greater understanding of the human condition as a whole. As we utilize the changes in society and technology and more individuals seek alternative medicine as a solution, it is likely that we will advance toward better health care for all.

ASK YOURSELF

1. What key study revealed how many Americans were using complementary and alternative therapies?
2. Name at least one alternative therapy.
3. How much money are people spending on alternative therapies?
4. What are some of the reasons people go outside the parameters of conventional care to seek alternative care?
5. Are there state and regional differences in alternative care? If so, what are they?
6. Is there a role for healing in the arts? If so, how is it manifested?
7. How has technology and telemedicine made an inpact?

REFERENCES

Astin, J. A. (1998) Why patients use alternative medicine: Results of a national study. *Journal of the American Medical Association, 279*(19), 1548–1553.

Astin, J. A., Marie, A., Pelletier, K. R., Hansen, E., & Haskell, W. L. (1998). A review of the incorporation of complementary and alternative medicine by mainstream physicians. *Archives of Internal Medicine, 158*(21), 2303–2310

Barrett, M. J. (2000). Why doctors hate the net. *The Forrester Report.* Cambridge: Forrester Research, Inc.

Boulton, S. (1998). Abuse of drug prescriptions. *British Dental Journal,* 184(2), 56.

Carper, J. (1997). *Miracle cures.* New York: HarperCollins.

Chabal, C., Erjavec, M. K., Jacobson, L., Mariano, A., & Chaney, E. (1997). Prescription opiate abuse in chronic pain patients: Clinical criteria, incidence, and predictors. *Clinical Journal of Pain,* 13(2), 150–155.

Chin, T. (2000, January 31). Internet health care business on verge of boom. *American Medical News,* p. 23.

Editor. (1999a). Chronic conditions spur use of alternative medicine in the U.S. *Geriatrics, 54*(1), 15–16.

Editor. (1999b). More HMOs are covering alternative medicine. *Healthcare Financial Management, 53*(4), 24.

Eisenberg, D. M., Kessler, R. C., Foster, C., Nortack, F. E., Calkins, D. R., & Delbanco, T. L. (1993).Unconventional medicine in the United States: Prevalence, costs, and patterns of use. *New England Journal of Medicine, 328* (Suppl. 4), S246–S252.

Eisenberg, D. M., Davis, R. B., Ettner, S. L., Appel, S., Wilkey, S., Van Rompay, M., & Kessler R. C. (1998).Trends in alternative medicine use in the United States, 1990-1997: Results of a follow-up national survey. *Journal of the American Medical Association, 280*(18), 1569–1575.

Foltz-Gray, D. (2000, February 15). Virtual healthcare. *American Way,* pp. 74–77.

Gemignani, J. (1999). Alternative care wins the day. *Business and Health, 17*(4), 9.

Gordon, N. P., Sobel, D. S., & Tarazona, E.Z. (1998). Use of and interest in alternative therapies among adult primary care clinicians and adult members in a large health maintenance organization. *Western Journal of Medicine 169*(3), 153–161.

Hansen, J. P., & Futch, D. B. (1997). Chiropractic services in a staff model HMO: Utilization and satisfaction. *HMO Practice, 11*(1), 39–42.

Johnson, M. (1999). Complementary therapies. *Imprint, 46*(2), 28+.

Kaptchuk, T. J., & Eisenberg, D. M. (1998). The persuasive appeal of alternative medicine. *Annals of Internal Medicine, 129*(12), 1061–1065.

Krauss, H. H., Godfrey, C., Kirk, J., & Eisenberg, D. M. (1998). Alternative health care: Its use by individuals with physical disabilities. *Archives of Physical Medicine and Rehabilitation, 79*(11), 1440–1447.

Landmark Healthcare. (1998).

Mitka, M. (1999). Futurists see longer, better life in the third millennium. *Journal of the American Medical Association, 281*(18), 1685–1686.

Morrison, I. (1999). Leadership and white space: The struggle for strategy innovation in health care. *Health Forum Journal, 42*(3), 18.

Parran, T. Jr. (1997). Prescription drug abuse. A question of balance. *Medical Clinics of North America, 81*(4), 967–978.

Plank, D. (1999). Alternative medicine comes of age. *Vegetarian Times, 260*(18), 18.

Rauber, C. (1998). Open to alternatives. *Modern Healthcare, 28*(36), 50–52, 54, 56–57.

Simoni-Wastila, L. (2000). The use of abusable prescription drugs: The role of gender. *Journal of Women's Health, Gender Based Medicine, 9*(3), 289–297.

Simpson, C. A. (1996). Integrating chiropractic in managed care. *Management Care Quarterly, 4*(1), 50–58.

Snyder, M., & Lindquist, R. (1998). *Complementary/alternative therapies in nursing.* New York: Springer.

Winters, R. (2000). Your vital signs online. *Time, 155*(8), G4–G9.

Complementary and Alternative Approaches to Healing

CHAPTER 4

Alternative and Complementary Therapies

Chapter Objectives

- Identify alternative and complementary health care therapies.
- Learn classification of different therapies and techniques.
- Develop strategies for use and practice.
- Understand the safety and effectiveness of alternative therapies.

NATURE OF ALTERNATIVE AND COMPLEMENTARY THERAPIES

Alternative therapies have been around since people began caring for one another, but the modern renaissance began in the 1960s. Only a few therapies were revived or invented then, but by the 1980s and the 1990s the movement had found its home. The terms *alternative, complementary,* and *unconventional* are sometimes used interchangeably, but there is a distinction between them. *Alternative therapy,* sometimes referred to as an *unconventional therapy,* pertains to a therapy that is used instead of a conventional, orthodox, or mainstream therapy. These therapies range from A (aromatherapy) to Z (zinc supplementation). Other examples of alternative therapies include modalities such as acupuncture, acupressure, herbs, guided imagery, touch, biofeedback, music, and relaxation.

Complementary therapy refers to an alternative therapy that is used in conjunction with conventional therapy. What is considered alternative and/or complementary care depends on the current accepted standards of medical practice (see Figure 4-1). For example, hypnosis and dietary manipulations were once considered outside the mainstream but are now mainline medical practice. Alternative therapies can also be described as those that exclude therapies common to conventional medicine, specifically prescription medications and surgery. More positively, alternative therapies include the view that the real power for healing comes from within, rather than outside of, the self.

Complementary and alternative medicine (CAM) assumes that disease is a complex, multifaceted state of imbalance and requires an approach that utilizes several strategies for facilitating healing. A second assumption suggests that individuals

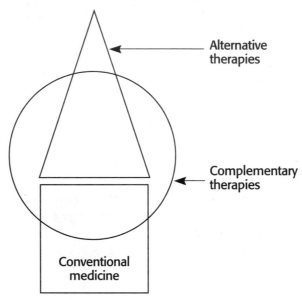

Figure 4-1 Relationship between alternative, complementary, and conventional therapies

can facilitate their own healing process by engaging their inner resources and becoming active participants in promoting their health.

Micozzi (1996) proposed a functional definition that departs from the idea that alternative medicine is everything not presently promoted in mainstream medicine:

> Complementary/alternative medical systems are characterized by a developed body of intellectual work that underlies the conceptualization of health and its precepts; that has been sustained over many generations by many practitioners in many communities; that represents an orderly, rational, conscious system of knowledge and thought about health and medicine; that relates broadly to a way of life (or lifestyle); and that has been widely observed to have definable results as practiced.

This definition speaks to the practice of these therapies as well as the ongoing research to establish efficacy and understanding. It also suggests we may have some responsibility for our own health and wellness (Johnson, 1999).

OFFICE OF ALTERNATIVE MEDICINE

In an effort to explore this new field widely referred to as CAM, the Office of Alternative Medicine (OAM) was established in late 1992 by the National Institutes of Health (NIH).

History of the OAM

The OAM was initiated through Congressional mandate under the 1992 NIH Appropriations Bill. The NIH is an agency of the U.S. Public Health Service and is part of the U.S. Department of Health and Human Services (DHHS). The NIH is one of the world's foremost biomedical research institutions and the federal focal point for biomedical research in the United States. It is comprised of 25 separate institutes, centers, and divisions (e.g., the National Eye Institute, the National Institute on Drug Abuse, and the National Institute on Aging) and is one of eight health agencies making up the DHHS. The OAM was originally organized under the Associate Director of Disease Prevention within the Office of the Director of the NIH. With the passage of the federal government's FY99 Omnibus appropriations bill, the OAM was elevated to freestanding center status. The OAM, now called the National Center for Complementary and Alternative Medicine (NCCAM), is able to fund its own research grants without partnering with other NIH institutes, something it could not do previously.

The OAM's first year was devoted to identifying the alternative medicine community and barriers to the evaluation of complementary and alternative medical practices. The OAM supported its first pilot grant in 1993, its first center grant in 1994, and its first investigator-initiated grant in 1996.

Its initial report, *Alternative Medicine, Expanding Medical Horizons,* presented a context for the need for a different approach to health care. It contends that while the dominant system of health care in the United States, often called conventional medicine or biomedicine, is extremely effective for treating infectious diseases and traumatic injuries, it is often ill equipped to handle complex, multifaceted chronic conditions. One reason is that, over the years, conventional medicine has increasingly emphasized finding a single "magic bullet" solution for each condition or disease it confronts. The reality is that many chronic conditions are not amenable to such one-dimensional solutions.

The 1999 Omnibus bill also provided $1 million to support the creation of a White House commission on CAM policy, which will study and make recommendations to Congress on appropriate policies on research, training, insurance coverage, licensing, and other health care issues affecting the future of CAM. The establishment of the NCCAM in 1999 and its appropriated annual budget of $50 million provide greater autonomy to initiate research projects at a time when the public is increasingly interested in CAM therapies. This will ultimately result in the expansion of clinical research in this field.

Like the OAM, the NCCAM is committed to conducting and supporting basic and applied research and training and disseminates information on CAM to practitioners and the general public. It will also set up and carry out other programs to further the investigation of CAM treatments proven efficacious in clinical settings.

Purpose of the OAM/NCCAM

The Congressional mandate establishing the OAM stated that the office's purpose is to facilitate fair, scientific evaluation of those therapies that could improve the public's health and well-being. The mandate also provides for a public information clearinghouse and a research training program. The OAM does not serve as a referral agency for either alternative medical treatments or individual practitioners. The OAM facilitates research on complementary and alternative medicine. The office is located on the NIH campus in Bethesda, Maryland; the OAM Clearinghouse is located in Silver Spring, Maryland.

Mission of the OAM/NCCAM

The OAM identifies and evaluates unconventional health care practices. This mission is operationalized via funding of an ongoing call for research proposals. In addition, the OAM has funded 11 research centers to study alternative and complementary treatments for specific health conditions. The office supports research and research training on these practices and disseminates information.

Budget of the OAM/NCCAM

The OAM's initial budget was $2 million in 1992 and $3.5 million per year in 1993 and 1994. The budget was increased to $5.4 million in 1995, $7.4 million in 1996, $12 million in 1997, and $20 million in 1998. Perhaps most significantly, the NCCAM's initial 1999 budget was 250% that of the OAM: $50 million.

OAM Programs

The OAM has six functional areas as detailed in Table 4-1.

PARTNERSHIP PROGRAMS

Since the creation of the OAM, progress has been made in the evaluation and, where appropriate, the clinical and scientific acceptance of CAM. This progress is due in part to initiatives jointly conducted by the NIH and the U.S. Food and Drug Administration (FDA). In particular, advances in the evaluation and acceptance of two CAM practices, acupuncture and botanical medicine, have resulted from ongoing cooperation between the two agencies. The regulation of the use of acupuncture needles in 1996 came as a result of a workshop sponsored by the OAM with the participation of the FDA, which explored key regulatory issues. Prompted by similar regulatory issues, as well as by the initiation of NIH-funded research projects, the OAM sponsored an international symposium to

TABLE 4-1	The OAM's Six Functional Areas
FUNCTIONAL AREA	**ACTIVITIES WITHIN THE AREAS**
1. Extramural affairs	Oversees and directs all new research. Began funding grants up to $30,000 a year in 1993
2. Research data base and evaluation	Provides an infrastructure for identifying and organizing the scientific literature on complementary and alternative practices
3. OAM clearinghouse and media relations	Disseminates information to the public, media, and health care professionals to promote awareness and education about complementary and alternative medicine research
4. International and professional liaison	Supports and facilitates cooperative efforts in research and education in alternative and complementary approaches worldwide and with professional organizations across the United States
5. Research development and investigation	Screens, prioritizes, and provides technical support to the most promising domestic and international research opportunities in complementary and alternative medicine; provides technical assistance and brings together researchers to prepare for grant applications
6. Intramural research training	Provides a foundation for scientists to conduct basic and clinical research in complementary and alternative medicine; three to five years of postdoctoral training will give researchers the opportunity to execute basic and clinical research

examine the evidence for and the role of botanical medicine in the United States. This conference generated a series of workshops sponsored by the Drug Information Association in conjunction with the NIH and FDA, which explored the scientific, regulatory, and policy issues of heterogeneous botanical products. These efforts resulted in the initiation of a large randomized multicenter clinical trial (sponsored by the National Institute of Mental Health) of the botanical St. John's wort for the treatment of depression. They also formed internal working groups within the FDA that are drafting a guidance policy for the development of botanicals as drugs in the United States (Eskinazi & Hoffman, 1998).

Sponsored Research

The OAM issued its first request for applications (RFA) in 1993, for grants of up to $30,000 each to fund exploratory pilot projects to identify promising areas of future research. The RFA was unusual in allowing any practitioner, with or without the backing of a conventional research institution, to apply. Collaboration between orthodox research investigators and alternative medical practitioners was encouraged. More than 800 letters of intent were received, and 452 applications were reviewed, the largest response to a single RFA in NIH history. Thirty awards were made in September 1993 and another 12 in September 1994. Each year since, increasing numbers of grant awards are made. The OAM continues to cofund research grants as appropriate applications for research into CAM are received and reviewed through the NIH peer review process.

Research Centers

The OAM/NCCAM has funded 11 research centers to study complementary and alternative treatments for specific health conditions. The centers form the foundation for conducting ongoing CAM research through the NIH. Each center develops a prioritized research agenda, provides technical assistance, provides mechanisms for research development, and conducts collaborative research. Average funding for each center is approximately $850,000 over three years.

In the fall of 1999, the NIH and the NCCAM awarded a grant of nearly $8 million to Maharishi University of Management to establish the first research center specializing in natural preventive medicine for minorities in the United States. This newest research institute, called the Center for Natural Medicine and Prevention, is at the University's College of Maharishi Vedic Medicine in Fairfield, Iowa. It is the newest of the NIH-supported centers in the country for studying natural medicine and the only one with specialization in minority health. It will study the effectiveness of alternative medical approaches for the treatment and prevention of cardiovascular disease in African Americans and other high-risk groups.

Studies published in the American Heart Association's journal *Hypertension* have shown that high blood pressure, which afflicts over 40 million Americans, can be effectively treated using transcendental meditation (TM). Other published findings have indicated that the TM program reduces heart disease, decreases stress hormones, promotes longevity, and reduces health care utilization.

The initial focus of the Iowa center will be to evaluate the effects of the TM program and antioxidant herbal preparations on the treatment and prevention of cardiovascular disease in at-risk African Americans. However, the center's scope will expand to include research on other serious chronic diseases, such as cancer, and will study other modalities of prevention-oriented health care. The center will involve the collaboration of four other major medical institutions, including the University of Iowa College of Medicine, Morehouse School of Medicine, Charles R. Drew University of Medicine and Science, and Cedars-Sinai Medical Center.

Research Database and Evaluation

The Research Database Program provides an infrastructure for identifying and organizing the scientific literature on CAM practices. Its goal is to establish a comprehensive electronic bibliographic database of this literature. This effort entails examining and further developing the classification system used to categorize information about CAM practices, maintaining a comprehensive list of journals that publish research on these practices, and expanding the terminology used to classify this research.

The literature identified from the database serves as an ongoing source of information for scientists, researchers, practitioners, and the public. The OAM has an internal research database with more than 100,000 specific citations on CAM topics.

The Evaluation Program develops rigorous techniques and applies them to the appraisal of CAM scientific literature. It details systematic evaluation methods appropriate for studies of CAM practices. These methods are applied to evaluate bodies of scientific evidence on these practices. The program is implementing a process for developing systematic reviews and meta-analyses of CAM scientific literature.

CLASSIFICATION OF CAM PRACTICES

The following classification system was designed by the OAM to assist in prioritizing applications for research grants in CAM. It is divided into seven major categories and includes examples of practices or preparations in each category (Alternative Medicine, 1992). Table 4-2 describes the seven categories.

TABLE 4-2	Description of NCCAM Classification System Categories

CATEGORY	DESCRIPTION
I. Mind-body medicine	Involves behavioral, psychological, social, and spiritual approaches to health
II. Alternative medical systems	Involves systems of theory and practice that have been developed outside of the Western biomedical approach
III. Lifestyle and disease prevention	Involves theories and practices designed to prevent the development of illness, identify and treat risk factors, or support the healing and recovery process
IV. Biologically based therapies	Includes natural and biologically based practices, interventions, and products
V. Manipulative and body-based systems	Refers to systems that are based on manipulation and/or movement of the body
VI. Biofield	Involves systems that use subtle energy fields in and around the body for medical purposes
VII. Bioelectromagnetics	Refers to the unconventional use of electromagnetic fields for medical purposes

Within each category, medical practices that are not commonly used, accepted, or available in conventional medicine are designated as CAM. Those practices that fall mainly within the domains of conventional medicine are designated as *behavioral medicine*. Practices that can be either CAM or behavioral medicine, depending on their application, are designated as *overlapping*.

I. Mind-Body Medicine

Mind-body medicine involves behavioral, psychological, social, and spiritual approaches to health. It is divided into four subcategories: mind-body systems, mind-body methods, religion and spirituality, and social and contextual areas.

1. The subcategory *mind-body systems* involves whole systems of mind-body practice that are used largely as primary interventions for disease. They are rarely delivered alone; instead they are usually in combination with lifestyle interventions or are part of a traditional medical system.

2. The subcategory *mind-body methods* contains individual modalities used in mind-body approaches to health. These approaches are often considered conventional practice and overlap with CAM only when applied to medical conditions for which they are not usually used (e.g., hypnosis for genetic problems) (see Table 4-3).

3. The subcategory *religion and spirituality* deals with those nonbehavioral aspects of spirituality and religion that examine their relationship to biological function or clinical conditions (see Table 4-4).

4. The subcategory *social and contextual areas* refers to social, cultural, symbolic, and contextual interventions that are not covered in other areas (see Table 4-5).

TABLE 4-3	**Individual Modalities Used in Mind-Body Approaches to Health**

CAM	BEHAVIORAL MEDICINE	OVERLAPPING
Yoga	Psychotherapy	Art therapy
Internal qigong	Meditation	Music therapy
Tai chi	Imagery	Dance therapy
	Hypnosis	Journaling
	Biofeedback	Humor
	Support groups	Body psychology

TABLE 4-4	**Modalities Used in Nonbehavioral Aspects of Spirituality and Religion**

CAM	OVERLAPPING
Confession	Prayer
Nonlocality	Consciousness studies
Nontemporality	Spirituality constructs (e.g., love, hope, faith, joy)
Soul retrieval	
Spiritual healing	
"Special" healers	

TABLE 4-5	**Interventions Used in Miscellaneous Areas**

CAM	OVERLAPPING
Caring-based approaches	Placebo
(e.g., holistic nursing, pastoral care)	Explanatory models
Intuitive diagnosis	Community-based approaches (e.g., Alcoholics Anonymous, Native American "sweat" rituals)

II. Alternative Medical Systems

This category involves complete systems of theory and practice that have been developed outside of the Western biomedical approach. It is divided into four subcategories: acupuncture and Oriental medicine, traditional indigenous systems, unconventional Western systems, and naturopathy.

    1. Table 4-6 includes the subcategory *acupuncture and Oriental medicine.*

TABLE 4-6	**Acupuncture and Oriental Medicine Systems of Theory and Practice Developed Outside of the Western Biomedical Approach**

ACUPUNCTURE	TAI CHI	HERBAL FORMULAS	DIET
Massage and manipulation	External and internal qigong	(Tui na)	Acupotomy

2. Table 4-7 includes the subcategory *traditional indigenous systems* other than acupuncture and traditional Oriental medicine.

TABLE 4-7	Traditional Indigenous Systems other than Acupuncture and Traditional Oriental Medicine
Native American medicine Kampo medicine Traditional aboriginal medicine	Curanderismo Psychic surgery Central and South American practices	Ayurvedic medicine Unani-tibbi, siddhi Traditional African medicine

3. The subcategory *unconventional Western systems* includes alternative medical systems developed in the West that are not classified elsewhere (see Table 4-8).

TABLE 4-8	Alternative Medicines Developed in the West Not Classified Elsewhere
CAM Homeopathy Functional medicine Environmental medicine Radiesthesia, psionic medicine Cayce-based systems Kneipp "classical" homeopathy Orthomolecular medicine Radionics	**OVERLAPPING** Anthroposophically extended medicine

4. The subcategory *naturopathy* is an eclectic collection of natural systems and therapies that has gained prominence in the United States. Treatments often consist of a combination of such things as juices, vitamin and mineral supplements, dietary changes, and other therapies with the intention to strengthen the immune system.

III. Lifestyle and Disease Prevention

This category involves theories and practices designed to prevent the development of illness, identify and treat risk factors, or support the healing and recovery process. Lifestyle and disease prevention is concerned with integrated approaches for the prevention and management of chronic disease in general or the common determinants of chronic disease. It is divided into three subcategories: clinical preventive practices, lifestyle therapies, and health promotion.

1. The subcategory *clinical preventive practices* refers to unconventional approaches to screen for and prevent health-related imbalances, dysfunction, and disease (see Table 4-9).

TABLE 4-9	**Unconventional Approaches to Screen for and Prevent Health-Related Imbalances, Dysfunction, and Disease**	
Electrodermal diagnostics	Medical intuition	Panchakarma
Chiriography	Functional cellular enzyme measures	

2. The subcategory *lifestyle therapies* deals with complete systems of lifestyle management that include behavioral changes, dietary changes, exercise, stress management, and addiction control. To be classified as CAM, the changes in lifestyle must be based on a nonorthodox system of medicine, be applied in unconventional ways, or be applied across non-Western diagnostic approaches.

3. The subcategory *health promotion* involves laboratory and epidemiological research on healing, the healing process, health-promoting factors, and autoregulatory mechanisms.

IV. Biologically Based Therapies

This category includes natural and biologically based practices, interventions, and products. Many overlap with conventional medicine's use of dietary supplements. This category is divided into four subcategories: phytotherapy or herbalism, special diet therapies, orthomolecular medicine, and pharmacological, biological, and instrumental interventions.

1. The subcategory *phytotherapy or herbalism* addresses plant-derived preparations that are used for therapeutic and preventive purposes.

2. The subcategory *special diet therapies* includes dietary approaches and special diets that are applied as alternative therapies for risk factors or chronic disease in general. Examples of diets included in this subcategory are Pritikin, Atkins, vegetarian, Ornish, and macrobiotic.

3. The subcategory *orthomolecular medicine* refers to products used as nutritional and food supplements (and not covered in other categories). These products are used for preventive or therapeutic purposes. They are usually

used in combinations and at high doses. Examples include niacinamide for arthritis and melatonin to prevent breast cancer.

4. The subcategory *pharmacological, biological, and instrumental interventions* includes products such as bee pollen and cartilage and procedures such as iridology and neural therapy applied in an unconventional manner that are not covered in other categories.

V. Manipulative and Body-Based Systems

This category refers to systems that are based on manipulation and/or movement of the body. It is divided into three subcategories (see Table 4-10).

TABLE 4-10	Subcategories of Manipulative Body-Based Systems

CHIROPRACTIC MEDICINE	MASSAGE AND BODY-WORK	UNCONVENTIONAL PHYSICAL THERAPIES
Encompasses many of the massage, body-work, and other unconventional physical therapies	Osteopathic manipulative therapy (OMT)	Hydrotherapy
	Cranial-sacral OMT	Diathermy
	Swedish massage	Light and color therapies
	Applied kinesiology	Colonics
	Reflexology	Alternate nostril breathing
	Acupressure	Heat and electrotherapies
	Pilates method	
	Body psychology	
	Alexander technique	
	Feldenkreis technique	
	Chinese tui na massage	
	Rolfing	

VI. Biofield

Biofield medicine involves systems that use subtle energy fields in and around the body for medical purposes. These systems include:

- Therapeutic touch
- Reiki
- Healing science
- Mariuel
- Healing touch
- Huna
- Natural healing

- SHEN
- External qigong
- Biorelax

VII. Bioelectromagnetics

Bioelectromagnetics refers to the unconventional use of electromagnetic fields for medical purposes.

Other Classification Systems

The OAM is not the only classification system (see Table 4-11) (Jacobs, 1996).

TABLE 4-11	*Encyclopedia of Alternative Medicine Classification System*

CLASSIFICATION	MODALITIES AND THERAPIES
Natural healing	Color therapy
	Homeopathy
	Iridology
	Polarity therapy
Plant medicine	Flower essence therapy
	Herbal medicine
Nutrition and diet	Diet therapies
	Naturopathic medicine
Mobility and posture	Alexander technique
	Chiropractic
	Osteopathy
	Cranial osteopathy
	Rolfing
	Dance therapy
	Yoga
The mind	Psychotherapy
	Hypnotherapy
	Meditation
	Autogenic training
	Visualization therapy
	Music therapy
Massage and touch	Massage therapy
	Aromatherapy
	Reflexology
Eastern therapies	Acupuncture
	Acupressure
	Shiatsu
	Tai chi chuan
	Chinese herbal medicine

Another classification system describes Ayurveda, Chinese medicine, and naturopathy. The difference between these three systems is shown in Table 4-12.

TABLE 4-12	Differences between Ayurveda, Chinese Medicine, and Naturopathy	
AYURVEDA	**CHINESE MEDICINE**	**NATUROPATHY**
Basic Premise		
Illness results from imbalances in the person's constitution. Good health results from restoring and maintaining proper balance.	Health is based on a balance between the five elements and between yin and yang, as well as on unblocked flow of energy (chi).	The body's natural healing abilities can be restored and supported by blending allopathic medicine and alternative therapies.
What Happens in an Average Visit		
The practitioner checks pulse, tongue, and eyes and takes a complete emotional and medical history.	The practitioner checks pulse and tongue and takes a complete emotional and medical history.	The practitioner takes a complete medical history, evaluates diet and lifestyle, and conducts a physical examination.
Common Kinds of Cures Prescribed		
Herbal pills, powders and pastes for detoxification, digestion and cleansing; diet and lifestyle changes; massage; yoga	Herbal remedies, acupuncture, massage, moxibustion (heat therapy), qigong, diet and lifestyle changes	Herbs, allopathic remedies, homeopathic remedies, diet and lifestyle changes

STRATEGIES FOR USE AND PRACTICE

The decision to use complementary and alternative treatments is an important one for practitioners and patients alike. The following are topics to discuss with clients who express interest in or who may already be using an alternative therapy:

- Safety and effectiveness of the therapy or treatment
- Expertise and qualifications of the health care practitioner
- Quality of the service delivery

Safety and Effectiveness of Alternative Therapies

Generally, safety means that the benefits outweigh the risks of a treatment or therapy. A safe product or practice is one that does no harm when used under defined conditions and as intended. Effectiveness is the likelihood of benefit from a practice, treatment, or technology applied under typical conditions by the average practitioner for the typical patient. Many people find that specific information about the safety and effectiveness of an alternative and complementary therapy may be less readily available than information about conventional medical treatments.

Practitioners who counsel clients planning to use one of the therapies should tell them to ask the health care practitioner, whether a physician or a practitioner of complementary and alternative health care, about the safety and effectiveness of the therapy or treatment he or she uses. The client should tell the practitioner about any alternative or conventional treatments or therapies they are already receiving, as this information may be used to consider the safety and effectiveness of the entire treatment plan.

The practitioner may have literature with information about the safety and effectiveness of the therapy. Credible information may be found in scientific research literature obtained through public libraries, university libraries, medical libraries, on-line computer services, and the U.S. National Library of Medicine (NLM) at the NIH.

For general, nonscientific information, thousands of articles on health issues and CAM are published in books, journals, and magazines every year. Articles that appear in popular magazines and journals may be located by using the *Reader's Guide to Periodical Literature* available in most libraries. For articles published in more than 3000 health science journals, the *Index Medicus,* found in medical and university libraries and some public libraries, should be consulted.

The client should be encouraged to be as informed as possible and continue gathering information even after a practitioner has been selected. Have the client ask the practitioner about specific new research that may support or not support the safety and effectiveness of the treatment or therapy. They should ask about the advantages and disadvantages, risks, side effects, expected results, and length of treatment that can be expected.

Suggest that the client speak with people who have undergone the treatment, preferably both those treated recently and those treated in the past. Optimally, they should look for people with the same health condition. Tell clients to remember that patient testimonials used alone do not adequately assess the safety and effectiveness of an alternative therapy and should not be the exclusive criteria for selecting a therapy. Controlled scientific trials usually provide the best information about a therapy's effectiveness and should be sought whenever possible.

Practitioner's Expertise

Health consumers should be advised to take a close look into the background, qualifications, and competence of any potential health care practitioner, whether a physician or a practitioner of alternative and complementary health care. First, they should contact a state or local regulatory agency with authority over practitioners who practice the therapy or treatment they seek. The practice of complementary and alternative medicine usually is not as regulated as the practice of conventional medicine. Licensing, accreditation, and regulatory laws, however, are increasingly being implemented.

Local and state medical boards, other health regulatory boards or agencies, and consumer affairs departments provide information about a specific practitioner's license, education, and accreditation and whether there are any complaints lodged against the practitioner. Check to see if the practitioner is licensed to deliver the services the practitioner says he or she delivers.

Appropriate state licensing of education and practice is the only way to ensure that the practitioner is competent and provides quality services. Most types of complementary and alternative practices have national organizations of practitioners that are familiar with legislation, state licensing, certification, or registration laws.

Some organizations will direct medical consumers to the appropriate regulatory agencies in their state. These organizations also may provide referrals and information about specific practitioners. The organizations usually do not function as regulatory authorities but promote the services of their members.

Second, they talk with those who have had experience with the practitioner, both health practitioners and other patients. They should find out about the confidence and competence of the practitioner in question and whether there have ever been any complaints from patients.

Third, they should talk with the practitioner in person and ask about the practitioner's education, additional training, licenses, and certifications, both unconventional and conventional. The practitioner's approach to treatment should be checked as well as how open the practitioner is to communicating with patients about technical aspects of methods, possible side effects, and potential problems.

When selecting a health care practitioner, many medical consumers seek someone knowledgeable in a wide variety of disciplines. Suggest that your client look for a practitioner they can talk to; they should feel comfortable asking questions. After selecting a practitioner, the education process and dialogue between the client and the practitioner should become an ongoing aspect of complementary health care.

Service Delivery

The quality of the service delivery, or how the treatment or therapy is given and under what conditions, is an important issue. However, quality of service is not necessarily related to the effectiveness or safety of a treatment or practice.

Suggest that your client visit the practitioner's office, clinic, or hospital. They should ask the practitioner how many patients he or she typically sees in a day or week and how much time the practitioner spends with the patient. The conditions of the office or clinic should be evaluated.

Many issues surround quality of service delivery and each one individually does not provide conclusive and complete information. For example, are the costs of the service excessive for what is delivered? Can the service be obtained only in one place, requiring travel to that place? These issues may serve as warning signs of poor service. The primary issue to consider is whether the service delivery adheres to regulated standards for medical safety and care.

Regulatory boards or agencies described in the previous section should be contacted to obtain objective information. The client can also gather information by talking with people who have used the service and through health care consumer organizations.

Costs

Costs are an important factor to consider, as many complementary and alternative treatments are not currently reimbursed by health insurance. Many patients pay directly for these services. Suggest that the client ask the practitioner and their health insurer which treatments or therapies are reimbursable. Find out what several practitioners charge for the same treatment to better assess the appropriateness of costs. Regulatory agencies and professional associations also may provide cost information.

Discussing All Issues with Your Client

All issues concerning complementary and alternative treatments and therapies should be discussed with the client. Competent health care management requires that the primary provider have knowledge of the client's conventional and alternative therapies to have a complete picture of the overall treatment plan. Figures 4-2 and 4-3 contain ideas to share with clients who seek additional information about complementary and alternative practices.

Alternative medical therapies, such as chiropractic, acupuncture, homeopathy, and herbal remedies, are in great public demand. Because the safety and efficacy of many of the alternative practices remain largely unknown, advising patients who use or seek alternative treatments presents a professional challenge. A step-by-step strategy is proposed whereby conventionally trained medical providers and their patients can proactively discuss the use or avoidance of alternative therapies. When you work with patients or clients, try the following strategy:

- Have a formal discussion of the patient's preferences and expectations.
- Ask the patient to keep a symptom diary: Suggest use of columns to record symptom, therapy used, and results.

How can I find more information about complementary and alternative therapy medical practices?

- Ask and read about CAM treatments and practices in general and about those particular practices used for specific health problems. Increasingly, health care providers are becoming familiar with alternative treatments or are able to refer you to someone who is. Other sources of more information include medical libraries, public libraries, and book stores.

- Ask practitioners of complementary and alternative health care about their practices. Many practitioners belong to a growing number of professional associations, educational organizations, and research institutions that provide information about CAM practices. Many organizations are developing Internet Home Pages. Any Internet browser software will have a mechanism for searching the World Wide Web by keyword or concept. Remember that these organizations may advocate a specific therapy or treatment and may be unable to provide complete and objective health information.

- If you have access to a computer with an Internet connection, you may be able to search university or medical libraries on specific conditions and alternative medical treatments. You also may try accessing and searching MEDLINE, one of the many computer databases available from the NLM.

Figure 4-2

How can I find a practitioner in my area?

- Contact medical regulatory and licensing agencies in your state. These agencies may be able to provide information about a specific practitioner's credentials and background. Many states license practitioners who provide alternative therapies such as acupuncture, chiropractic services, naturopathy, herbal medicine, homeopathy, and massage therapy.

- Ask other health care professionals or contact a professional association or organization. These organizations can provide names of local practitioners and provide information about how to determine the quality of a specific practitioner's service.

- Ask people you trust for recommendations. Colleagues, friends, and family members may have had experiences they can share.

Figure 4-3

■ Contact an alternative provider and get information from them.

■ Schedule a follow-up visit to monitor results.

In the absence of professional medical and legal guidelines, the proposed management plan emphasizes patient safety, the need for documentation in the patient record, and the importance of shared decision making (Eisenberg, 1997).

SUMMARY

The Office of Alternative Medicine (OAM) was established in 1992 to explore the new field of CAM. In 1999 the name was changed to the National Center for Complementary and Alternative Medicine (NCCAM). The primary mission of the office is to fund and evaluate promising research to validate the effectiveness of promising therapies and to disseminate information to the public about them. Multiple classification systems are used to help organize the plethora of new modalities.

ASK YOURSELF

1. What is the relationship between alternative, complementary, and conventional therapies?
2. What is the mission and purpose of the NCCAM?
3. What are some of the various classification systems for CAM?
4. Describe some of the strategies for use and practice of CAM.
5. How can I find out more about CAM?

REFERENCES

Alternative medicine: Expanding medical horizons. (1992). Washington, DC: U.S. Government Printing Office.

Eisenberg, D. M. (1997). Advising patients who seek alternative medical therapies. *Annals of Internal Medicine, 127*(1), 61–69.

Eskinazi, D., & Hoffman, F. A. (1998). Progress in complementary and alternative medicine: Contribution of the National Institutes of Health and the Food and Drug Administration. *Journal of Alternative and Complementary Medicine, 4*(4), 459–467.

Jacobs, J. (Ed.). (1996). *The encyclopedia of alternative medicine.* Boston: Carlton Books.

Johnson, M. (1999). Complementary therapies. *Imprint, 46*(2), 28+.

Micozzi, M. (Ed.). (1996). *Fundamentals of complementary and alternative medicine.* New York: Churchhill Livingstone.

Office of Alternative Medicine Clearinghouse. (1998). *Alternative Medicine Information Package.* Washington, D.C.: National Institutes of Health.

CHAPTER 5

Integrative Medicine

Objectives

- Learn the difference between conventional and integrative medicine.
- Vicariously experience an integrative health care center.
- Learn about the philosophical and operational aspects of wellness centers.
- Read the stories of providers who work in model centers.
- Apply principles of integrative medicine in clinical practice.

INTRODUCTION

Integrative medicine is evolving as a new direction in health care. This field of practice combines the concepts and practices of conventional and alternative medicine. Integrative medicine is healing-oriented care that draws upon all therapeutic systems to form a comprehensive approach to the art and science of medicine. The delivery of this kind of health care is more than merely adding some new therapies, such as massage/aromatherapy or vitamin, mineral, and herbal products, to a conventional practice. The practice of integrative health care supports a philosophy of patient/client self-empowerment, prevention of illness, and self-care practices that support maximum health. When clients understand that they have a direct role in their health or illness, a cybernetic relationship begins between the proactive patient and the enlightened integrative medicine provider.

FACTORS INFLUENCING DEVELOPMENT OF INTEGRATIVE HEALTH CARE CENTERS

Many factors influence the development of integrative health care centers, including:

- *A satisfying professional practice.* Many providers are tired of the allopathic paradigm and seek the satisfaction of offering holistic care from a broader base.

82

■ *Escalating costs.* There is a correlation between increasing costs for acute care while there are increasing numbers of chronic conditions that require a different kind of management approach.

■ *Growing interest in health and wellness issues.* Consumers are becoming savvy about their health and are actively seeking ways to become more involved in their own care.

■ *Changing population demographics.* As people age and develop increasing numbers and frequency of chronic diseases, their interest in alternative care heightens. Table 5-1 shows changing population numbers.

TABLE 5-1	**Population Demographics**	
	1900	2000
World population (in billions)	1.6	6
U.S. population (in millions)	76	273
U.S. life expectancy (years)	47	77
Source: U.S. Bureau of Census.		

Prior to the Industrial Revolution, at the beginning of the last century, less than 3% of the world's population was over 65. Currently 14% are over 65, and by 2030, the number may be around 25%.

In 1998, 66 million persons in the world were aged 80 or over. This number is expected to increase almost six-fold by 2050, to 370 million persons. Those aged 80 or over are often referred to as the oldest-old. They are still a small part of today's population (1.1% of the world's population is 80 years or older), but it is the fastest growing segment. For instance, while total population between 1970 and 1998 grew by 60%, the size of the oldest-old increased more than twofold, from 26.7 million to 66.0 million, or by 147%. Growth rates of the oldest-old will increase even more in the future; in 2050 this population group is expected to be almost 6 times as large as today.

The age group beginning to show the surge in chronic illnesses is the over-62-year-olds, and the projections are for almost doubling numbers of Americans in this age group over 30 years, from 33.5 million in 1995 to 61.9 million by 2025. The implications of these data are that more and more senior citizens, along with the rest of the population base, are going to seek increasing numbers of healing therapies in access friendly environments.

MODEL CENTERS

Many contemporary consumers of care are looking beyond the traditional hospital and clinic walls seeking a different kind of care. Patients with chronic diseases that cannot be remedied with conventional surgery and pharmaceutical agents are embracing integrative medicine centers and wellness centers. Some of these new establishments are within existing institutions while others are emerging as freestanding centers. These centers are different than traditional settings because their approach is multifaceted. For example, a cancer patient receiving chemotherapy and/or radiation may also receive nutritional counseling, relaxation therapy, massage, music and meditation classes, and support groups. Generally, the settings are esthetic in comparison to the businesslike appearance of most medical centers. For centers in your area check the telephone yellow page directory and Internet Web sites and seek word-of-mouth referrals. A sampling of a few of the literally hundreds of integrative centers and what they offer is in the Appendix.

Wellness Centers

Wellness centers may or may not vary much from an integrative medical center. Many wellness centers are nurse run while others are physician directed. See the Appendix for an example of a full-service, multidimensional wellness center.

Related Practices

Self-care and wellness are rapidly becoming mainstays of practice for many, including pharmacists. Consumer confidence and trust in pharmacists provide continuing opportunities for pharmacists to create products and services to satisfy consumer demands related to disease prevention and health care delivery (Srnka & Portner, 1997). Many previously solo practitioners are joining with others to partner integrated practices.

FOCUS OF CARE

The three foci of care in integrative health care are (a) health promotion, (b) illness, disease, or disability prevention, and (c) illness care (Laffrey & Kulbok, 1998). Health promotion is the center of the model, signifying that all measures are aimed, either directly or indirectly, at optimizing health potential in a way that is realistic at each level of both health status and complexity of the client system. The practitioner's primary concern is promotion of optimal health as it is defined with and by the client. Alternative and complementary therapies may be used in any of the three areas.

An important aspect of health promotion is that it also encompasses the other foci of care. Even when care is directed toward alleviating or preventing illness or disability, it will still contribute to health promotion. One of the defining characteristics of health promotion is that it goes beyond the alleviation of a specific illness or risk to maximize overall health. For example, providing symptom relief to the individual with pain leads to better health relative to that specific problem but may contribute little to alleviating other illnesses or risks. The use of broader measures, such as regular meditation or relaxation, reduces specific pain and also contributes to reducing risks of other conditions, such as cardiovascular disease, and increases general well-being over a longer term.

The second focus of care is illness or disease prevention. At times, the client's health may require protection because of an existing or potential threat. Illness and disease prevention strategies are those that aim to reduce the likelihood that an actual illness, disease, or injury will occur. The strategies aimed at reducing the threat of a disease are usually specific to that disease. Examples of preventive care include immunizing a child to prevent rubella or mumps or communicating information about risks of exposure to contaminants when handling food.

The third focus of care is illness care, in which assessments and interventions are provided for alleviating symptoms, illness, disease, or injury. This care can be provided directly to a patient, and it includes measures applied to the immediate environment, such as removing sources of excess noise or disruptions that would interfere with healing. Both direct and indirect measures are aimed at resolving an existing disease or illness.

The core of the model (see Figure 5-1) is health promotion. Although resolving and preventing an illness or a disease are important aspects of health care, facilitating the client's greatest health potential completes the process. This attention to health promotion is an important aspect of integrative care.

HEALERS WORKING IN WELLNESS CENTERS

Karen is a counselor who works at a center in the central eastern region of the United States. Like others who work in these settings, her journey began and continues to be her own healing journey. Although her path began two decades ago,

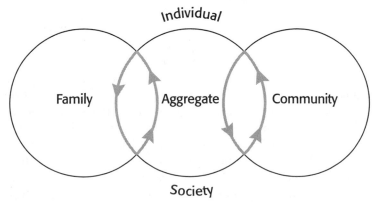

Figure 5-1 Model of integrative practice

the realization of the educational accomplishment became reality only 10 years ago when she was in her late thirties. The desire to learn how the body and the mind communicate with each other was the motivation to return to school. After working in an acute care setting and in home care, her dream of working in a wellness center came true. Personal life experiences had taught her that the integration of mind, body, and spirit is essential to maintaining wholeness. At the wellness center, her role is to help nurture that process in others. This is accomplished through educational programs, discussion groups, activities for support groups, and ongoing communication with patients, family members, and other members of the health care team. The professionals she works with include physicians, licensed social workers, a registered dietitian, a massage therapist, a physical therapist, and others. The stimulating environment of the center is what appeals to her sense of adventure.

Karen's role at the wellness center is to promote wholeness by guiding others to discover insights about their own belief systems, creating an awareness of our conditioned responses, and encouraging lifestyle changes. To be present at the moment when it all comes together is the most rewarding aspect of her job. When the "light" goes on in the soul, it is at that moment when the heart, mind, body, and spirit are open to maximum healing potential. Karen believes that these moments occur frequently if we are attuned to their existence. One such example is when a participant in a cancer program at the center experiences the state of complete peace of mind, body, and spirit as a result of a guided imagery. The mental and sensory images, coupled with the physical cues of relaxation, create an opportunity for the physiology to change. It is during these quiet moments when one senses the divine intervention that allows one to take a step on the path to healing.

CONTINUING EDUCATION IN INTEGRATIVE MEDICINE

Many innovative programs have been spawned by the integrative health approach. For example, in one program physicians can earn up to 52 Continuing Medical Education (CME) credits. They go to the world-renowned Canyon Ranch Health Resort in Tucson, Arizona, while expanding their knowledge of integrative medicine with experts in the field. *Examining Integrative Medicine* is a unique weeklong program specially designed for physicians to experience and explore this new direction in health care. This one-of-a-kind program was designed by Canyon Ranch Health Resort and the University of Arizona Program in Integrative Medicine to combine solid, practical information that can be applied to a practice. The primary limitation is that the program is for physicians only. However, there are many other wonderful continuing education programs in excellent vacation locales for all levels of health care practitioners.

In continuing education workshops, lectures, and group activities there is the opportunity to examine such topics as:

- Botanical medicine
- Nutritional medicine
- Mind/body medicine
- Chinese medicine
- Meditation
- Philosophy of science
- Energy medicine
- Personal healing
- Tai chi
- Future trends
- Acupuncture, bodywork, water therapies, and a host of other modalities
- Integrative medicine approaches to clinical conditions

EXISTING HOSPITAL PRACTICE IMPLICATIONS

Bringing alternative and complementary therapies to your place of practice can be very exciting. However, it is not always possible to develop a freestanding facility on your own, but almost anyone can use the following information to develop a center where they currently work. Table 5-2 details a six-step plan of how to proceed to develop a complementary/alternative practice in your existing agency.

TABLE 5-2	**Six-Step Plan for Establishing an Environment for Practice of Alternative and Complementary Therapies in an Existing Health Care Agency**

1. Learn about the laws and regulations of complementary/alternative practice (CAP) in your state.
   - Talk with your state health commissioner and learn about CAP policy mandates and/or legislation.
   - Find out about your state medical and nursing associations positions.
   - Ascertain if there are any centers/schools that offer credentialing courses; assess range of offerings and activity level.
   - Find out person(s) responsible for strategic planning, health plan administration, or growth strategic group.

(Continued on next page)

2. Assess local activity with regards to CAP.
    - Find out if there are freestanding CAP centers in your community.
        1. How do they operate?
        2. Who are their practitioners/clients?
        3. What is their fiscal management/collection plan?
    - Visit other centers.
        1. Be prepared to see many different kinds of centers and practices.
        2. Observe and analyze the operations of both uncredentialed and credentialed centers.
3. Conduct formal marketing research to "test" the marketplace.
    - Assess the results to measure community/hospital "readiness."
        1. Community:
            (a) Ascertain the level of acceptance and interest among the community, physicians, and providers in the area.
            (b) Assess the number and frequency of community education, conferences, seminars, and CME Continuing Education Units (CEU).
        2. Ascertaining the hospital's cultural acceptance and views toward the following methods of care can help you assess and measure the institution's readiness to institute CAP:
            (a) Wellness/preventative services and programs
            (b) Hospice
            (c) Midwifery
            (d) Osteopathy
            (e) Chiropractors
            (f) Role of dietitians/nutritional service
            (g) Chaplaincy service
    - Learn about the political/administrative situation and any other considerations that may have posed a delay to previous attempts to implement CAP.
4. If the preceding steps produce a favorable response, then proceed to delineate and choose among the many modalities of care.
    - Consider placing therapies on a spectrum encompassing "conservative," "controversial," and "esoteric" (perhaps using different colors to represent in-house practitioners, area practitioners, etc.).
5. Compile and present results to hospital administration with a proposed plan of action as to how to proceed:
    - Integrate the responses to address the measured political and marketplace readiness results.
    - Be aware that every hospital has its nuances and "the best approach" may differ widely.
    - Discuss the plan of action as to which CAPs will best adopt to and/or align within your hospital.
6. Following the assessment and analysis, if there is an embracing response, return to the spectrum of modalities of care created earlier in the process.
    - Take the steps to consider the viability of creating an on-site complementary and/or alternative therapy treatment room as a pilot project.
        1. Allocate funding.
        2. Begin offering services.
        3. Evaluate after a pilot period.
    - Revamp and/or alter the program based on the pilot project.
    - Institute a full-fledged hospital program of CAP.

Advantages to Hospital for Implementing a CAP Program

Any individual or group can seek to evolve the practices at an existing hospital or health care agency. There are several advantages for doing so:

■ Improved client satisfaction—the hospital is viewed as innovative.

■ Enhanced community outreach and publicity for the hospital.

■ Increased ability for consumers to become involved in their own health care.

■ Cost-effective benefits of greater wellness and early prevention for patient populations.

BUSINESS ASPECTS OF INTEGRATIVE HEALTH CARE PROGRAMS

A strong business plan is essential for new integrative programs to sustain themselves. Leadership commitment to the program is essential. Leaders need to believe in the philosophical principles of integrative care and the use of the emerging modalities and be able to articulate these beliefs when in public meetings. Superior management skills are needed to guide these programs through adolescence into clinical and business maturity. By carefully considering the staffing, team building, compensation methods, marketing, and program evaluation and development issues, health care executives should be able to steer between the rocks on their way to integrative medicine decisions that are right for their organizations. Many claim that integrative medicine has the potential to reshape health care delivery in a more patient-centered direction. While this may be true, such programs must prove themselves from financial and clinical operational perspectives in order to achieve this potential. Luminary clinical skills are not enough to guarantee the survival of such programs—a strong clinical base of expertise in alternative therapies is a key success factor. As with any health care venture, there are no substitutes for clinical excellence or sound management (Berndtson, 1998).

Integrative program structures are multifaceted and are comprised of the following (Milton & Benjamin, 1999):

■ *Political climate.* For many it may be necessary to initially organize the integrative center apart from the existing organization.

■ *Physical environment.* Best to begin with a small independent site or a subset of an existing site.

■ *Practitioners.* Programs can begin with providers in the community who are already providing alternative and complementary care and expand to recruit new providers as the need occurs. Another excellent source of providers is already employed individuals who want in-house education to improve and expand their skills.

- ■ *Practice environment.* There are many side aspects to a successful program. Such things as the type and quality of piped-in music, types of reading material and videos, availability of purified water and caffeine-free teas, aroma of the environment, clothing worn by the personnel, non-clinical-appearing bathrooms, examination rooms decorated with inviting colors, and examination tables with wide, comfortable cushions are but a part of an environment that conveys the message "we really care for you."

This desire for health and well-being is driving the rapid growth of the CAM industry and points to a new role for health care professionals, including business opportunities for medical groups. Complementary and alternative medicine represents the opportunity to grow practice revenues, expand a group's tool kit for assisting patients with health care issues, and retain or increase market share by proactively responding to consumers (Hofgard & Zipin, 1999).

Budgetary Considerations

The most successful budget planning seems to be one that is divided into three phases:

- ■ Planning—including exploration costs
- ■ Implementation—including marketing costs
- ■ Evaluation—including costs related to publicizing the project and its outcomes

For a complete budgetary analysis see Milton and Benjamin (1999).

PROJECTIONS FOR THE FUTURE

Dramatic changes are in the making for how health care is delivered. There will be increasing numbers of freestanding integrative health clinics and wellness centers, hospitals will move to develop in-house alternative care programs, and individual practitioners will upgrade and augment their alternative/complementary skills with continuing education programs. The twenty-first century will be an exciting time for many innovative changes looming on the horizon.

SUMMARY

Integrative medicine utilizing a wellness approach is here to stay. As increasing numbers of practitioners and consumers learn about alternative and complementary therapies, private, group, and hospital practices will change to meet the new demands. The innovative integrative medicine and wellness centers that developed at the end of the twentieth century will provide the basis for others that will be developed in the twenty-first century.

ASK YOURSELF

1. What are some characteristics of integrative care?
2. What are some factors influencing the development of an integrative care center?
3. Is there a place for integrative care in my practice? If so how might I go about establishing an integrative care center?
4. Whose approval is necessary to move forward in building an integrative care or wellness center?
5. What are the important steps to follow to establish an integrative care or wellness center?
6. What are some of the budgetary considerations in establishing a new center?
7. How would my professional practice change in integrative care?

REFERENCES

Berndtson, K. (1998). Complementary and alternative medicine. Integrative medicine: Business risks and opportunities. *Physician Executive, 24*(6), 22–25.

Hofgard, M. W., & Zipin, M. L. (1999). Complementary and alternative medicine: A business opportunity? *Medical Group Management Journal, 46*(3), 16–24, 26–27.

Laffrey, S., & Kulbok, P. (1998). An integrative model for holistic community health nursing. *Journal of Holistic Nursing, 17*(1), 88–103.

Milton, D., & Benjamin, S. (1999). *Complementary and alternative therapies: An implementation guide to integrative health care.* Chicago, IL: American Hospital Association Press.

Srnka, Q., & Portner, T. S. (1997). Exploring self-care and wellness: A model for pharmacist compensation by managed care organizations. *American Journal of Managed Care, 3*(6), 943–952, 955–957.

SUGGESTED READINGS

Casey, M. M. (1997). Integrated networks and health care provider cooperatives: New models for rural health care delivery and financing. *Health Care Management Review, 22*(2), 41–48.

Cotroneo, M., Outlaw, F. H., King J., & Brince, J. (1997). Integrated primary health care. Opportunities for psychiatric-mental health nurses in a reforming health care. *Journal of Psychosocial Nursing Mental Health Services, 35*(10), 21–27.

Dill, B. (1998). Integrated health care: Working together across specialties. *Journal of Psychosocial Nursing Mental Health Services, 36*(2), 9–10.

Gordon, J. (1996). *Manifesto for a new medicine: Your guide to healing partnerships and the wise use of alternative therapies.* Reading, MA: Addison-Wesley.

Hoffman, E., Maraldo, P., Coons, H. L., & Johnson, K. (1997). The women-centered health care team: Integrating perspectives from managed care, women's health, and the health professional workforce. *Womens Health Issues, 22*(6), 362–374, 375–379.

Morton, M. (1997). *Five steps to selecting the best alternative medicine.* Novato, CA: New World Library.

Phalen, K. (1998). *Integrative medicine: achieving wellness through the best of Eastern and Western medicine.* Boston, MA: Journey Editions.

Quinn, J. F. (1997). Summer healing: A model for an integrative health care system. *Advances in Practical Nursing Quarterly, 3*(1), 1–7.

Sinclair, B. P. (1997). Advanced practice nurses in integrated health care systems. *Journal of Obstetric, Gynecologic, and Neonatal Nursing, 26*(2), 217–223.

Sinclair, B. P. (1996). Integration of health care delivery. Report of a WHO study group. *World Health Organization Technical Report Series, 26*(2), 1–68.

Swartz, K., & Brennan, T. A. (1996). Integrated health care, capitated payment, and quality: The role of regulation. *Annals of Internal Medicine, 26*(4), 442–448.

PART III

Healing Modalities

INTRODUCTION

The increasing development and use of complementary and alternative (CAM) therapies has changed the way many Americans think of health care. Concepts of self-care and self-responsibility have impacted how both professionals and consumers live. The chapters in this section represent many of the most widely used modalities and include:

Herbal medicine and nutrition

Homeopathy

Naturopathy

Mind-body therapies

Posture and mobility

Touch therapies and bodywork

Chiropractic

Energetic therapies

Eastern therapies

Other therapies that do not fit in the above categories

Part 3 of this book is designed to lead the reader to:

◼ Explore the complex array of alternative and complementary therapeutic modalities.

◼ Analyze the different ways that therapies are classified.

◼ Understand that some therapies are validated with scientific research while others are based on anecdotal claims and personal belief systems.

Healing involves a multiplicity of approaches. Often healing is related to a philosophical orientation, the phenomenon of presence, attitudes and behaviors, and beliefs and values. In many instances, however, one or more of the above are coupled with a therapeutic modality. For example, the attitude of joyful service is coupled with therapeutic massage, resulting in a calm, poised, and pleasant therapist who applies skilled hands to a recipient's body.

The chapters on healing philosophies and modalities in this section do not present the entire scope of alternative and complementary therapies, but the material does describe a comprehensive range of what a number of therapies purport to accomplish. Some of the therapies are briefly described while others are more fully explained and illustrated. Many of the cited therapies have entire books devoted to them. Therefore, the purpose of this book is not to extensively detail each therapy, but rather to introduce the concepts and stimulate the reader to discover more about the particular modalities and/or philosophies explained.

Some alternative and complementary therapies are investigated. In many instances a research box that validates the effectiveness of the therapy accompanies these modalities. These evidenced-based modalities often have more than one study and thus additonal studies are provided in the Appendix. Occasionally a controversial therapy is not substantiated, but often both the advocate's and critic's perspectives are given.

The practitioners of these alternative and complementary modalities range from the self-trained layperson to professionals with graduate school degrees and advanced certification. As you read about these broad array of modalities, it may be valuable to be aware of the range and type of modality providers and the broadest national training standards. These practitioners are the colleagues to whom you will refer and will have referrals from. Table 1 describes the many types of health care providers and the broadest national training standards for each. Often practitioners are unaware of the types of education and standards that their peers have achieved. For example, registered nurses may not know about the training of chiropractors and visa versa. Therefore, this table serves as a guide to learn more about the training and education of a variety of health care practitioners.

TABLE 1	**Type of Health Care Provider and Broadest National Training Standards**
TYPE OF PRACTITIONER	**BROADEST NATIONAL TRAINING STANDARD**
Advanced nurse practitioner	Passing scores on the National Council Licensure Examination for Registered Nurses (NCLEX- RN), further certification by the American Academy of Nurse Practitioners Certification Program, and current licensure, registration, or certification as Nurse Practitioner in the state, territory, or possession of the United States where practicing. Pharmaceutical prescriptive authority documentation from appropriate issuing state agency, as required by law.

Clinical nurse specialist	Passing scores on the NCLEX-RN, a Master's Degree in Nursing, current national certification in the Advanced Practice Specialty area, and approval by the Board of Nursing in the state, territory, or possession of the United States where practicing. Pharmaceutical prescriptive authority documentation from appropriate issuing state agency, as required by law.
Doctor of chiropractic	Certification and passing scores on parts I, II, III, and IV of the National Board of Chiropractic Examiners as a doctor of chiropractic or current licensure, registration, or certification as a doctor of chiropractic in the state, territory, or possession of the United States where practicing.
Doctor of osteopathy performing holistic medicine	Passing scores on the National Board of Osteopathic Medical Examiners Exam (NBOME) for osteopathic physician in the state, territory, or possession of the United States where practicing.
Licensed massage therapist	If practicing in a regulated state, territory, or possession of the United States, licensure, certification, or registration as required by law. If practicing in an unregulated jurisdiction, a minimum of 500 hours of training from a Commission on Massage Therapy Accreditation (COMTA)-approved school and/or passing scores on a National Certification Examination (NCE).
Naturopathic doctor or physician	If practicing in a regulated state, territory, or possession of the United States, licensure, certification, or registration as required by law. If practicing in an unregulated jurisdiction, current active certification by and passing scores received on Naturopathic Physicians Licensing Exam (NPLEX) in Naturopathic Medicine or current, active licensure, registration, or certification as a naturopathic physician in another state, territory, or possession of the United States.
Certified nurse midwife	Successful completion of a nurse midwifery program or an educational program accredited by the American College of Nurse Midwives or successfully completed certification process of the American College of Nurse Midwifery Certification Council and current active licensure certification or registration in the state, territory, or possession of the United States where practicing.
Doctor of Oriental medicine and/or licensed acupuncturist	If practicing in a regulated state, territory, or possession of the United States, licensure, certification, or registration as required by law. If practicing in an unregulated jurisdiction, current active National Certification Commission for Acupuncture and Oriental Medicine (NCCAOM) certification in acupuncture or current active licensure, registration, or certification as an acupuncturist or as an Oriental medicine provider in another state, territory, or possession of the United States.
Physician's assistant	Passing scores on the Physician Assistant National Certifying Examination (PANCE) or the Physician Assistant National Recertifying Examination (PANRE) as well as certification by the National Commission on Certification of Physician Assistants (NCCPA) or current active licensure, registration, or certification as a physician assistant in the state, territory, or possession of the United States where practicing.

(Continued on next page)

Licensed practical nurse (also licensed vocational nurse)	Passing scores on the National Council Licensure Examination for Registered or Practical Nurse (NCLEX-PN) and current, active licensure, registration, or certification as a practical nurse in the state, territory, or possession of the United States where practicing.
Registered midwife	If practicing in a regulated state, territory, or possession of the United States, licensure, certification, or registration as required by law. If practicing in an unregulated jurisdiction, current, active certification as a certified professional midwife (CPM) by the North American Registry of Midwives or certification by the American College of Nurse Midwife Certification Council (ACC) or current licensure, registration, or certification as a midwife in another state.
Registered nurse	Passing scores on the NCLEX-RN and current, active licensure, registration, or certification as a registered nurse in the state, territory, or possession of the United States where practicing.

Source: Alternative Link, LLC. Copyright 1999. Used with permission.

Table 2 details a key to the provider abbreviations that are used for state licenses as well as to describe the individual practitioners. For example, it is common within the professional field to refer to a certain level of social worker as an MSW.

TABLE 2   Health Care Provider Abbreviations Used for State Licenses

ABBREVIATION USED FOR STATE LICENSE	NAME OF PRACTITIONER
CNS	Clinical nurse specialist
NS	Nurse specialist
DC	Doctor of chiropractic
DO	Doctor of osteopathy
DDS	Doctor of dental surgery
MD	Medical doctor
CPC	Certified professional counselor
MFCC	Marriage and family counselor
MSW	Master of social work
PhD, EdD, PsyD, LCP, MFCC, MA	Psychologist
MT	Massage therapist
CMT	Certified massage therapist
LMP	Licensed massage practitioner
LMT	Licensed massage therapist
MP	Massage practitioner
ND	Naturopathic doctor
CNM	Certified nurse midwife

NM	Licensed nurse midwife
ANP	Advanced nurse practitioner
APN	Advanced practice nurse
APRN	Advanced practice registered nurse
ARNP	Advanced registered nurse practitioner
CNP	Certified nurse nractitioner
CRNP	Certified registered nurse nractitioner
RN, NP, C	Registered nurse, nurse practitioner, certified
RNP	Registered nurse practitioner
DOM	Doctor of Oriental medicine
AcT	Acupuncture therapist
AP	Acupuncture physician
CA	Certified acupuncturist
DAc	Doctor of acupuncture
Lac	Licensed acupuncturist
OT	Occupational therapist
PA	Physician's assistant
LPN	Licensed practical nurse
LVN	Licensed vocational nurse
PT	Physical therapist
RM	Registered midwife
CM	Certified midwife
CPM	Certified professional midwife
DEM	Direct entry midwife
GM	Granny midwife
LLM	Licensed lay midwife
LM	Lay midwife
LM	Licensed midwife
RN	Registered nurse, professional nurse, professional registered nurse

Source: Alternative Link, LLC. Copyright 1999. Used with permission.

SUMMARY

Chapters 6–15 cover an extensive array of complementary and alternative therapies. Some are very old and are substantiated with scientific research while others are too new or undeveloped to have been studied yet. It is important to remember that the field of complementary and alternative therapies is ever expanding and a source of comfort and healing to many.

CHAPTER 6

Herbal Medicine, Nutrition, and Supplements

with Lennie Martin

Chapter Objectives

- Become familiar with a variety of herbal medicines, nutrition, and supplement therapies used in some alternative and complementary practices.
- Understand the background and heritage from which herbal medicine arise.
- Be able to describe what herbal medicine is and who uses it.
- Learn what nutritional supplements are and the theory behind them.
- Learn about special diet therapies.
- Compare and contrast the quality of various nutrition therapies.

HERBAL MEDICINE

Herbal medicine is the use of unrefined plant-based products to treat, prevent, or cure disease (Glisson, Crawford, & Street, 1999). Herbal products may also be used to promote optimal health and reduce the effects of chronic conditions (Tyler, 1996). *Phyto* means plant, and phytochemicals or phytonutrients are biologically active plant molecules that are used to promote health and prevent disease (Smith, 1998). The term *phytomedicine* refers to therapeutic use of plants. *Phytotherapy*, a term derived from European literature, involves using standardized herbal products therapeutically.

Herbs are plants that grow from seeds and whose stems wither away after each season's growth. In common usage, herb refers to any useful plant (Gundling, 1999). *Botanical medicine* is a more inclusive term, as it encompasses both herbs and woody plants with therapeutic uses.

Overview

Herbs and other plants have been used medicinally since ancient times, predating recorded history. Native cultures held their medicine women and men in respect, as these healers knew the secrets of the plant world. The potency of many herbs became documented as Western science developed skills of chemical analysis. Herbs and medicinal plants such as belladonna for cardiac arrhythmia, foxglove (digitalis) for cardiac insufficiency, opium for sedation and pain, warfarin

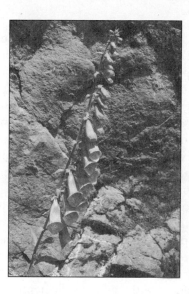

Figure 6-1 *Digitalis purpurea,* or foxglove, has a long history of medicinal use. (Photo courtesy of Photodisc.)

for blood thinning, chamomile for digestive upsets and menstrual problems, and sassafras for blood cleansing and urinary diuresis were used well into the past century by physicians (see Figure 6-1).

Climate and ecology support growth of various herbs in different areas of the world. Throughout the South Pacific islands, a drink called kava, made from the rhizomes and roots of the perennial shrub *Piper methysticum,* was used to induce relaxation and sleep, soothe nerves, and relieve headaches, stomach and urinary problems, asthma, and rheumatism (Singh, 1992). Kava has been extensively studied over the past 130 years, and its effects on muscular relaxation, sedation, sleep induction, anxiety reduction, and anticonvulsant properties are well documented (Bloomfield, 1998; Lehmann, Kinzler, & Friedemann, 1996; and Volz & Kieser, 1997). Vitex (*Vitex agnus castus),* named chaste tree by the Greeks, has been used since ancient times by temple priestesses to suppress libido and by monks and priests in medieval times to reduce sexual desire. Extracts made from the berries of this small tree, indigenous to the Mediterranean region, have been used medicinally in Europe for years to treat premenstrual syndrome (PMS), breast pain, and menopausal symptoms (Martin & Jung, 2000). Black cohosh (*Cimicifuga racemosa),* native to North America, has a long history of traditional use by Native Americans for female conditions, rheumatism, and snake bites and as an insect repellent. Clinical studies have demonstrated the effectiveness of extracts from the dried root of this herb in reducing hot flashes, insomnia, depression, and vaginal dryness during menopause (Warnecke, 1985; Stoll, 1987).

Herbal medicine is extensively used in Europe. Up to 40% of physicians in Germany and France use botanicals in daily practice, having received formal training in phytotherapy during medical school (Glisson et al., 1999). In Germany, herbs are classified as drugs and are regulated by the German Commission E, which has produced over 300 monographs on the benefits and dangers of herbal products. About 65% of herbs have positive health benefits. Commission E monographs provide accurate information about pharmacology, dosing, and adverse effects, with guidelines for appropriate use. Herbal product manufacturers are allowed to place medical claims on the label if they follow monograph guidelines and present data supporting safety and efficacy (Tyler & Foster, 1996).

In the United States, herbs are classified as dietary supplements and are unregulated. Sales of medicinal herbs in this country have exploded since the Dietary Supplement Health and Education Act was passed by Congress in 1994. In addition to the dietary supplement classification, this act permitted manufacturers to make statements about physiological effects of herbs but not about preventing or curing disease (Gundling, 1999). Ginsing can be promoted as an "immune system enhancer" but not as a cure for chronic fatigue syndrome and palmetto to "improve urinary flow" but not to cure enlarged prostate glands. Suggested doses are allowed. The law does not require premarket testing for safety and efficacy, has no stipulation for using standardized manufacturing methods, and does not require FDA approval.

Many clinicians and scientists concerned with herbal medicines have suggested that the United States adopt a Commission E type program to provide herbal monographs and better regulate the herbal industry (Marwick, 1995). However, many consumers and manufacturers of herbal and nutritional products do not want government regulation. They are concerned that regulation will drive prices up, decrease competition, reduce consumer choice, and possibly lead to medical control by requiring prescriptions.

Some principles in rational, reliable phytotherapy include:

1 *Standardization.* A standardized product or extract will have a certain percentage or quantity of active ingredients. For example, ginko biloba preparations are standardized to contain at least 6% terpene lactones and 24% flavone glycosides; black cohosh to contain 5% triterpene glycosides; and kava to contain 30–55% kavalactones. Another term for standardized extracts is *guaranteed potency herb,* meaning scrutiny through the harvesting and manufacturing process so the end product will have the proper percentage of active ingredients from the raw herb. The quality of herbal products can be affected by climate, fertilization, soil, disease, harvest time, and storage conditions. Variations in these factors can alter the chemical composition of the raw herb (Ogletree & Fischer, 1997).

2 *Regulation.* An oversight agency can hold manufacturers to quality standards for growing, harvesting, and production. It can require purity and guaranteed quantity of active ingredients and studies to justify claims made for products. Self-regulation by the herbal industry has led to some very poor quality products. Some companies make products with little or no active ingredients, use parts of the plant that do not contain active ingredients, or substitute a similar plant to decrease expense. Products may be contaminated with other herbs or chemicals, leading to adverse

effects (Cetaruk & Aaron, 1994; Larrey, 1997). Companies manufacturing these products do not have to document injuries or report incidences of contamination (Thompson, 1997).

3 *Quality control.* Currently herbal manufacturers do not have to validate the quality and quantity of ingredients. Studies have shown that many ginseng products contain no or minimal amounts of ginsenosides or oleanolic acids (Cui, Garle, Eneroth, & Bjorkhem, 1994) and that the hormone dehydroepian drosterone (DHEA) products contained from 0% to 150% of the amount of dehydroepiandrosterone stated on the label (Parasrampuria, Schwartz, & Petesch, 1998). Some reputable herbal companies are listed in the resource section at the end of the chapter.

Practitioners

PATIENTS

Self-medication with herbal products is widespread. It is estimated that about 80% of people worldwide use herbal remedies (Glisson et al., 1999). Over one-third of Americans use herbs for health purposes (Miller, 1999). Sales of herbal products are increasing in the United States by 15% per year, with annual sales projected to exceed $5 billion in 2000 (Tyler, 1996). The rapidly growing interest in herbal products among consumers has been spurred by an explosion of literature about the beneficial components of plants. Scientific insights about the structure and function of healing nutrients, with evidence that phytochemicals enhance the molecular processes of cellular biochemistry, has produced a "phytochemical revolution" among consumers and health practitioners (Smith, 1998, pp. 286–307).

PHYSICIANS

Medical doctors now represent the fastest growing group selling dietary supplements and natural products. In 1999, the *Nutrition Business Journal* reported that over $350 million of these products were sold directly to conventional or alternative medical practitioners, who in turn sold $700 million in products to their patients (*UCB Wellness Letter* (b), 1999). That represents a 100% markup and raises issues about conflict of interest. The Federation of State Medical Boards is examining this issue as potential exploitation of the physician-patient relationship.

NURSES

Many nurses have expanded practice through use of a wide variety of healing modalities, such as therapeutic touch, jin shin jyutsu, polarity therapy, massage, acupressure, healing touch, and other forms of body- and energy-balancing work. Patients seek assistance with nutrition and supplements from nurses, who are increasingly expected to be knowledgeable about herbs, vitamins, nutrition, and dietary supplements. Nurses are among the ranks of midlevel marketers, buying private labels not available in drugstores and reselling these to patients. Some of the same issues around exploitation of the nurse-patient relationship arise as for physicians.

HERBALISTS AND NATUROPATHS

These practitioners focus upon nutrition and dietary supplements as treatment modalities. Their use of herbal medicine is extensive, and most are well trained in their educational programs. Often naturopaths utilize sublingual forms of hormones and herbs.

Training Requirements

People generally learn about therapeutic and medicinal use of herbs by attending continuing education courses or seminars taught by experienced herbalists. There are no formal training programs, and often the ancient apprenticeship system is used, where students spend months working with master herbalists to learn herbal lore and techniques by practice and observation.

Naturopathic physicians study herbal medicine as part of their curriculum for licensure/certification by the profession. There is no state licensure or certification for herbalists.

Treatment

PHYSICIANS AND NURSES

Many physicians and nurses incorporate herbal and nutritional interventions into their regular practices. The practitioner-patient encounter usually involves an initial visit for assessment, then a series of follow-up visits to review effects of therapies and make adjustments. Diagnostic testing including blood chemistry, lipids, thyroid studies, and complete blood count is usually ordered. Numerous diseases have significant nutritional components, such as diabetes, hyperlipidemia, cardiovascular disease, obesity, allergic conditions, arthritis, and gastrointestinal problems. Diet history is an important part of patient assessment, to identify foods that provoke or worsen symptoms, or put the patient at increased risk. While diet and nutrition advice has long been standard in medical and nursing practice, certain herbal therapies are now being included as an expected part of the treatment regimen.

For example, vitamin E, 400–800 mg daily, has protective effects against cardiovascular disease (Rapola, Virtamo, Haukka, et al., 1996). Elevated homocysteine levels and low folic acid levels in serum have been associated with increased risk of coronary artery disease (Hopkins et al., 1995; Morrison, Schaubel, Desmeules, & Wigle, 1996). In chronic smokers, vitamin C (usual dose 1000–2000 mg) improves endothelial dysfunction (Heitzer, Just, & Munzel, 1996) and reduces oxidant stress as measured through urinary prostaglandins (Reilly,

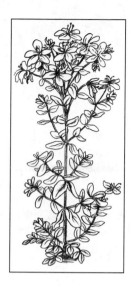

Figure 6-2 *Hypericum perforatum,* or St. John's wort, has been used to treat depression and anxiety.

Delanty, Lawson, & FitzGerald, 1996). Garlic, 900 mg (active ingredient *allocin*), reduces total cholesterol and low-density lipoprotein (LDL-C) in patients with hypercholesterolemia (Adler & Holub, 1997).

St. John's wort (*Hypericum perforatum*) has been traditionally used in Europe to treat mild to moderate depression and anxiety (see Figure 6-2). Its use in the United States is increasing, usually standardized to hypericin, 300 mg (containing 5% hyperforin), taken three times daily. This dosage of St. John's wort was found superior to placebo in alleviating depressive symptoms (Laakmann, Schule, Baghai, et al., 1998). Multicenter clinical trials are under way to compare St. John's wort with selective serotonin reuptake inhibitor (SSRI) antidepressants for moderate to severe depression. Millions of Americans take St. John's wort, which contains at least 10 compounds with pharmacological action and may interact with other drugs (*UCB Wellness Letter* (a), 1999). See Table 6-1.

Estrogenic herbs such as black cohosh and red clover and progestogenic herbs such as vitex and wild yam (disogenin) or soy-derived progesterone are becoming expected options for treating PMS and menopausal symptoms in women. Physicians such as Christiane Northrup (1998) and many nurse practitioners offer specialized care to women in natural phytotherapy and bioidentical hormones for women's health and menopause (Martin & Jung , 1999).

Ginko biloba is frequently used to enhance memory and mental function, primarily through its action in dilating capillaries and inhibiting platelet aggregation. It also scavenges free radicals, which has a protective effect on vascular walls. Ginko's antioxidant properties result from synergistic actions of bioflavonoids, terpenoids, and organic acids. These antioxidant compounds can ameliorate the cell damage and excessive lipid peroxidation seen in Alzheimer's disease (Kanowski, Herrmann, Stephan, et al., 1996).

TABLE 6-1

HERB	BOTANICAL NAME	USE	RISKS AND INTERACTIONS
Cascara sagrada	*Rhamnus purshiana*	Laxative	Severe vomiting or diarrhea, hypocalcemia, electrolyte loss, potentiates cardiac glycosides and thiazide diuretics
Feverfew	*Tanacetum parthenium*	Migraines, headaches	Gastrointestinal disturbances, apthous ulcers, inhibits platelets, avoid with anticoagulants, induces menses, avoid during pregnancy
Garlic	*Allium sativum*	Improves lipids, antibacterial	Inhibits platelets, reduces serum glucose, avoid with anticoagulants
Hawthorne	*Crataegus laevigata*	Heart function, angina	High doses cause central nervous system (CNS) depression, hypotension, may interact with heart medications
Licorice	*Glycyrrhiza glabra*	Gastritis, ulcers, cough, menopause (isoflavones)	Prolongs action of corticosteroids, may cause hypokalemia, hypertension, edema, contraindicated in liver disease, potentiates digitalis
Ma huang	*Ephedra sinica*	Bronchitis, cough, asthma	CNS stimulation, headaches, nausea, irritability, tachycardia, insomnia, high blood pressure, arrhythmias; interacts with cardioglycosides, guanethidine, MAO inhibitors, oxytocin, alkaloids
Milk thistle	*Silybum marianum*	Liver disease, gallbladder	Mild diarrhea, allergic rash (rare)
Purple coneflower	*Echinacea purpurea*	Infections, cold, cough, urinary tract infections, wounds	Activation of autoimmune diseases, overreactive immune responses, avoid with multiple sclerosis, AIDS, collagen and leukoses diseases, tuberculosis
St. John's wort	*Hypericum perforatum*	Depression, anxiety	Indigestion, constipation, photodermatitis; reduces effects of HIV drugs, coumadin, digoxin, cyclosporin; may reduce effectiveness of oral contraceptives; dizziness in elderly
Valerian	*Valeriana officinalis*	Insomnia, anxiety, restlessness	Gastrointestinal symptoms (rare), drowsiness, headache, mydriasis, cardiac dysfunctions (long-term use)

HERBALISTS AND NATUROPATHS

These practitioners often have extensive intake interviews that may last 1–2 hours. A holistic approach is taken, including questions about the patient's lifestyle, stress factors, relationships and family, work situation, habits, hobbies and pleasure activities, as well as dietary and nutritional practices. The encounter may be for only one visit or there may be follow-up visits. Naturopaths may order blood or saliva tests, if allowed in their states. Both practitioners may use "muscle testing" to assess patient's sensitivities to various foods and herbs. This involves having the patient hold an extended arm up against pressure by the practitioner while the test substance is held in the other hand beside the body or a small amount of the substance is placed on the tongue. Weak muscle resistance by the patient is thought to indicate sensitivity to the substance, which means the patient should not ingest the substance, as it may be detrimental.

A wide variety of herb products are recommended by herbalists and naturopaths, sometimes especially formulated on site or by private companies. Patients should be aware that these practitioners may be selling a line of product as part of their business practice and use judgment in buying products. Reputable practitioners will usually offer the choice of shopping in local health food stores or drugstores for competitive products at lower prices.

Advice to Patients

Probably the best advice a health care practitioner can give their patients interested in herbal therapy is to locate an experienced herbalist who will work with their health needs. Self-medication with herbal products, while very common, does have some risks. Patients taking prescription drugs, especially anticoagulants and monoamine oxidase (MAO) inhibitors, should seek medical advice before self-medicating with herbs (see Table 6-1). Patients can be informed about the lack of regulation and standardization of herbal products. Practitioners should become familiar with two or three reputable companies and suggest that patients use their products. Patients should report any unusual symptoms at once to their health practitioner.

Benefits of herbal medicine are many, and patients can be informed about reliable information sources. As with any medication, herbal products should be used for the shortest time necessary to obtain the desired results. Patients can be encouraged to keep track of which herbs they have taken, for what purposes, and the outcome in terms of symptom relief. This allows documentation of effective herbal therapies or provides data for analyzing which herbal approaches were not effective.

Research

Research on medicinal use of herbs is rapidly expanding. Several herbs have been studied in randomized clinical trials, with some currently under way. The journals and newsletters that publish substantial numbers of articles on herbal medicine include:

Alternative and Complementary Medicine	*Pharmacopsychiatry*
Alternative Medicine Review	*Holistic Nursing Update*
Alternative Medicine Alert	*Integrative Medicine Consult*
Phytomedicine	*Journal of Holistic Nursing*
Herbalgram	

Outcomes of research on herbal products are often contradictory, with some studies finding symptom relief or improvement while other studies do not demonstrate significant results. The quality, strength, and specific components of herbs used in the studies have an impact on results. Other factors such as study length, herb dosage levels, and measurement tools also affect results.

RESEARCH ON SELECTED HERBS

Saw palmetto (*Serenoa repens*) is used to treat benign prostatic hyperplasia (BPH). Extracts of saw palmetto berries contain fatty acids, phytosterols, polysaccharides, diterpenes, triterpenes, and alcohols. These compounds exert an antiandrogenic and antiexudative action, largely by inhibiting testosterone receptor binding and reducing inflammatory responses in the prostate gland. One randomized, placebo-controlled trial of one week duration showed no significant difference between saw palmetto and placebo (Strauch, Perles, Vergult, et al., 1994). An earlier clinical trial resulted in significant improvements in dysuria, nocturia, urinary flow, and residual urinary flow (Champault, Patel, Bonnard, et al., 1984). A large open study (no controls) demonstrated significant improvements in dysuria, nocturia, quality of life scores, urinary flow and residual urinary flow, and prostate size, with 88% of both patients and physicians rating palmetto as effective (Braeckman, 1994).

Evening primrose oil (*Oenothera biennis*) has been used for many years to relieve breast pain and symptoms of PMS. This oil contains high concentrations of *cis*-linoleic acid and *cis*-y-linolenic acid (GLA), two fatty acids that the human body produces in limited amounts. One study found that supplementation of 2.4–3.2 g/day of EPO in divided doses led to decreased pain in 44% of women with cyclical breast pain and 27% of women with noncyclical breast pain (Gateley & Mansel, 1991). Another study found that taking four capsules containing 72% linoleic acid and 9% GLA twice daily during the last 14 days of the menstrual cycle relieved PMS symptoms (Larsson, Jonasson, & Fianu, 1989). However, other studies have shown that EPO has no effect on relieving PMS symptoms (Budieri, Li Wan, & Dornan, 1996).

Vitex agnus-castus (chasteberry) is another herb with a traditional reputation for treating menstrual abnormalities and PMS. Its use has been especially widespread in European countries. A recent German study compared Vitex with pyrodoxine (vitamin B_6) since earlier research indicated the latter could improve symptoms of nervousness, irritability, depression, bloating, breast tenderness, weight gain, and skin and digestive problems. This controlled, double-blind study of 175 women with PMS found standardized Vitex extract to be superior to pyridoxine in alleviating typical PMS complaints (Lauritzen, Reuter, Repges, Bohnert, Schmidt, 1997).

The most extensive study of ginko biloba performed in the United States assessed the efficacy and safety of ginko for Alzheimer's disease and multi-infarct dementia. The 52-week, randomized, double-blind, placebo-controlled study ended with 202 patients completing the data. The researchers used a German preparation of ginko, Schwabe's EGb761 (40 mg three times daily, before meals). Outcome was measured by a cognitive impairment scale, a daily living and social behavior rating scale, and a general psychopathology clinical scale. The study found slight improvement in the study group on the cognitive impairment scale, with significant worsening of the placebo group. The study group showed improvement in daily living and social behavior, while the placebo group deteriorated. There was no significant difference between groups on the clinical psychopathology scale (Le Bars, Katz, Berman, et al., 1997).

NUTRITION AND SPECIAL DIET THERAPIES

The field of clinical nutrition has been available as a professional specialty for many years in universities and colleges. Many hospitals, large clinics, and schools employ clinical nutritionists who design menus for patients with special dietary needs or for students in school. Sometimes the term *dietician* is used for this specialty.

Nurses and physicians have courses in nutrition included in their basic education, but this ranges from one or two lectures to two full semesters. With nursing's emphasis on health promotion, interest in nutrition tends to be quite high. Most physicians focus more on pathophysiology and disease diagnosis and management and often do not keep current on nutrition research. Several physicians, however, have become internationally known for their unique nutritional programs, such as Robert Atkins, Nathan Pritikin, Dean Ornish, Barry Sears, and Andrew Weil. Their approaches are discussed below.

In recent years, a wide variety of practitioners have jumped into the field of nutrition, presenting an array of theories about the best diet for health, weight loss, vitality, and longevity. Consumers and patients often become confused about contradictory recommendations, and fad diets spin by at a dizzying pace. The FDA periodically issues dietary guidelines that can be useful, but these, too, change over the years as new data change our understanding of nutrients and metabolism.

Overview

The field of nutrition has greatly proliferated in recent years and good nutrition has finally been recognized as a primary source of good health. Nutrition constitutes the food we eat as well as how the food is selected, prepared, served, and eaten. Vegetarianism and macrobiotics are two of the more popular varieties of alternative food choices.

Though opinions vary among nutritionists as to what constitutes a healthy, balanced diet, there is a general consensus on following the food pyramid guidelines: Eat mostly grains, followed by vegetables and fruit, followed by fish, eggs, and dairy, and, lastly, by poultry and meat (see Figure 6-3). When in doubt, variety counts. According, to many in the alternative field of nutrition, Americans eat excessive amounts of meat and protein. Therefore, vegetarian, vegan, macrobiotic, raw food, and "live food" (sprouted and fermented foods) diets are often recommended. Special diets included in this section are macrobiotic, soy food, vegetarian, Pritikin, Ornish, and high fiber.

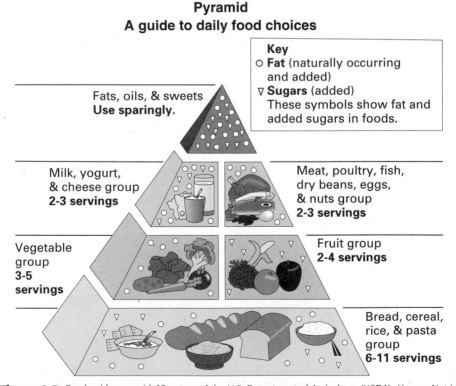

Figure 6-3 Food guide pyramid. [Courtesy of the U.S. Department of Agriculture (USDA), Human Nutritional Information Service, 1992. Food Guide Pyramid (*Home and Garden Bulletin*, No. 252) Washington, DC: USDA.]

MACROBIOTICS

The macrobiotic way of living and eating originated in Japan and maintains that health is a natural birthright and the natural state of the human being. The human being is unique physically, emotionally, and consciously. To best develop, nourish, and sustain these unique human qualities, we must understand what is real human food. In the macrobiotic view, human food must be good not only for the human being but also for society, the environment, and the economy. It makes no sense to consume foods that appear to be nutritionally correct but pollute the environment, waste natural resources, feed fewer people, and are costly to produce, manufacture, store, and transport.

Macrobiotics is based on a worldview of life and health that includes diet, bodywork, self-expression, and cooking. The first step in the macrobiotic way of living is to learn the application of these principles to daily food selection and preparation. The macrobiotic way is not a rigid dietary formula that condemns or accepts any food blindly, but rather one that encourages people to understand not only the value and proportion of nutritional factors but also the "life quality" of the food chosen.

The macrobiotic way encourages an approach to eating that provides complex carbohydrates, quality protein, and fat through the use of whole grains as a main food and vegetables and other supplemental foods. A low-fat, high-fiber "macrobiotic" diet is based on whole grains, vegetables, sea vegetables, and seeds. A diet of these natural foods, cooked in accordance with macrobiotic principles designed to synchronize one's eating habits with the cycles of nature, is used to promote health. Macrobiotic cookbooks can be found at most health food stores.

VEGETARIANISM

Vegetarians follow a meatless diet. There are three primary categories of vegetarians:

- **Vegans** eat exclusively plant products, and no meat, dairy, or fish products.
- **Lactovegetarians** also eat dairy products, but not eggs, meat, or fish.
- **Ovolactovegetarians** include both eggs and dairy products in the menu, but no meat or fish.

There are a number of variations on these themes. Some vegetarians (called "fruitarians") eat only raw fruits, sometimes supplemented with vegetables and nuts. Others may be part-time vegetarians or may eat no red meat but include white meat such as chicken or fish in their diet. Some vegetarian diets restrict products such as alcohol, sugar, caffeine, or processed foods.

Although the benefits of a low-fat, high-fiber, vitamin-rich diet are not restricted to vegetarianism, the type of menu that vegetarians favor can promote health in a number of ways, reducing the risk of heart disease, liver and gallbladder disease, cataracts, and stroke. Many studies have found a link between reduced cancer rates and diets rich in fruits, vegetables, and grains: The American Cancer Society recommends five or more servings of fruits and vegetables and six or more servings of grain (bread, cereal, rice, and pasta) daily.

The American Dietetic Association has declared that vegetarian diets can be healthy and nutritionally complete when properly planned. However, it is unwise to be too restrictive with children under two years of age; they need liberal amounts of the essential fatty acids found primarily in meat. Likewise, during pregnancy and breastfeeding, consult a dietitian to make sure that a vegetarian diet is complete and balanced.

SOY FOODS

A whole school of thought revolves around the consumption of soy foods. These foods include such items as tofu, tempeh, and miso, used both alone and in multiple combinations. Among the legumes, soybeans are very high in protein, with oils that include omega-3 fatty acids. They contain isoflavones, which are phytochemicals with hormonal effects (see the section on phytoestrogen, below). The amazing versatility of soy has been used to advantage by Western technology, which has fashioned numerous processed foods from soy, including powdered protein drinks, nondairy frozen desserts, vegetarian hot dogs, burgers, and pepperoni, cheese, and a plethora of meat substitutes such as "Tofurkey" for vegetarians to use at Thanksgiving.

Many contemporary health professionals encourage the substitution of soy proteins for some of the animal foods in the standard Western diet. By using soy products, you can decrease intake of saturated fat and increase omega-3 essential fatty acids (EFAs), fiber, and protective phytochemicals. There would be less exposure to environmental toxins, drugs, and hormones often found in meats. Highly processed soy foods made with "isolated soy protein" may not contain the isoflavones, fiber, and healthful oils of the whole bean.

There are many brands of soy milk on the market, ranging from full fat to nonfat, plain, sweetened, flavored, and calcium fortified. Soy milk may be substituted for cow's milk in most recipes, and it is often used for children who do not tolerate lactose. Roasted soy nuts are flavorful substitutes but may be cooked in unhealthy oils. Soy butters are also available, but many people do not care for the taste. Mixing soy butter with peanut butter often improves taste.

Soybeans and soy products may upset digestion and produce gas in some people. Textured vegetable protein (TVP), soy flour, and soy grits are the worst offenders. Fermented forms such as tempeh and miso are less likely to cause unpleasant digestive effects. People can become acclimated to eating soy by taking a small amount daily for several weeks, then gradually increasing the amount.

The epidemiological evidence for health protective effects of soy is positive. Countries whose populations eat a lot of soy have low rates of breast cancer, menopausal problems, and prostate cancer. Soy isoflavones can possibly protect people from hormonally driven cancers, coronary heart disease, and osteoporosis.

ATKINS DIET

New York cardiologist Robert Atkins developed this low-carbohydrate, high-fat diet over 25 years ago, and it is enjoying a resurgence. His theory is that carbohydrates, not fat, underlie obesity, hypertension, heart disease, fatigue, and energy problems. All forms of carbohydrates, both simple and complex, are restricted while ample servings of fats (meat, butter, cream, cheese) are allowed. People do lose weight on this diet, but questions have been raised about long-term effects of high protein and fat intake.

PRITIKIN DIET

The Pritikin diet was developed to treat people with high blood pressure, heart disease, adult-onset diabetes, and other chronic diseases. It is based on the premise that fat is the important underlying factor in causing these conditions. The diet is restricted to no more than 10% of total calories as fat, and good results in correcting or controlling these conditions have resulted. Pritikin meals emphasize grains—including bread and pasta—fish, and chicken.

ORNISH DIET

Ornish, a California cardiologist, developed his diet to prevent and reverse coronary heart disease. Fat calories are restricted to 10%–20%, with emphasis on vegetables, fruit, legumes, and whole grains. In a program that includes a low-fat vegetarian diet, stress reduction, exercise, and group support, Ornish has demonstrated through studies that coronary artery disease can actually be reversed within a relatively short period of time.

ZONE DIET

Biochemist Barry Sears developed a modified Atkins regimen that distinguishes among types of fats and carbohydrates. His theory is that various foods act chemically to affect hormones that regulate metabolism. Each meal should consist of 40% carbohydrates, 30% protein, and 30% fat. This 4:3:3 ratio maintains a balance of eicosanoids that provide a system of checks and balances that will put people in "the zone." This properly regulates their metabolism, so they will lose weight, maintain energy and vitality, and be healthier. Certain carbohydrates support balance; apples and black beans will put you in "the zone" while carrots or pasta will cause a glucose-insulin cascade that leads to depositing fatty cells and depleted energy.

HIGH-FIBER DIET

Fiber is the indigestible part of food that makes up most of the bulk in the stool, also called roughage. Fiber comes from resistant carbohydrates, which are too complex for human digestive systems to break down. Insoluble fiber comes from whole grains (especially wheat bran), and soluble fiber comes from whole grains, nuts, seeds, fruits, and vegetables. Vegetarians eat a lot of fiber, but people eating mainly meat, potatoes, and white bread have low fiber intake. The average American diet includes 20 g of fiber daily. According to Andrew Weil (2000), an optimum diet should provide 40 g of fiber daily. Good sources of fiber include raw fruits (especially berries), vegetables (especially beans), and whole grains. High-fiber diets are protective against constipation, irritable bowel, colitis, colon cancer, and hypercholesterolemia.

Practitioners

It seems as if everyone is a self-styled nutritionist. Few topics call forth such a wide range of strongly held opinions as what constitutes the best diet. Patients certainly take initiative in their dietary practices and are being exposed to many conflicting ideas through written and broadcast media and the Internet. As new research is published about nutrition, we are learning more about micronutrients and the complex mechanisms by which the body metabolizes, utilizes, and excretes foods. One primary function of health care praciticners is to support patients in becoming better informed and finding reliable, scientific sources of information to counter the influence of faddists and entrepreneurs with a market in mind.

Nutritionists with university education offer counseling on a broad range of diet-related health issues, including weight loss, food allergies, and dietary supplementation with vitamins, minerals, or food concentrates.

Naturopaths often include nutritional therapies in their treatment regimens, along with herbs and supplements. The field of "functional medicine" uses primarily dietary interventions, along with vitamin-mineral supplements. Many practitioners such as chiropractors, massage therapists, osteopathic physicians, physical therapists, and other energy workers incorporate principles of functional medicine in their work. Jeffrey Bland (2000) is one of the best known proponents of functional medicine and provides a product line intended to assist the body in correcting metabolic and nutritional deficiencies that underlie chronic illness.

AMERICAN DIETETIC ASSOCIATION

The American Dietetic Association (ADA), founded in 1917, has nearly 69,000 members in the United States and abroad that help shape the food choices and impact the nutritional status of the public. The membership includes dietitians, dietetic technicians, students, and others holding baccalaureate and advanced degrees in nutrition and dietetics. The ADA and its foundation established the National Center for Nutrition and Dietetics (NCND) as an easily accessible objective source of scientifically based food and nutrition information. The NCND continues to showcase ADA and its members as the most valued source of this information.

The NCND offers objective nutrition information to the public through ongoing programs such as National Nutrition Month and the Consumer Nutrition Hot Line. An 800/900 service offers consumers the opportunity to listen to timely nutrition messages, talk with registered dietitians, and receive answers to their food and nutrition questions. The NCND's Information Center provides members with the latest information on nutrition-related topics.

Members of the ADA build skills and stay current in their specialty area through 29 dietetic practice groups that offer vital networking contacts, practice-related publications, and continuing professional education workshops. The *Journal of the American Dietetic Association* and the *ADA Courier* supply members with current food and nutrition research and practice information as well as association news.

Treatment

Nutritional counseling ideally is an ongoing process, taking place over several visits. An assessment is needed to determine the patient's current dietary practices, including eating habits, snacking, and types and amounts of foods. A diet log is often used as a take-home assignment, in which patients record the time of eating, foods, amounts, circumstances, and sometimes feelings associated with eating. On a follow-up visit, the practitioner reviews this log, using it to both educate the patient and plan objectives of nutrition therapy. Written educational materials are helpful to patients in learning nutritional and caloric contents of foods and habits associated with eating that will promote digestion and absorption. Additional visits provide for reassessment, education, and evaluation of meeting goals.

Advice to Patients

Nutrition is a complex subject, with many strongly held opinions among patients and practitioners. Patients should become well informed about current knowledge in the field, rather than accepting one viewpoint. Understanding the meaning of food and awareness of the behavior patterns leading to poor nutritional practices will help patients maintain a healthy diet.

In recent years, a number of diets have swept the country promising to control weight, increase energy, promote health, and extend longevity. Many have conflicting recommendations on amounts of carbohydrates, fats, and proteins, and some purport to contain special supplements with wondrous properties. Patients must be wary of the promises and claims made by proponents of fad diets. They should seek advice of trained nutritional counselors or talk with their health provider about research that supports or contradicts these claims.

For example, a few years ago two best-selling diet books took the country by storm: Covert Bailey's *Fit or Fat?* and Harvey and Marilyn Diamond's *Fit for Life.* These authors advocate never mixing protein and carbohydrates at the same meal. Barry Sears, in his book *The Zone,* advocates a specified 4:3:3 ratio of carbohydrates, protein, and fats at every meal. Robert Atkins recommends high-fat, low-carbohydrate meals to promote health and vitality, while Dean Ornish calls this approach irresponsible, since his research has shown that high-fat diets increase the risk of coronary heart disease.

Any diet that recommends a narrow range of foods or extreme amounts of any food type or supplement should be viewed with suspicion. No one approach will be best for everyone because of metabolic and digestive uniqueness. However, some principles of good nutrition and proper eating can provide guidelines through this dietary morass.

Principles of Optimum Diet

The optimum diet should:

- Supply all needs for calories, macronutrients, and micronutrients.
- Support general health throughout life and maximize longevity.
- Provide pleasure in eating.
- Promote social interaction and reinforce personal and cultural identity.

The diet should provide a variety of foods, with a high percentage of fresh, unprocessed foods. It should be abundant in fruits and vegetables, grown and produced with a minimum of harmful elements. It should supply:

- Calories: 2000–3000 calories daily, depending on gender, body size, and activity level.
- Calorie distribution: 50%–60% carbohydrates, 30% fat, 10%–20% protein.
- Carbohydrates: about 250 g for women and 300 g for men, most from less refined and processed foods with a low-glycemic-index (below 60). Eat some low-glycemic-index foods with each meal (whole grains, beans, vegetables, nontropical fruits), and include some low-glycemic-index

foods with high-glycemic-index foods (wheat, corn, sugars, some rice, potatoes, pasta, tropical fruits).

■ Fat: 600 calories from fat in a 2000-calorie/day diet, in a 1:2:1 ratio of saturated to monounsaturated to polyunsaturated fat. No more than 100 calories from saturated fat (butter, cream, cheese, full-fat dairy, un-skinned chicken, fatty meats, products with palm and coconut oil). Have a 2–4:1 ratio of omega-6 to omega-3 EFAs. This can be done by increasing amounts of oily fish, soybeans, walnuts, hemp or flax seeds, or oils. Avoid margarine, all products made with partially hydrogenated oils, and fried foods, especially in fast-food restaurants.

■ Protein: 50–100 g protein in a 2000-calorie/day diet. Eat more vegetable protein, especially from beans, and less animal protein, except for fish and reduced-fat dairy products.

■ Vitamins and minerals: a diet high in fresh foods with plenty of fruits and vegetables provides most of the necessary micronutrients. These supplements are recommended:

(a) Vitamin C, 100 mg twice daily

(b) Vitamin E, 400–800 IU of natural d-alpha-tocopherol

(c) Selenium, 200 μg (yeast bound)

(d) Mixed carotenoids, 25,000 IU

(e) B-complex vitamin with 400 μg folic acid

(f) Calcium, 1200–1500 mg (calcium carbonate if under age 65, calcium citrate if over 65 or having digestive problems)

■ Fiber: 40 g daily. Good sources are fruits, especially berries, vegetables, especially beans, and whole grains.

■ Protective phytochemicals: for additional protection against environmental toxicity and cancer, eat a variety of fruits, vegetables, mushrooms, and tea (especially green tea).

■ Water: drink six to eight glasses of water daily, as pure as possible. Use bottled water or a home water purifier if tap water tastes of chlorine or you live in areas where contaminants are suspected.

■ Stimulants: avoid or minimize alcohol and caffeine (Weil, 2000).

Research

The Lifestyle Heart Trial study by Ornish, Scherwitz, Billings, et al. (1999) was extended from one to five years to further assess the effect of 10% fat, a vegetarian diet, aerobic exercise, stress management, and group psychosocial support on the course of coronary heart disease (CHD). Although the groups were small (20 experimental, 15 control), the results of the randomized controlled trial were significant, showing that patients can maintain comprehensive diet and lifestyle changes that stop or reverse the progression of CHD. The average percent diameter coronary artery stenosis decreased in the experimental group by 1.75 percentage points at one year and 3.1 percentage points at five years. In dramatic contrast, this measure increased in the control group by 2.3 percentage points at one year and 11.8 percentage points at five years. The LDL levels of the experimental group showed improvement over the control group who took lipid-lowering drugs and even more improvement compared with controls who took no drugs. Among patients in the experimental group there were 0.89 cardiac events per patient, with 2.25 cardiac events per patient in the control group. These results demonstrate the effectiveness of diet and lifestyle in reducing cardiac events by stopping or reversing CHD and improving LDL levels (Ornish et al., 1999).

The relationship between diet and breast cancer has spurred considerable research as well as popular books. Popular literature suggests that low-fat diets can reduce breast cancer risk. Bob Arnot's recent book, *The Breast Cancer Prevention Diet*, claiming that breast cancer can be prevented or even treated by consuming olive oil, soy protein, fish oil, flaxseed, and a low-calorie diet, was countered by an analysis in the *UCB Wellness Letter* (a), (1999), which provided evidence that these measures had no proven relationship on breast cancer. A longitudinal investigation analyzed dietary fat intake in 88,795 women free of cancer in 1980 who were then followed for 14 years as part of the Nurses' Health Study. Fat intake was assessed by food frequency questionnaires. Average total fat intake declined from 39% of total calories in 1980 to 31% in 1990. No correlation was found between total fat intake and risk for breast cancer, in either pre- or postmenopausal women. Separate analyses were done for breast cancer risk and intakes of animal fat, vegetable fat, polyunsaturated fat, saturated fat, monounsaturated fat, trans-unsaturated fat, omega-3 fat, and cholesterol. The study found that women who had greater intake of vegetable, polyunsaturated, monounsaturated, and trans-unsaturated fats had lower breast cancer risk. These data indicate that women are unlikely to reduce breast cancer risk by lowering fat intake in midlife (Holmes et al., 1999).

Interest in antiaging regimens has focused attention on diet and supplements. Timothy Smith (1998) presents these principles for an antiaging diet: About 80% of calories should come from complex carbohydrates, with 10% each from protein and fat, emphasizing plant-derived foods, 40–60 g fiber, very low fat with adequate EFAs, very low protein mainly from plant sources, fresh foods grown without pesticides, antioxidants, vitamin and mineral supplements, very low/no caffeine, alcohol, and simple sugars. Research has found the best way to delay aging in animals is dietary restriction, consisting of reducing calories without decreasing intake of essential nutrients (Lee et al., 1999). Numerous studies have shown that dietary restriction can slow functional deterioration and retard onset of age-related diseases. The antiaging effect of food restriction is attributed to reduction of oxidation damage to cells by decreasing the action of free radicals (Yu, 1998).

NUTRITIONAL SUPPLEMENTS

Supplements are vitamins, minerals, enzymes, and other food products, derivatives, additives, and ingredients that are used to potentiate the use of food intake. Controversy abounds about whether supplements can help prevent illness and disease or treat them once diagnosed. What we do know is that supplements have helped people with vitamin deficiency diseases, such as beri beri or scurvy. There is controversy about whether people in developed countries who eat a diet with a wide variety of foods, especially fruits and vegetables, need any type of supplementation. Some contend that soils have become depleted of vitamins, mineral, and other micronutrients because of large-scale farming with chemical fertilizers. No conclusive evidence has been provided to date to substantiate that contention.

Many leaders in the nutritional field do recommend supplements, however. This is largely based on the inadequate diet of most Americans, which fails to provide a well-rounded intake of enough nutrients from a variety of sources.

Overview

In the past people obtained vitamins, minerals, and other micronutrients from whole foods. The ability to refine and concentrate specific micronutrients became available early in the twentieth century, starting with vitamins. As science has delved more deeply into the chemical and molecular structures of micronutrients, there has been an explosion of knowledge about many specific enzymes, hormones, neurotransmitters, amino acids, fatty acids, peptides, and other substances. Research is discovering the complex, minute functions of many micronutrients in the body. Capitalizing on this, pharmaceutical and nutriceutical companies have developed many products that claim to improve specific body functions or prevent malfunctioning of body systems.

Some traditional herbals and plants do have micronutrient effects (see Table 6-2). For example, evening primrose can be converted in the body to the prostaglandin precursor DGLA and has GLA (gamma linoleic acid) effects, which lowers serum cholesterol. Psyllium is still used as a bulk-forming laxative for constipation and irritable bowel syndrome. Senna is a strong cathartic, while cascara is a gentle laxative. Cranberry juice has been used to relieve urinary tract infections. A recent study pinpointed the condensed tannins (proanthocyanidins) in cranberries as the compounds responsible for inhibiting the adherence of *Escherichia coli* to uroepithelial cells. This makes the bacteria more easily excreted through urine, thus less likely to cause symptoms (Howell, Vorsa, Der Marderosian, et al., 1998).

TABLE 6-2	**Common Micronutrients**

VITAMINS

A, 1000–10,000 IU

Beta-carotene, 25000–50000 IU

Thiamin (B_1), 100–250 mg

Riboflavin (B_2), 50–250 mg

Niacinamide (B_3), 50–250 mg

Pantothenic acid (B_5), 60–2000 mg

Pyridoxine (B_6), 25–250 mg

B_{12}, 500–500 µg

Biotin, 200–800 µg

Folic acid, 400–800 µg

C, 200–2000 mg

Bioflavonoids, 500–4000 mg

D, 200–1000 IU

E, 400–800 IU

MINERALS

Calcium, 600–1500 mg

Magnesium, 300–500 mg

Potassium, 100–200 mg

Manganese, 5–15 mg

Iron, 0–40 mg,

Chromium, 100–600 µg

Selenium, 100–300 µg

Boron, 1–3 mg

Iodine, 100–225 µg

Copper, 1–3 mg

Zinc, 15–50 mg

Molybdenum, 75–250 mg

Vanadium, 25–100 mcg

ESSENTIAL FATTY ACIDS (EFAs)

Alpha-linolenic acid (omega-3), 2000–10,000 mg (flaxseed oil)

Gamma-linolenic acid (omega-6), 250–500 mg (borage, black current oil)

HORMONES, OTHERS

Dehydroepiandrosterone (DHEA, use controversial), 10–100 mg

Pregnenolone (steroid precursor), 25–200 mg (as indicated)

Estrogen (as indicated)

Progesterone (as indicated)

Testosterone (as indicated)

Melatonin, 0.5–10 mg (as indicated)

Coenzyme Q10 (use controversial), 50–300 mg

Proflavonol (grapeseed extract), 10–20 mg

Phosphatidylserine (brain nutrient), 100–300 mg (as indicated)

Acetyl-L-carnitine (brain nutrient), 500–3000 mg (as indicated)

Sources: Smith, 1998; Weil, 2000.

PHYTOESTROGENS

Phytoestrogens are common dietary compounds. They are present in all plants in one form or another, so unless you are eating a totally plant-free diet, you are exposed to them every day. There are many different types of phytoestrogens. Some plants have only one type, but most contain several different types. The five most common types of phytoestrogens in the human diet and their common plant sources are:

- Flavones: most red/yellow colored fruits and vegetables
- Flavonols: most red/yellow colored fruits and vegetables
- Flavanones: citrus fruits
- Isoflavones: legumes
- Lignans: most cereals, fruits, and vegetables

Isoflavones have emerged as the most interesting phytoestrogens because:

1. They have the most potent estrogenic activity of all of the common phytoestrogens.
2. They have an extensive range of biological activity in the body.

There are over 1000 different isoflavones in the plant kingdom, and they are found almost exclusively in legumes. Legumes are vegetables that have high levels of protein; they are consumed widely in many traditional cultures as a source of protein instead of meat. Legumes include chick peas, soy, clover, lentils, and beans. Most Americans obtain their dietary protein from meat, not legumes, so the level of isoflavones in their diet is usually very low compared to people in other cultures.

There is mounting scientific evidence that the health benefits enjoyed by people with traditional legume-based diets (Asians and Latin Americans) are due to the presence of isoflavones. Of the considerable range of isoflavones consumed by humans, only a small proportion are estrogenic.

Practitioners

Practitioners who recommend supplements are naturopaths, physicians, nurses, dieticians and nutritionists, chiropractors, and self-trained individuals.

Advice to Patients

It is important to tell your clients that supplements, herbs, and special diets may have side effects or untoward consequences. They should check the credentials of the provider as well as learn all they can about the product.

Research

Dietary micronutrients are an area of intense research at present. These food constituents allow more focused studies than do general diets and macronutrients. Patients and professionals need to find a good source that summarizes research studies (see Resources section). As with any scientific research, findings are often contradictory.

Antioxidants are the focus of considerable research. Oversupplementation of rats with vitamin C and a separate group with vitamin A led to improved auditory sensitivities and a trend for fewer mitochondrial DNA deletions associated with hearing loss in aging. In this same study, the group of rats given 30% caloric reduction maintained the most acute auditory sensitivities and lowest quantity of mitochondrial DNA deletions. The study concluded that nutritional strategies may limit the age-associated increase in reactive oxygen metabolites that lead to DNA damage and reduce the degree of hearing loss in aging (Seidman, 2000). In 30 top-class endurance training cyclists, five months of vitamin E supplementation led to significant reduction in creatine kinase and malondialdehyde serum levels. This suggests a protective effect of vitamin E against oxidative stress caused by strenuous exercise (Rokitzki, Lothar, et al., 1994). A randomized, double-blind, placebo-controlled trial over 4.7 years studied the effects of vitamin E and beta-carotene on risk for developing angina in male smokers age 50–69 who were initially free of CHD. Vitamin E compared with no vitamin E led to decreased risk for angina (RR 0.91). The incidence of angina per 1000 patient years was 19.6 for the vitamin E group and 21.5 for those not receiving vitamin E. Beta carotene was not associated with a change in angina risk (RR 1.06) (Rapola et al., 1996).

Other vitamin studies have had variable results. Prior studies have shown that taking vitamin B_6 supplements could relieve symptoms of carpal tunnel syndrome (CTS). Researchers at the University of Michigan measured serum levels of vitamin B_6 in a group of workers in several automobile parts plants performing repetitive-motion work that led to CTS in one-third of the group. No correlation was found between low serum vitamin B_6 levels and CTS. The study concluded that use of vitamin B_6 was unwarranted for CTS (Franzblau et al., 1996). Nearly 50 years ago, some doctors started using large doses of niacinamide (vitamin B_3) for osteoarthritis. A recent double-blind, randomized study of 72 osteoarthritis patients found that those taking 500 mg niacinamide three times daily for three months had significant improvements in joint mobility and overall severity of arthritis and reduction of erythrocyte sedimentation rate in comparison to the placebo group. The niacinamide group was able to reduce use of anti-inflammatory medicines (Jonas et al., 1996).

Hormones are another area of research interest. Blood levels of melatonin have been found to be low in patients with cluster headaches, especially during attacks. A double-blind study was done of 20 patients with cluster headaches who were treated with melatonin, 10 mg, or placebo once daily for 14 days. Headache frequency was significantly reduced in the melatonin group, but no improvement was seen in the placebo group. Of the 10 patients receiving melatonin, headaches stopped after three to five days of treatment and did not recur until melatonin was discontinued (Leone et al., 1996). Dioscorea, an extract of wild yams containing several steroid molecules, has been marketed for several years for estrogenic and DHEA raising effects. A study of seven healthy people, average age 73, administered dioscorea tablets two per day for one week, four per day for one week, and eight per day for one week. Ingestion of dioscorea had no effect on serum DHEA levels (Araghiniknam et al., 1996).

Research on osteoporosis has found that a number of different micronutrients and supplements can have beneficial effects on preventing or reversing bone loss. Fatty acids were studied over a period of 18 months by randomly assigning 65 women (average age 79.5 years) into two groups: one taking a fatty acid supplement containing gamma-linolenic acid and eicosapentaenoic acid and a placebo group. All women received 600 mg/day calcium. In the placebo group, bone density of the lumbar spine declined and of the hip was unchanged. In the fatty acid group, bone density increased at both sites, with significantly lower risk of hip fracture (Kruger et al., 1996). Clinical trials of ipriflavone, a synthetic isoflavone, have found increased or stable bone mineral density in experimental groups, while placebo groups had declines in bone density (Adami, Bufalino, Cervetti, et al., 1997; Agnusdei, Crepaldi, Isaia, et al., 1997). Ipriflavone appears particularly effective in older women (over 65), resulting in 6% increase in bone mineral density after one year and decreased fracture rates (Agnusdei et al., 1997).

SUMMARY

Herbal medicine is the use of unrefined plant-based products to treat, prevent, or cure disease. This focus of treatment has been used since antiquity, but has experienced a recent renaissance. Each year, more data is being accumulated about various herbs and how they are used to treat a plethora of conditions. Likewise, nutrition and special diet therapies have mass appeal as the U.S. population in general is paradoxically both obese and keenly interested in personal fitness. A substantial portion of Americans use a variety of nutritional supplements to enhance and preserve health.

ASK YOURSELF

1. What kind of practioner uses herbs to treat others?
2. What foods would be included in a macrobiotic diet?
3. Name at least three special diets and what they accomplish.
4. What are some research studies that support supplements as effective?
5. Are there any precautions to follow when taking an herb, special diet, or supplement?

REFERENCES

Adami, S., Bufalino, l., Cervetti, R., DiMarco, C., DiMarco, O., Fantasia, L., Isaia, G. C., Serni, U., Vecchiet, L., Passeri, M. (1997). Ipriflavone prevents radial bone loss in postmenopausal women with low bone mass over 2 years. *Osteoporosis International, 7*, 119–125.

Adler, A. J., & Holub, B. J. (1997). Effect of garlic and fish-oil supplementation on serum lipid and lipoprotein concentrations in hypercholesterolemic men. *American Journal of Clinical Nutrition, 65,* 445–450.

Agnusdei, D., & Bufalino, L. (1997). Efficacy of ipriflavone in established osteoporosis and long-term safety. *Calcified Tissue International 61,* S23-S27.

Agnusdei, D., Crepaldi, G., Isaia G., et al. (1997). A double blind, placebo-controlled trial of ipriflavone for prevention of postmenopausal spinal bone loss. *Calcified Tissue International 61,* 142–147.

Araghiniknam, M., Chung, S., Nelson-White, T., Eskelson, C., Watson, R. R. (1996). Antioxidant activity of dioscorea and dehydroepiandrosterone (DHEA) in older humans. *Life Science 11,* 147–157.

Bland, J. S. (2000). *Nutritional management of the underlying causes of chronic disease.* Gig Harbor, Wa: Institute for Functional Medicine.

Bloomfield, H. H. (1998). *Healing anxiety with herbs.* New York: HarperCollins.

Braeckman, J. (1994). The extract of *Serenoa repens* in the treatment of benign prostatic hyperplasia: A multicenter open study. *Current Therapeutic Research 55,* 776–784.

Budieri, D., Li Wan Po, A., Dornan, J. C. (1996). Is evening primrose oil of value in the treatment of premenstrual syndrome? *Controlled Clinical Trials 17,* 60–68.

Cetaruk, E. W., & Aaron, C. K. (1994). Hazards of nonprescription medications. *Emergency Medicine Clinics of North America, 12,* 483–510.

Champault, G., Patel, J. C., Bonnard, A. M., et al. (1984). A double–blind trial of an extract of the plant *serenoa repens* in benign prostatic hyperplasia. *British Journal of Clinical Pharmacology, 18,* 461–462.

Cui, J., Garle, M., Eneroth, P., & Bjorkhem, I. (1994). What do commercial ginseng products contain? *Lancet, 344,* 134.

Franzblau, A., Rock, C. L., Werner, R. A., Albers, J. W., Kelly, M. P., & Johnson, E. C. (1996). The relationship of vitamin B6 status to median nerve function and carpal tunnel syndrome among active industrial workers. *Journal of Occupational and Enviromental Medicine, 38,* 485–491.

Gateley, C. A., & Mansel, R. E. (1991). Management of the painful and nodular breast. *British Medical Bulletin, 47,* 284–294.

Glisson, J., Crawford, R., & Street, S. (1999). Review, critique, and guidelines for the use of herbs and homeopathy. *Nurse Practitioner 24,* 44–67.

Gundling, K. (1999, Nov. 13) *Medicinal botanical agents.* Paper presented at the Women's Health Symposium, University of California, Davis Women's Center for Health, Sacramento, CA.

Heitzer, T., Just, H., & Munzel, T. (1996). Antioxidant vitamin C improves endothelial dysfunction in chronic smokers. *Circulation, 94,* 6–9.

Holmes, M. D., Hunter, D. J., Colditz, G. A., Stampfer, M. J., Hankinson, S. E., Speizer, F. E., Rosner, B., Willett, W. C. (1999). Association of dietary intake of fat and fatty acids with risk of breast cancer. *Journal of the American Medical Association, 281,* 914–920.

Hopkins, P. N., et al. (1995). Higher plasma homocysteine and increased susceptibility to adverse effects of low folate in early familial coronary artery disease. *Arteriosclerosis, Thrombosis and Vascular Biology, 15,* 1314–1320.

Howell, A., Vorsa, N., Der Marderosian, A., & Foo, L. Y. (1998). Inhibition of the adherence of P-finbriated *Escherichia coli* to uroepithelial-cell surfaces by proanthocyanidin extracts from cranberries. *New England Journal of Medicine, 339,* 1085–1086.

Jonas, W. B., Rapoza, C. P., Blair, W. F. (1996). The effect of niacinamide on osteoarthritis: A pilot study. *Inflammation Research, 45,* 330–334.

Kanowski, S., Hermann, W. M., Stephan, K., Wierich, W., Horr, R. (1996). Proof of efficacy of the ginko biloba special extract EGb 761 in outpatients suffering from mild to moderate primary degenerative dementia of the Alzheimer type of multi-infarct dementia. *Pharmacopsychiatry, 29,* 47–56.

Kruger, M. C., et al. (1996). Calcium, gamma-linolenic acid (GLA) and eicosapentanoic acid (EPA) supplementation in osteoporosis. *Osteoporosis International, 6* (1, Suppl.), 250.

Laakmann, G., Schule, C., Baghai, T., & Keiser, M. (1998). St. John's wort in mild to moderate depression: The relevance of hyperforin for the clinical efficacy. *Pharmacopsychiatry, 31,* S54–S59.

Larrey, D. (1997). Hepatotoxicity of herbal remedies. *Journal of Hepatology, 26* (1, Suppl.), 47–51.

Larsson, B., Jonasson, A., & Fianu, S. (1989). Evening primrose oil in the treatment of premenstrual syndrome. *Current Therapy Research, 46,* 58–63.

Lauritzen, C., Reuter, H. D., Repges, R., Bohnert, K., Schmidt, U. (1997). Treatment of premenstrual tension syndrome with Vitex agnus castus. Controlled, double-blind study versus pyridoxine. *Phytomedicine, 4*(3), 183–189.

Le Bars, P. L., Katz, M. M., Berman, N., Itil, J. M., Freedman, A. M., & Schatzberg, A. F. (1997). A placebo-controlled, double-blind, randomized trial of an extract of ginko biloba for dementia. *Journal of the American Medical Association, 278,* 1327–1332.

Lee, C. K., et al. (1999). Gene expression profile of aging and its retardation by caloric restriction. *Science, 285,* 1390–1393.

Lehmann, E., Kinzler, E., & Friedemann, J. (1996). Efficacy of a special kava extract (*Piper methysticum*) in patients with states of anxiety, tension and excitedness of nonmental origin—a double-blind placebo-controlled study of four weeks treatment. *Phytomedicine, 3*(2), 113–119.

Leone, M., D'Amico, D., Moschiano, F., Fraschini, F., & Bussone, G. (1996). Melatonin versus placebo in prophylaxis of cluster headaches: A double-blind pilot study with parallel groups. *Cephalagia, 16*(7), 494–496.

Martin, L., & Jung, P. (1999). *Taking charge of the change: Self-care guide for the mid-life woman in the new millennium.* Nevada City, CA: Women at the Gateway.

Martin, L., & Jung, P. (2000). Herbs for menopause. *Holistic Nursing Update, 1,* 28–31.

Marwick, C. (1995). Growing use of medicinal botanicals forces assessment by drug regulators. *Journal of the American Medical Association, 273,* 607–609.

Miller, D. (1999, Oct.). Nutriceutical review: A review of commonly used medicinal herbs. *Vital Signs*, pp. 4–6.

Morrison, H. I., Schaubel, D., Desmeules, M., & Wigle, M. D. (1996). Serum folate and risk of fatal coronary heart disease. *Journal of the American Medical Association, 275,* 1893–1896.

Northrup, C. (1998). *Women's bodies, women's wisdom: Creating physical and emotional health and healing.* New York: Bantam.

Ogletree, R. L., & Fischer, R. G. (1997). *Physicians and pharmacists guide to the top 10 scientifically proven natural products* (2nd ed., pp. 1–95). Brandon, MS: Natural Source Digest.

Ornish, D., Scherwitz, L. W. , Billings, J. H., Brown, S. E., Gould, K. L., Merritt, T. A., Sparler, S., Armstrong, W. T., Ports, T. A., Kirkeeide, R. L., Hogeboom, C., Brand, R. J. (1998). Intensive lifestyle changes for reversal of coronary heart disease. *Journal of the American Medical Association, 280,* 2001–2007.

Parasrampuria, J., Schwartz, K., & Petesch, R. (1998). Quality control of dehydroepiandrosterone dietary supplements. *Journal of the American Medical Association, 280,* 1565.

Rapola, J. M., Virtamo, J., Haukka, J. K., Heinonen, O. P., Albanes, D., Taylor, P. R., Huttunen, J. K. (1996). Effect of vitamin E and beta carotene on the incidence of angina pectoris. *Journal of the American Medical Association, 275,* 693–698.

Reilly, M., Delanty, N., Lawson, J. A., & FitzGerald, G. A. (1996). Modulation of oxidant stress in vivo in chronic cigarette smokers. *Circulation, 94,* 19–25.

Rokitzki, L., Logemann, E., Huber, G., Keck, E., Keul, J. (1994). Alpha–tocopherol supplementation in racing cyclists during extreme endurance training. *International Journal of Sports and Nutrition, 4,* 253–264.

Seidman, M. D. (2000). Effects of dietary restriction and antioxidants on presbyacusis. *Laryngoscope, 110,* 727–738.

Singh, Y. N. (1992) Kava: An overview. *Journal of Ethnopharmacology, 37*(1); 13–45.

Smith, T. J. (1998) *Renewal: The anti-aging revolution* (pp. 286–307). Emmaus, PA: Rodale.

Stoll, W. (1987). Phytotherapy influences atrophic vaginal epithelium. *Therapeutikon, 1,* 23.

Strauch, G., Perles, P., Vergult, G., Gabriel, M., Gibelin, B., Cummings, S., Malbeeq, W., & Malice, M. P. (1994). Comparison of finasteride (Proscar) and *Serenoa repens* (Permixon) in the inhibition of 5a-reductase in healthy male volunteers. *European Urology, 26,* 247–252.

Thompson, C. A. (1997). Adverse reactions to alternative medicine. *American Journal of Health Systems Pharmacy, 54,* 1707.

Tyler, V. E. (1996). *Herbs of choice: The therapeutic use of phytomedicinals.* New York: Pharmaceutical Products.

Tyler, V. E., & Foster, S. (1996). Herbs and phytomedicinal products. In T. R. Covington (Ed.), *Handbook of nonprescription drugs* (11th ed., pp. 695–713). Washington, DC: American Pharmaceutical Association.

UCB Wellness Letter (1999a, May). Wishful thinking about diet and breast cancer. School of Public Health, University of California, Berkeley, CA.

UCB Wellness Letter (1999b, June). Doctors "supplement" their income. School of Public Health, University of California, Berkeley, CA.

UCB Wellness Letter (2000, May). Worry wort. School of Public Health, University of California, Berkeley, CA.

Volz H. P., Kieser, M. (1997). Kava-kava extract WS 1490 versus placebo in anxiety disorders: A randomized placebo-controlled 25-week outpatient trial. *Pharmacopsychiatry, 30*, 1–5.

Warnecke, G. (1985). Using phyto-treatment to influence menopause symptoms. *Medizinische Welt, 36*, 87.

Weil, A. (2000). *Eating well for optimum health.* New York: Knopf.

Yu, B. P. (1996). Aging and oxidative stress: Modulation by dietary restriction. *Free Radical Biology and Medicine, 21*, 651–668.

RESOURCES

For those practitioners interested in herbal medicine, it is important that the sources used be reliable. The following ones are recommend:

Associations

American Dietetic Association and National Center for Nutrition and Dietetics
216 W. Jackson Boulevard
Chicago, IL 60606–6995
312-899-0040, ext. 4750
Fax: 312-899-4739
www.eatright.org

American Society for Clinical Nutrition (ASCN)
American Journal of Clinical Nutrition
9650 Rockville Pike
Bethesda, MD 20814-3998
ASCN phone: 301-530-7110
ASCN fax: 301-571-1863
AJCN phone: 301-530-7038
AJCN fax: 301-571-8303

Books

Blumenthal, M., Goldberg, A., Gruenwaid, J., et al. (Eds.), (1997). *German Commission E Monograph* (S. Klein & R. S. Rister (Trans.) Austin, TX: American Botanical Council.

Duke, J. A. (1987). *Handbook of medicinal herbs.* Boca Raton, FL: CRS Press.

Duke, J. A. (1992). *Handbook of edible weeds.* Boca Raton, FL: CRS Press.

Duke, J. A. (1997). *Green pharmacy.* Emmaus, PA: Rodale Press.

Herbal PDR. (1998). Montvale, NJ: Medical Economics Co.
Tyler, V. E. (1993). *The honest herbal: A sensible guide to the use of herbs and related reme-dies.* Binghamton, NY: Pharmaceutical Products Press.
Tyler, V. E. (1994). *Herbs of choice: The therapeutic use of phytomedicinals.* Binghamton, NY: Pharmaceutical Products Press.
Weiss, R. F. (1988). *Herbal medicine.* Portland, OR: Medicina Biologica.

Herbal Product Companies

N.S.D. Products
Natural Products for a Healthy Lifestyle
P.O. Box 880
Brandon, MS 39043
Phone: 601-825-6811

Physiologics
6565 Odell Place
Boulder, CO 80301-3330
Phone: 800-765-6775

PhytoPharmica
825 Challenger Drive
Green Bay, WI 54311
Phone: 800-553-2370

Journals and Newsletters

HerbalGram, American Botanical Council, Austin, TX 78720
Holistic Nursing Update, American Health Consultants, Atlanta, GA; Web address: www.ahcpub.com
Lawrence Review of Natural Products, Facts & Comparisons, St. Louis, MO

Internet

American Botanical Council
http://www.herbalgram.org/

A Web site with links to many herbal resources.

Ask Dr. Weil
http://www.hotwired.com/drweil/

Offers advice on a wide variety of herbal topics.

Phytochemical Database
http://www.ars-grin.gov/ngrlsb/

Developed by James A. Duke, PhD, a former USDA researcher and consultant. Offers a comprehensive source of information on the biochemical and clinical effects of botanical extracts and preparations.

U.S. Department of Agriculture Agricultural Genome Information System
http://probe.nalusda.gov

Provides information on taxonomy and worldwide use of herbs.

Homeopathy

Chapter Objectives

- Learn about the theory and practice of homeopathy.
- Learn about the educational preparation and contrast the preparation of practitioners of homeopathy and conventional medicine.
- Discover what therapies homeopathic practitioners use.
- Know what kinds of advice to offer to patients when they ask about referral to a homeopathic practitioner.

OVERVIEW

Homeopathy is a system of medicine and healing that attempts to stimulate the body to heal itself. Homeopathy is a nontoxic approach used worldwide that embraces a person-oriented philosophy, versus the disease-oriented approach common in conventional medicine. It is based on the law of similarities: like heals like.

In the late 1700s, the most popular therapy for most ailments was bloodletting. Some doctors had so much faith in bleeding that they were willing to remove up to four-fifths of the patient's blood. Other therapies of choice included blistering, placing caustic or hot substances on the skin to draw out infections, and administering dangerous chemicals to induce vomiting or purge the bowels. Massive doses of a mercury-containing drug called calomel cleansed the bowels but at the same time caused teeth to loosen, hair to fall out, and other symptoms of acute mercury poisoning.

Samuel Hahnemann, a German physician disenchanted with these methods, began to develop a theory based on three principles: the law of similars, the minimum dose, and the single remedy (Burton Goldberg Group, 1993). The word *homeopathy* is derived from the Greek words for "like" (*homoios*) and "suffering" (*pathos*). With the law of similars, Hahnemann theorized that if a large amount of a substance caused certain symptoms in a healthy person, smaller amounts of the same substance could treat those symptoms in someone who is ill. The basis of his theory took shape after a strong dose of the malaria treatment quinine caused his healthy body to develop symptoms similar to ones caused by the disease. He continued to test his theory on himself as well as family and friends by administering varying doses of different herbs, minerals, and other substances. He called these experiments "provings." However, at first, the intensity of the symptoms caused by the original proving was harrowing. So Hahnemann began decreasing the doses to see how little of a substance could still produce signs of healing.

With the minimum dose, or law of infinitesimals, Hahnemann believed that a substance's strength and effectiveness increased the more it was diluted. Miniscule doses were prepared by repeatedly diluting the active ingredient by factors of 10. A "6X" preparation (the X is the Roman numeral for 10) is a 1-to-10 dilution repeated six times, leaving the active ingredient as one part per million. Essential to the process of increasing potency while decreasing the actual amount of the active ingredient is vigorous shaking after each dilution.

Some homeopathic remedies are so dilute that no molecules of the healing substance remain. Even with the sophisticated technology now available, analytical chemists may find it difficult or impossible to identify any active ingredient. But the homeopathic belief is that the substance has left its imprint or a spiritlike essence that stimulates the body to heal itself.

Finally, a homeopathic physician generally prescribes only a single remedy to cover all the patient's symptoms, mental as well as physical. However, the use of multiingredient remedies is recognized as part of homeopathic practice.

According to the National Center for Homeopathy, homeopathy is based on the following:

1. The acceptance that all symptoms represent the body's attempt to restore itself to health.

2. Instead of viewing symptoms as something wrong (which must be set right), they are considered signs of the way the body is attempting to help itself.

3. Instead of trying to stop a cough, for example, with a suppressant (the common treatment of choice in conventional medicine), homeopaths would recommend a remedy that would cause a cough in a healthy person, thus stimulating the ill body to restore itself.

4. The individual and the totality of symptoms must be considered. A cough, for example, in one individual might need a different remedy than one in another individual, depending on the characteristics of the cough and the totality of the individual's symptoms. Homeopaths do not consider a cough to be a single illness. Rather, they might consider coughs to be different illnesses in different people.

5. Health is not considered to be only the absence of illness. Rather, a healthy person is one who is considered free on all levels: physical, emotional, and mental.

6. A remedy is considered to be homeopathic only if it is taken based upon the similar nature of the effect of the medicine to the illness. A medicine labeled "homeopathic" will work only if it is homeopathic (or similar) to the symptoms presented.

History

Homeopathy was brought to the United States from Europe in the early 1800s. By the mid-1800s, several medical colleges, including the New England Female Medical College, taught homeopathy. By the early 1900s, there were 22 homeopathic medical colleges and one out of five doctors used homeopathy. The decline of homeopathy in the United States followed medical science's move toward a mechanical model of the body and of disease. By 1920, only 15 colleges remained, and by the late 1940s, no courses in homeopathy were taught.

The American Foundation for Homeopathy began teaching homeopathy as a postgraduate course for doctors in 1922. Today, the courses are offered by the National Center for Homeopathy. Slowly, homeopathy is having a renaissance and is embraced as the healing philosophy of choice by a segment of the population.

In other parts of the world homeopathy is more popular. Forty percent of general practitioners in The Netherlands practice homeopathy. India has over 100 homeopathic medical schools, and it is practiced along with conventional Western medicine in government clinics.

Regulation

The FDA regulates homeopathic remedies under provisions of the Food, Drug, and Cosmetic Act. The FDA regulates homeopathic drugs in several significantly different ways from other drugs. Manufacturers of homeopathic drugs are deferred from submitting new drug applications to the FDA. Their products are exempt from good manufacturing requirements related to expiration dating and from finished product testing for identity and strength. Homeopathic drugs in solid oral dosage form must have an imprint that identifies the manufacturer and indicates that the drug is homeopathic. The imprint on conventional products, unless specifically exempt, must identify the active ingredient and dosage strength as well as the manufacturer. The reasoning behind the difference is that homeopathic products contain little or no active ingredients. From a toxicity, poison control standpoint, the active ingredient and strength were deemed to be unnecessary. Interest in homeopathy is growing because of the costs and impersonality of modern medical care and the increase in infectious diseases that do not respond to allopathic medicine. However, extreme dilutions are the main reason many scientists doubt the effectiveness of homeopathic products.

Scientists have petitioned the FDA to hold homeopathic products to the same standards as other drugs. While some studies support the efficacy of homeopathy, controlled clinical studies determining effective levels of dilution for these substances are needed (Der Marderosian, 1996).

Another difference between pharmaceuticals and homeopathic preparations involves alcohol. Conventional drugs for adults can contain no more than 10% alcohol, and the amount is even less for children's medications. But some homeopathic products contain much higher amounts because the agency has temporarily exempted these products from the alcohol limit rules.

Homeopathic products are not exempt from all FDA regulations. If a homeopathic drug claims to treat a serious disease such as cancer, it can be sold by prescription only. Only products sold for so-called self-limiting conditions such as colds, headaches, and other minor health problems that eventually go away on their own can be sold without a prescription (over the counter). Requirements for nonprescription labeling include:

- An ingredients list
- Instructions for safe use
- At least one major indication
- Dilution (e.g., 2X for one part per hundred, 3X for one part per thousand)

Over the past several years, the agency has issued about 12 warning letters to homeopathic marketers. The most common infraction was the sale of prescription homeopathic drugs over the counter. Other problems include:

- Products promoted as homeopathic that contain nonhomeopathic active ingredients, such as vitamins or plants not listed in homeopathic references
- Lack of tamper-resistant packaging
- Lack of proper labeling
- Vague indications for use that could encompass serious disease conditions

In addition to enforcement, the agency is also focusing on preventing problems by educating the homeopathic industry about FDA regulations.

PRACTITIONERS

The practice of homeopathy is regulated by each individual state. Usually, it can be employed legally by individuals whose degrees entitle them to practice medicine in the state. This may include doctors of medicine, doctors of osteopathy, doctors of naturopathy, dentists, nurse practitioners, and veterinarians.

TABLE 7-1	Certification for Homeopathic Practitioners	
MEDICAL LICENSE	**CERTIFYING ORGANIZATION**	**CREDENTIAL**
Doctor of medicine, doctor of osteopathy	American Board of Homeotherapeutics	DHt
Nurse practitioner	Homeopathic Academy of Naturopathic Physicians	DHANP
All practitioners	Council for Homeopathic Certification	CHC

Medical doctors and osteopaths in Arizona and Nevada and medical doctors in Connecticut who want to practice homeopathy must be licensed by the state homeopathic licensing board. In some states, doctors of chiropractic are permitted to administer homeopathic remedies. While the practice of medicine is regulated under the law, the use of homeopathic medicines for self-care of acute (short-term) illnesses is permitted in most states.

No diploma or certificate from any school or program is recognized as a license to practice homeopathy. Certification of competency to practice homeopathy for medical practitioners is as shown in Table 7-1.

Training Requirements

Formal training in homeopathy can be pursued in an alternative school such as a school of naturopathy, homeopathy, or acupuncture. There are also correspondence and required-attendance schools. Training can also be informal. Informal training can be as simple as self-study through books or seminars or correspondence courses. This is an acceptable route for learning homeopathy for personal use, first aid, et cetera. Even for professional study, many students begin with self-study or long-distance study as there is no hands-on or laboratory work involved. Even some professionals choose this route.

There are homeopathy courses specifically geared to medical doctors or other practitioners with medical training. These courses spend less time on the basics of health care and more time on specific applications of homeopathy. Among the schools offering classes specifically geared to licensed medical professionals are the Hahnemann College of Homeopathy, Albany, CA; the International Foundation for Homeopathy, Edmonds, WA; the National Center for Homeopathy, Alexandria, VA; and the Canadian Academy of Homeopathy, Toronto, ON.

In the United States, the American Board of Homeotherapeutics certifies medical doctors or osteopaths who meet their educational standards and pass both oral and written exams. Successful candidates are awarded the designation of diplomate in homeopathy (DHt).

Educational programs vary in length from two-day seminars to four-year courses. Tuition depends on the length of the program. Weekend or week-long seminars usually run between $200 and $1000. Longer programs can be as high as $5000 per year. Prerequisites vary by school. Some courses are structured only for medical practitioners. These professional seminars require students to already have a medical degree/license or to be enrolled in a recognized college. Other courses are open to any interested student and have no formal prerequisites.

Homeopathy is regulated by each state. However, anyone calling him or herself a "homeopathic doctor" implies that they are practicing medicine and must follow the laws governing the practice of medicine in that state. In all states, one cannot practice medicine without a license. But laws vary widely from state to state. A few states, like Arizona, state that homeopathy belongs under the jurisdiction of licensed medical doctors. Some state laws allow homeopathy within the scope of practice for certain other health professionals, such as acupuncturists.

TREATMENT

Homeopathy consists of highly individualized treatments based on a person's genetic history, personal health history, body type, and present status of all physical, emotional, and mental symptoms. Treatments generally consist of homeopathic medicines. According to the National Center for Homeopathy, homeopathic medicines are drug products made by homeopathic pharmacies in accordance with the processes described in the *Homeopathic Pharmacopoeia of the United States*. Medicines may be made from plants, animals, animal substances (such as the ink of the cuttlefish), or chemicals (such as penicillin). These substances are diluted carefully, following a specific process, until very little of the original remains.

A plant substance, for example, may be mixed in alcohol to obtain a tincture. One drop of the tincture is then mixed with 99 drops of alcohol (to achieve a ratio of 1:100), and the mixture is vigorously shaken. The shaking process is called succussion. The final bottle of this mixture would be labelled as "1C." One drop of the 1C is then mixed with 100 drops of alcohol and the process of succussion is repeated to make a 2C. The entire dilution and shaking process is again repeated to make a 3C. By the time a 3C is reached, the dilution is 1 part in 1 million. Small globules made from sugar are then saturated with the liquid dilution. These globules are what constitute homeopathic medicine.

Some homeopathy preparations are derived from substances that people find desirable, such as chamomile, marigold, and daisy flowers. However, even toxic

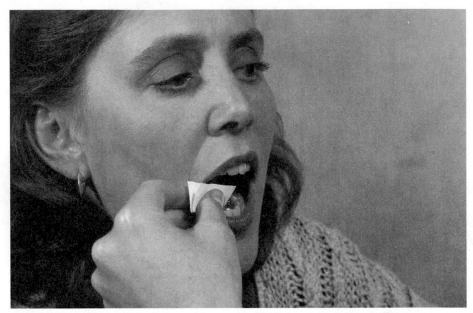

Figure 7-1 A patient taking a homeopathic preparation. (Photo courtesy of Photodisc.)

substances such as poison ivy, mercury, arsenic, pit viper venom, and hemlock are part of homeopathic care.

Patients receiving homeopathic care frequently feel worse before they get better because homepathic medicines often stimulate, rather than suppress, symptoms. This seeming reversal of logic is a relevant part of homeopathy because symptoms are viewed as the body's effort to restore health (see Figure 7-1).

The different homeopathy therapies are:

■ *Constitutional.* One dose is given, usually of a high potency. Then one waits up to six months to see if there is a shift in symptoms. The disadvantage is that there is no immediate relief of acute symptoms (e.g., how long can one wait for disabling migraines or diarrhea to disappear?). However, this approach has proven to be good for deep-seated, chronic, inherited predispositions such as allergies, familial asthma, cancer, depression, old vaccination damage, and chemical exposures (e.g., pesticides, drugs used during pregnancy).

■ *Classical: single remedies used.* The practitioner takes a detailed history and asks a lot of questions (see Figure 7-2). From those answers and by observation, the practitioner attempts to match the pattern of the patient's symptoms to the pattern of a single remedy. This can be chosen manually or by computer. The potency is usually determined by a number of factors, including severity of symptoms and how recent or old the problem is. This approach is closest to the one developed by Hahnemann and it is the most common form of practice. It is most popular in England, India, the United States, and Canada and is good for home and first-aid use.

- *Combination: remedies contain two to four ingredients.* The diagnostic approach may be the same as for the classical therapies. Other diagnostic styles may include kinesiology (muscle testing) or electrodermal biofeedback. This style is extensively used in France, Canada, and the United States.

- *Complex: uses remedies with up to 25 ingredients.* The diagnostic approach may be the same as the combination approach. Multiple ingredients are used to encourage what is known as homeopathic or lymphatic drainage. This is best for complex, difficult cases where multiple problems occur simultaneously. Drainage helps remove toxicity from organs or systems that are overloaded due to chronic, genetic, or environmental factors. Used extensively in Germany with electronic diagnostic equipment, but it can be used with kinesiology.

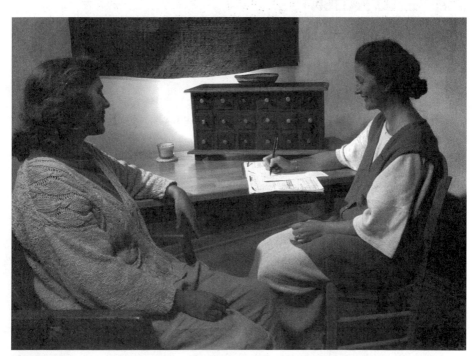

Figure 7-2 A homeopathic practitioner begins treatment by taking a detailed patient history. (Photo courtesy of Photodisc.)

After a patient receives treatment (been given a constitutional remedy), he or she may be told the following:

1. Do not eat or drink anything for 20 minutes before or after taking the remedy.
2. Store the remedy in a cool, sunless location, and take the small pills sublingually.
3. Avoid consumption of coffee and mint products when taking remedies.
4. Avoid contact with camphor and napthalene (found in mothballs) and other strong smelling substances or environments.
5. If the physical condition temporarily worsens, it means that the body is processing its relationship to the cause of the problem and the remedy is working.
6. Any changes in health experienced over the next several weeks are most likely due to the remedy.
7. Call the homeopathy practitioner with any questions or concerns or if considering an adjunctive medical intervention.

ADVICE TO PATIENTS

There are several questions that patients may want to ask a homeopath before beginning treatment. They should take time to research and interview practitioners. Some questions to ask a practitioner are:

- Where and how long they studied?
- With whom did they study (teachers, schools, apprenticed with other practitioners)?
- Are they board certified? If so, by what board?
- What style(s) of homeopathy do they practice?
- How will the style(s) match a particular patient or condition?
- Have they treated this particular condition before?
- What is their experience with chronic (long-term) or serious conditions?
- What other therapies are available in their office?
- What is the practitioner's success rate?
- What are the charges?

Before taking any homeopathic, over-the-counter, or prescription medications, the health provider should be asked to fully explain the substance's or medication's benefits, risks, and costs as well as about alternatives to the medication or substance.

Many who do not believe in the effectiveness of homeopathy say any successful treatments are due to the placebo effect, or, in other words, positive thinking. But supporters counter that their medicine works in groups like infants and even animals.

The American Medical Association (AMA) does not accept homeopathy, but it does not reject it either. The AMA encourages doctors to become aware of alternative therapies and use them when and where appropriate. Similarly, the American Academy of Pediatrics has no specific policy on homeopathy.

Findings from a study of the types of patients seen by homeopathic physicians indicate that they were younger, more affluent, and more likely to present with long-term complaints. Physicians using homeopathic medicine surveyed spent more time with their patients, ordered fewer tests, and prescribed fewer pharmaceutical medications than physicians practicing conventional medicine (Jacobs, Chapman, & Crothers, 1998).

RESEARCH

Recent research on homeopathy is controversial, and double-blind, controlled studies are scarce. A number of supportive studies were published in the 1980s, but there were more challenging reports in the 1990s.

Studies Supporting Use of Homeopathy

In a meta-analysis review of 107 controlled clinical studies performed between 1966 and 1990, 81 of the studies showed that homeopathic medicines were beneficial in treating headaches, postoperative symptoms, and other health-related disorders (Kleignen, 1991). In a double-blind study on the effects of homeopathic remedies on influenza, twice as many patients taking the homeopathic remedy were cured in 48 hours as compared to those who took placebo (Ferley, 1989). One study indicated positive results for homeopathy and hay fever (Reilly, 1986), while another found homeopathy effective with dental neuralgic pain following tooth extraction (Albertini, 1985). Others report homeopathy successful for Parkinson's disease, bronchitis, sinusitis, and migraine headaches (Gerhard, 1988) and influenza and motion sickness (Zenner, 1990).

Studies Not Supporting Use of Homeopathy

A recent study was aimed at assessing whether the clinical effect reported in randomized controlled trials of homeopathic remedies is equivalent to that reported for placebo. Researchers sought studies from computerized bibliographies and contracts with researchers, institutions, manufacturers, individual collectors, homeopathic conference proceedings, and books. All languages were included. Double-blind and/or randomized placebo-controlled trials of clinical conditions were considered. The review of 185 trials identified 119 that met the inclusion criteria, 89 had adequate data for meta-analysis, and two sets of trials were used to assess reproducibility. Two reviewers assessed study quality with two scales and extracted data for information on clinical condition, homeopathy type, dilution, "remedy," population, and outcomes. The findings were that the combined odds ratio for the 89 studies entered into the main meta-analysis was 2.45 [95% confidence interval (CI) 2.05, 2.93] in favor of homeopathy. The odds ratio for the 26 good-quality studies was 1.66 (1.33, 2.08), and that corrected for publication bias was 1.78 (1.03, 3.10). Four studies on the effects of a single remedy on seasonal allergies had a pooled odds ratio for ocular symptoms at four weeks of 2.03 (1.51, 2.74). Five studies on postoperative ileus had a pooled mean effect size difference of -0.22 standard deviations (SDs) (95% CI -0.36, -0.09) for flatus and -0.18 SDs (-0.33, -0.03) for stool (both with $p < 0.05$). The interpretation of results of the meta-analysis are not compatible with the hypothesis that the clinical effects of homeopathy are completely due to placebo. However, the researchers found insufficient evidence from these studies that homeopathy is clearly efficacious for any single clinical condition (Linde et. al., 1997).

One study used scientific methods to evaluate two claims made by practitioners of alternative medicine: a placebo-controlled, double-blind study of homeopathy in children with warts and a cohort study of the influence of lunar phases on postoperative outcome in surgical patients. Outpatients of a dermatology department were used for the homeopathy study and inpatients at an anesthesiology department for the cohort study. There were 60 volunteers for the homeopathy study and 14,970 consecutive patients undergoing surgery under general anesthesia for the lunar phase study. In the homeopathic study, the children with warts were treated with individually selected homeopathic preparations (homeopathic study); in the lunar phase study surgical procedures were performed, including abdominal, vascular, cardiac, thoracic, plastic, and orthopedic operations, and the lunar phase at the time of operation was assesed. The main outcome measures were a reduction of the area occupied by warts by at least 50% within eight weeks for the homeopathic study, and death from any cause within 30 days after surgery for the lunar phase study. Results were that 9 of 30 subjects in the homeopathy group and 7 of 30 subjects in the placebo group experienced at least 50% reduction in area occupied by warts ($\chi^2 = 0.34$; $p = 0.56$); the mortality rate was 1.20% in patients operated on during a waxing moon and 1.33% in patients operated on during a waning moon ($\chi^2 = 0.49$; $p = 0.50$). The conclusion of the study is that statements and methods of alternative medicine, as far as they concern observable clinical phenomena, can be tested by scientific methods. When such tests yield negative results, as in the studies presented herein, the particular method or statement should be abandoned. Otherwise one would run the risk of supporting superstition and quackery (Smolle, Prause, & Kerl, 1998).

The meta-analysis of homeopathy trials that appeared in *Lancet* in 1997 (Langman, 1997; Vandenbrouke, 1997) seemed to endorse the experience of practitioners and patients that homeopathic medicines have specific clinically relevant effects. However, results from later unsuccessful trials (Dean, 1998) and negative inferences from a review of trials for a condition excluded from the meta-analysis—delayed-onset muscle soreness (DOMS)—have since been presented to suggest that the meta-analysis may well have overestimated the positive effects of homeopathy and the "placebo question" is still not resolved. This article reviewed the evidence underlying this challenge to the meta-analysis and homeopathy and demonstrated that the analysis would be valid if it were based on a comprehensive literature search, appropriate classification of primary studies, clear discrimination between clinical effectiveness and placebo questions, sound and transparent review methods, and a reliable and unconfounded clinical treatment model for testing the ultramolecular hypothesis. It is suggested that different models are needed to answer different questions (Dean, 1998).

Studies with Neutral Conclusions

Linde and Melchart (1998) summarized the state of clinical efficacy research on individualized homeopathy. Electronic databases as well as other sources were searched for possibly relevant studies. Randomized or quasi-randomized controlled clinical trials comparing an individualized homeopathic treatment strategy with placebo, no treatment, or another treatment were eligible. Information on patients, methods, interventions, outcomes, and results was extracted in a standardized manner and quality was assessed using a checklist and two scoring systems. Trials providing sufficient data were pooled in a quantitative meta-analysis. The results showed a total of 32 trials (28 placebo controlled, 2 comparing homeopathy and another treatment, 2 comparing both) involving a total of 1778 patients met the inclusion criteria. The methodological quality of the trials was highly variable. In the 19 placebo controlled trials providing sufficient data for meta-analysis, individualized homeopathy was significantly more effective than placebo (pooled rate ratio 1.62, 95% CI 1.17–2.23), but when the analysis was restricted to the methodologically best trials, no significant effect was seen. The results of the available randomized trials suggest that individualized homeopathy has an effect over placebo. The evidence, however, is not convincing because of methodological shortcomings and inconsistencies.

In Britain, 42% of general practitioners refer patients to homeopaths. Two recent meta-analyses of homeopathy indicate that there is enough evidence to show that homeopathy has added effects over placebo (Vallance, 1998). Against this evidence is a backdrop of considerable scientific scepticism. Homeopathic remedies are diluted substances—some are so diluted that statistically there are no molecules present to explain their proposed biological effects (ultrahigh dilutions, or UHDs). Without knowledge of the evidence, most scientists would reject

UHD effects because of their intrinsic implausibility in the light of our current scientific understanding. The objective of this study is to critically review the major pieces of evidence on UHD effects and suggest how the scientific community should respond to its challenge. Such evidence has been conducted on a diverse range of assays—immunological, physiological, behavioral, biochemical, and clinical—in the form of trials of homeopathic remedies. Evidence of UHD effects has attracted the attention of physicists who have speculated on their physical mechanisms. Controversial phenomenon can split the scientific community. It is argued that if the phenomenon was uncontroversial, the evidence suffices to show that UHD effects exist. However, given that the observations contradict well-established theory, normal science has to be abandoned and scientists need to decide for themselves what the likelihood of UHD effects are. Bayesian analysis describes how scientists ought rationally to change their prior beliefs in the light of evidence. Theories indicate that whether UHD effects are proved or not depends on the beliefs and behaviors of scientists in their communities. This article argues that there is as yet insufficient evidence to drive rational scientists to a consensus over UHD effects, even if they possessed knowledge of all the evidence. The difficulty in publishing high-quality UHD research in conventional journals prevents a fair assessment of UHD effects. Given that the existence of UHD effects would revolutionize science and medicine and the considerable empirical evidence of their existence, the philosophies of science tell us that possible UHD effects warrant serious investigation by conventional scientists and serious attention by scientific journals (Vallance, 1998).

In a survey of clients entering care with nine practicing classical homeopaths in the Los Angeles metropolitan area between January 1994 and July 1995, participants completed a self-administered questionnaire before undergoing diagnosis by the homeopath (Goldstein & Glick, 1998). Follow-up interviews were conducted by phone one month after diagnosis and face-to-face four months after diagnosis, along with a self-administered questionnaire before the final interview. A total of 104 participants entered the study; 77 completed all data collection. Clients sought homeopathic care for a wide array of largely chronic conditions. Respiratory, gastrointestinal, and female reproductive problems were the most common primary complaints. Most clients were highly educated but had limited knowledge about homeopathy before entering treatment. Approximately 80% reported earlier, unsuccessful attempts to get relief from mainstream care. Four months after treatment, general measures of health status showed improvement, and only 29% of participants reported no improvement for the primary complaint leading to treatment. Satisfaction with homeopathic treatment was high regardless of outcome. Three outcome measures of perceived change—overall health status, primary condition for which treatment was sought, and outlook on life—were predicted by different combinations of study variables. The conclusion was that homeopathy does not divert people from seeking mainstream care. The use of alternative modes of care such as homeopathy can be understood as attractive and satisfying to educated individuals with chronic problems.

Homeopathic remedies are advocated for the treatment of postoperative ileus, yet data from clinical trials are inconclusive. Meta-analyses of existing clinical trials to determine whether homeopathic treatment has any greater effect than placebo administration on the restoration of intestinal peristalsis in patients after abdominal or gynecological surgery (Barnes, Resch, & Ernst, 1998). Meta-analyses were conducted using RevMan software. Separate meta-analyses were conducted for the homeopathic treatments versus placebo: homeopathic remedies of <12C potency versus placebo and homeopathic remedies of ≥12C potency versus placebo. A "sensitivity analysis" was performed to test the effect of excluding studies of low methodologic quality. The endpoint was time to first flatus. Meta-analyses indicated a statistically significant (p <0.05) weighted mean difference (WMD) in favor of homeopathy (compared with placebo) on the time to first flatus. Meta-analyses of the three studies that compared homeopathic remedies ≥12C versus placebo showed no significant difference (p >0.05). Meta-analyses of studies comparing homeopathic remedies <12C with placebo indicated a statistically significant WMD (p <0.05) in favor of homeopathy on the time to first flatus. Excluding methodologically weak trials did not substantially change any of the results. There is evidence that homeopathic treatment can reduce the duration of ileus after abdominal or gynecological surgery. However, several caveats preclude a definitive judgment. These results should form the basis for a randomized controlled trial to resolve the issue.

SUMMARY

Homeopathy was derived from care practices in the sixteenth and seventeenth centuries and is experiencing worldwide renewal. In the United States homeopathic care is rapidly expanding. Homeopathy is a system of medicine and healing that attempts to stimulate the body to heal itself. It is a nontoxic approach that embraces a person-oriented philosophy and is based on the law of similarities: Like heals like. Anyone can study, learn, and practice homeopathy, as training programs range from informal self-taught to on-site formal classroom settings. Research in the field is controversial as to the effectiveness of the therapy.

ASK YOURSELF

1. What is the nature of homeopathy therapy?
2. Where and how can students learn about this therapy?
3. What is the origin of homeopathy? Describe them.
4. What are some of the controversial research about homeopathy? Describe them.

REFERENCES

Albertini, H. (1985). Homeopathic treatment of neuralgia using arnica and hypericum: A summary of 60 observations. *Journal of the American Institute of Homeopathy,* 78, 126–128.

Barnes, J., Resch, K. L., & Ernst, E. (1998). Homeopathy for postoperative ileus? A meta-analysis. *Journal of Clinical Gastroenterology, 25*(4), 628-633.

Burton Goldberg Group. (1993). *Alternative medicine: The definitive guide.* Puyallup, WA: Future Medicine Publishing.

Dean, M. (1998). Out of step with the Lancet homeopathy meta-analysis: More objections than objectivity? *Journal of Alternative and Complementary Medicine, 4*(4), 389–398.

Der Marderosian, A. H. (1996). Understanding homeopathy. *Journal of the American Pharmaceutical Association (Washington), 24*(4); 317–321.

Ferley, J. P., Zmirou, D., D'Adehmar, D., & Balducci, F. (1989). A controlled evaluation of a homeopathic preparation in the treatment of influenza-like syndromes. *British Journal of Clinical Pharmacology, 27,* 329–335.

Gerhard, W. (1988). The biological treatment of migraines, based on experience. *Biological Therapy, 5*(3), 67–71.

Goldstein, M. S., & Glik, D. (1998). Use of and satisfaction with homeopathy in a patient population. *Alternative Therapies in Health and Medicine, 134*(2), 60–65.

Jacobs, J., Chapman, E. H., & Crothers, D. (1998). Patient characteristics and practice patterns of physicians using homeopathy. *Archives of Family Medicine, 7*(6), 537–540.

Kleignen, J. (1991). Clinical trials of homeopathy. *British Medical Journal,* 302; 316–323.

Langman, M. J. (1997). Homeopathy trials: Reason for good ones but are they warranted? *Lancet* 350 (9081), 825.

Linde, K., & Melchart, D. (1998). Randomized controlled trials of individualized homeopathy: A state-of-the-art review. *Journal of Alternative and Complementary Medicine, 4* (4), 371–388.

Linde, K., Clausius, N., Ramirez, G., Melchart, D., Eitel, F., Hedges, L. V., & Jonas, W. B. (1997). Are the clinical effects of homeopathy placebo effective? A meta-analysis of placebo-controlled trials. *Lancet, 350*(9081), 834–843.

Reilly, D. T., Taylor, M. A., McSharry, C., & Aitchison, T. (1986). Is homeopathy a placebo response: Controlled trial of homeopathic potency, with pollen in hayfever as model. *Lancet* 2, 881–886.

Smolle, J., Prause, G., & Kerl, H. (1998). A double-blind, controlled clinical trial of homeopathy and an analysis of lunar phases and postoperative outcome. *Archives of Dermatology, 134*(11), 1368–1370.

Vallance, A. K. (1998). Can biological activity be maintained at ultra-high dilution? An overview of homeopathy, evidence, and Bayesian philosophy. *Journal of Alternative and Complementary Medicine, 4*(1), 49–76.

Vandenbrouke, J. P. (1997). Homeopathy trials: Going nowhere. *Lancet* 350 (9081), 824.

Zenner, S., & Metelmann, H. (1990). Therapeutic use of lymphmyosot-results of a multi-center use observation study on 3,512 patients. *Biological Therapy* 8 (3), 49.

RESOURCES

American Association of Homeopathic Pharmacists
1441 West Smith Rd.
Ferndale, WA 98248
Phone: 800-478-0421

American Institute of Homeopathy
801 N. Fairfax Street, Suite 306
Alexandria, VA 22314
Phone: 703-246-9501
Web site: http://www.healthy.net/aih

The AIH is a trade association whose membership comprises medical and osteopathic physicians and dentists. The AIH is dedicated to the promotion and improvement of homeopathic medicine and the dissemination of pertinent medical knowledge. Established in 1844, one year after the death of homeopathy's German-born founder, Samuel Hahnemann, the AIH is the oldest national medical professional organization in the United States.

British Institute of Homeopathy (U.S.)
PMB 423
520 Washington Boulevard
Marina del Rey, CA 90292
Phone: 310-306-5408
Fax: 310-827-5766
E-mail: bihus@thegrid.net

Provides information and home study courses on homeopathy.

Homeopathic Academy of Naturopathic Physicians
12132 S.E. Foster Place
Portland, OR 97266
Phone: 503-761-3298
Fax: 503-762-1929
E-mail: hanp@igc.apc.org
Web site: http://www.healthy.netthanp

A professional association of naturopathic physicians certified in homeopathy.

Homeopathic Educational Services
2124 Kittredge Street
Berkeley, CA 94704
Phone: 510-649-0294
E-mail: mail@homeopathic.com
Web site: http://www.homeopathic.com

Provides a catalogue of homeopathic books, tapes, videos, and software.

National Center for Homeopathy
801 N. Fairfax Street, Suite 306
Alexandria, VA 22314
Phone: 703-548-7790
Fax: 703-548-7792
E-mail: nchinfo@igc.apc.org
Web site: http://www.homeopathic.org

Offers referrals to physicians and other licensed health practitioners who practice homeopathy and publishes a Directory of Homeopathic Practitioners *that lists practitioners, study groups, and pharmacies throughout the United States and Canada. Provides courses for lay-people and professionals and sponsors study groups throughout the United States.*

Internet

http://www.homeopathic.net

Naturopathy

Chapter Objectives

- To gain understanding of the nature and scope of naturopathy medicine.
- To learn how and where naturopathy doctors are educated.
- To discover what conditions naturopathy treats.
- To understand what substantiating research documents the effectiveness of naturopathy.

OVERVIEW

Naturopathic medicine treats health and illness conditions by utilizing the body's inherent ability to heal. Naturopathic physicians aid the healing process by incorporating a variety of alternative methods based on an assessment of the person's individual needs. A whole-person approach, including lifestyle, employment, diet, and past history, is taken when determining what treatments to use.

The naturopathic approach includes a host of healing practices and modalities, for example, herbal medicine, diet and dietary supplements, acupuncture, exercise, massage, homeopathy, pharmaceuticals, and some physical therapies such as ultrasound, electric current, and light therapy. Modern naturopathic physicians are primary health care providers who use therapies that are almost exclusively nontoxic and natural (hence the name naturopathic).

History

The history of naturopathy dates back to antiquity. Modern practices are derived from many cultures, including Chinese (traditional Chinese medicine), Indian (Ayurveda), Greek (Hippocratic medicine), and Native American. In contemporary times, the practice was consolidated and named in the late-nineteenth century. Naturopathic medicine was popular and widely available throughout the United States well into the early part of the twentieth century. By the 1920s, there were a number of naturopathic medical schools coast to coast, thousands of naturopathic physicians, and multiple thousands of patients using naturopathic therapies. Due to the rise of scientific medicine coupled with the discovery of miracle drugs such as sulfa in the 1930s and penicillin in the 1940s and the institutionalization of a large medical system, naturopathy began to fall out of favor with the population. As the use of advanced technology and pharmaceuticals increased during the 1950s, the use of naturopathic medicine and most other methods of natural healing declined.

In the 1970s and 1980s, the American public became increasingly curious about alternative options. People were living longer, with increasing numbers of chronic diseases and few conventional remedies for them. Naturopathy and all of complementary alternative medicine began to enter a new era of rejuvenation as the consumer began to explore new therapies for new problems.

Principles

The practice of naturopathy is based on six principles (Cassileth, 1999):

1. *The healing power of nature is powerful.* Naturopaths believe that the body has the power to heal itself, and the role of the practitioner is to facilitate this natural process with the aid and use of nontoxic therapies.

2. *Treat the cause rather than the effect.* Practitioners seek to discover the underlying cause of a disease rather than suppress symptoms. In contrast to allopathic medicine, naturopaths avoid suppression of the natural responses of the body, such as fever and inflammation. Symptoms are seen as manifestations of the body's natural healing process. While symptoms are present, an attempt is made to discover the cause, which can be any combination of body, mind, emotional, or spiritual stressors.

3. *First, do no harm.* Naturopaths use natural therapies and avoid invasive interventions that may harm the patient.

4. *Treat the whole person.* A holistic approach is used, with the understanding that individuals are complex beings of interacting body, mind, emotion, spiritual, social, environmental, cultural, and other factors. This belief dictates a therapeutic interaction in which no illness or disease is seen as incurable.

5. *The naturopath is a teacher.* Practitioners strive to motivate and teach patients to assume more personal responsibility for health by adopting an attitude of wellness that incorporates a healthy diet and lifestyle.

6. *Prevention is the best cure.* Naturopaths focus on preventive medicine.

PRACTITIONERS

The number of new naturopathic doctors is steadily increasing in the United States, and licensure of naturopathic physicians is expanding into new states. By 1996, 11 of the 50 states had naturopathic licensing laws; these states are Alaska, Arizona, Connecticut, Hawaii, Maine, Montana, New Hampshire, Oregon, Utah, Vermont, and Washington. Accreditation by the Council on Naturopathic Medical Education (CNME) affords naturopathic doctors eligibility for licensing in the 11 states that regulate naturopathic medicine.

Training Requirements

A naturopathic physician attends a four-year graduate-level naturopathic medical school and is educated in the same basic sciences as a medical doctor but also studies holistic and nontoxic approaches to therapy, with a strong emphasis on disease prevention and optimizing wellness. The naturopathic physician is required to complete four years of training in clinical nutrition, acupuncture, homeopathic medicine, botanical medicine, psychology, and counseling (to encourage people to make lifestyle changes in support of their personal health). Traditional schools of naturopathy require on-campus learning and some courses in minor surgery techniques. Nontraditional schools offer distance learning and do not necessarily award degrees. Table 8-1 lists both traditional and nontraditional schools of naturopathy.

TABLE 8-1	**Traditional and Nontraditional Schools of Naturopathy**
SCHOOL	DESCRIPTION
Traditional Schools	
Bastyr University, Bothell, WA	Founded in 1978, the leading residential school in naturopathic medicine, and one of three residential schools accredited by the CNME. Bastyr's curriculum includes studies in nutrition, acupuncture, and homeopathy as well as courses in minor surgery. This school established the first government-funded clinic for natural medicine as well as an AIDS research center.
Canadian College of Naturopathic Medicine (CCNM), Toronto, Canada	Officially recognized in North America by the CNME, its graduates are eligible to write licensing exams in all Canadian jurisdictions with regulatory legislation.

(Continued on next page)

Southwest College of Naturopathic Medicine (SCNM), Tempe, AZ	Founded in 1993, this residential school currently offers two programs of study, a master's certificate in acupuncture and a doctor of naturopathic (NP) program. The master's certificate is a three-year program, and the ND program is four years of study.
National College of Naturopathic Medicine (NCNM), Portland, OR	Established in 1956, this residential school is the oldest in the United States and is accredited by the CNME. Like Bastyr, NCNM requires minor surgical studies to obtain an ND.

Nontraditional Schools

Westbrook University, Aztec, NM	As a distance learning school, Westbrook's nontraditional program is accredited by the National Board of Naturopathic Examiners, and the American Naturopathic Medical Certification and Accreditation Board. Westbrook offers combination bachelor's of science (BS)–ND advanced degrees in natural health sciences, clinical nutrition, herbology/nutrition, holistic health science, and iridology. Their ND program includes instruction in medical sciences, physical medicine, and herbal and homeopathic medicine. Requirements for the ND program include two clinical externships. This program exceeds the 4100 study hours established for standardized naturopathy.
Clayton College of Natural Health (CCNH) Birmingham, AL	Established in the mid-1980s, it is accredited by the World Association of Universities and Colleges. The school offers advanced degree programs in natural health and in holistic nutrition, and a PhD program in holistic health sciences. Most graduates go into practice for themselves as naturopathic consultants.
Australasian College of Herbal Studies (ACHS) U.S. office located in Lake Oswego, OR	This school gives diplomas and certificates but no degrees. In 1998 it became the first state-licensed school to teach natural health by distance learning. The college originated in New Zealand in 1978; it was established in Hong Kong, Australia, and the United States in 1991. ACHS gives training in aromatherapy, herbal and homeopathic medicines, and nutrition.

As an example of the numbers of students enrolled in traditional programs, in 1996, Bastyr University alone had almost 1000 students in its various degree-granting programs. In addition to their formal education, many naturopathic doctors take additional training and certification in acupuncture and home birthing.

Licensure Requirements

All U.S. states and Canadian provinces with licensure laws require a resident course of study of at least four years and 4100 hours of study from a college or university recognized by the State Examining Board. Applicants for licensure must pass the Naturopathic Physicians Licensing Exam (NPLEX). This exam includes basic sciences, diagnostic and therapeutic subjects, and clinical sciences.

Regulation

In the United States, the naturopathic medical profession's infrastructure includes accredited educational institutions, professional licensing by a growing number of states, national standards of practice and care, peer review, and a commitment to scientific research.

The CNME is the only accrediting agency recognized by the U.S. Department of Education and by the American Association of Naturopathic Physicians (AANP) to accredit naturopathic programs and colleges. The CNME issues a bulletin twice a year giving the accrediting status of each institution it rates. At this time, there are three accredited institutions:

1. National College of Naturopathic Medicine, Oregon
2. Bastyr University, Washington
3. Southwest College of Naturopathic Medicine, Arizona

One institution is a candidate for accreditation status:

4. Canadian College of Naturopathic Medicine, Ontario, Canada

Through its efforts, the CNME has helped secure licensing and regulations for naturopathic doctors in Alaska, Arizona, Connecticut, Hawaii, Maine, Montana, New Hampshire, Oregon, Utah, Vermont, and Washington. The CNME states that only residential schools that require surgical studies as part of the ND program should be able to offer degrees that afford their graduates eligibility for licensing. Some argue, however, that the current regulations are too strict. Not all students of naturopathic medicine wish to study surgical procedures, and some practitioners do not think surgery is a true part of naturopathic medicine.

TREATMENT

Naturopathic medicine is defined primarily by its fundamental principles. Methods and modalities are selected and applied based upon these principles in relationship to the individual needs of each patient. The naturopathic physician meets with the patient and does a complete history and physical exam to identify what underlying conditions are manifesting in the illness (see Figure 8-1).

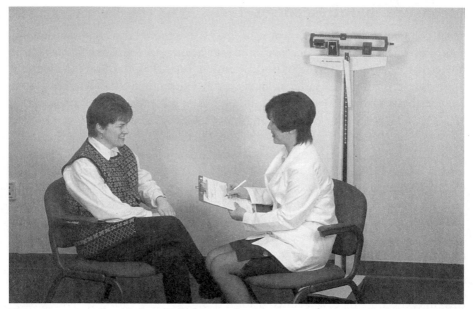

Figure 8-1 A naturopathic doctor meets with a patient prior to treatment to take a detailed patient history.

Diagnostic and therapeutic methods are selected from various sources and systems. Naturopaths use similar diagnostic and testing procedures, such as blood and urine analysis, as do medical doctors, although a naturopath will often address a broader range of lifestyle factors that may affect a patient's health than typical allopathic physicians might. A naturopath may spend an hour gathering a health history and pertinent lifestyle data. Naturopaths recommend appropriate lifestyle and dietary changes as well as encourage patients to play an active role in their own healing process and in disease prevention. Both homeopathy and acupuncture may be used to stimulate the system. Sometimes herbal medicines and supplements are used as tonics and nutrients to strengthen and support a weakened immune system. Ways are discussed to ease emotional stress and doctor and patient explore what changes are needed to create a relaxing environment. Since care is holistic in nature, naturopathic doctors explore the spiritual realm with patients, and when disharmony is discerned he or she guides patients to take an appropriate course of action. Naturopathic practice excludes major surgery and the use of most synthetic drugs. A typical clinical practice includes the following diagnostic and treatment modalities:

- Methods of clinical and laboratory diagnostic testing, including diagnostic radiology and other imaging techniques
- Nutritional medicine, dietetics, and therapeutic fasting
- Hygiene and public health measures

- Homeopathy
- Acupuncture
- Chinese medicine, psychotherapy, and counseling
- Minor surgery and naturopathic obstetrics (natural childbirth), naturo-pathic physical medicine, including naturopathic manipulative therapies
- Counseling about lifestyle modification
- Hydrotherapies (heat, cold, ultrasound) and therapeutic exercise

Naturopathic medicine is used for many conditions, but most people seek care for treatment of chronic and degenerative diseases. Severe trauma, emergency childbirth, or orthopedic problems requiring surgery are referred elsewhere. In acute cases, such as ear infection, bronchitis, and common illness, a natural approach is taken to symptom management. At the same time an exploration of the underlying physical, mental, spiritual, and environmental causes is done with the goal of helping the patient understand how these factors coalesce to cause the illness.

For many diseases and conditions, such as ulcerative colitis, headache, asthma, premenstrual syndrome (PMS), flu, obesity, and chronic fatigue, treatments used by naturopathic physicians can be primary and even curative. Naturopathic physicians also refer patients to an appropriate medical specialist such as an oncologist or a surgeon. Naturopathic therapies can be designed to complement the treatments used by conventionally trained medical doctors. The result is a team care approach that recognizes the needs of the patient to receive the best overall treatment most appropriate to his or her specific medical condition.

ADVICE TO PATIENTS

There are several things you may want to suggest your patient discuss with their naturopathic doctor. They include questions about their education, medical practices, and treatment regimens.

One question to ask is where the naturopath earned his or her degree. Most programs are on campus, but some off-campus (distance-learning) programs exist. While earning a naturopathy degree off campus does not necessarily mean the practitioner is lacking, the patient may want to investigate the school prior to beginning therapy with the naturopathic doctor. Your patient may want to look at the school's catalog to determine whether or not substantive and significant course work was required to earn the naturopathic degree in question.

Once your patient has established contact with a specific naturopathic doctor and has a consultation, they may be given a dietary and/or supplement regimen. Suggest that they review the therapy or therapeutic agents prescribed. They should be aware that graduates of naturopathic medical programs often prescribe "medications" that have failed to show any genuine efficacy in well-designed and executed laboratory and/or clinical trials. Some may prescribe megadose regimens of certain nutrients and amino acids without the benefit of long-term studies indicating safety. Tell them to ask their doctor the expected outcomes of any prescriptions and treatments. They may also want to ask the practitioner about journal citations and/or copies of papers published in reputable peer-reviewed journals indicating the safety and efficacy of the diet and/or supplements he or she has prescribed. It may be that no articles are available in the office, and then it is up to them to investigate the risks and benefits of the treatments and prescriptions.

Another area to have your patient question is whether or not they can get insurance coverage. They may have to be proactive and take the first step by telling their insurer that they are using a naturopathic doctor with good results and that they would like those services recognized and covered for reimbursement. They can ask their naturopathic doctor to give them a statement that details the specific charges. This will avoid any confusion of what their insurer may or may not cover. Members of the All-Natural Healthcare Association (ANHA) are provided with names of insurers who currently cover naturopathy. Their policy may or may not cover visits to naturopathic doctors. It is up to them to find out. If the visits are not covered, your patients will have to pay out of pocket for the coverage.

RESEARCH

Strong scientific evidence validating the effectiveness of naturopathy medicine as a whole is sparse. However, there are studies validating the effectiveness of some of the specific supplements or remedies. Many publications that support naturopathy are from Germany or Sweden, where naturopathy is popular.

An example of treatment with a natural product would be the use of glucosamine sulfate in the treatment of osteoarthritis. Most conventional practitioners would use nonsteroidal anti-inflamatory drugs (NSAIDs) to alleviate the pain of the arthritis. A naturopathic doctor, however, would look for a substance that would promote the healing process rather than suppress the symptoms—thus the use of the supplement glucosamine sulfate. A number of clinical studies have documented the long-term positive effects of glucosamine sulfate versus conventional drugs. In one six- to eight-week study of 12 patients on glucosamine and 12 on placebo, there was an 80% reduction in pain in the experimental group (Pujalte, Llavore, Ylescupidez, 1980). Another study reported decreased pain, decreased joint tenderness, and increased active and passive range of motion (Drovanti, Bignamini, Rovati, 1980). One study showed the ibuprofen group had faster pain relief, but the glucosamine group had longer lasting relief (Lopez, 1982). Similar investigations found quicker pain relief with ibuprofen but fewer side effects with glucosamine (Rovati, 1992). A study of the in vitro effects of exogenous glucosamine found it stimulated the repair and production of articular cartilage proteoglycans (Da Camara & Dowless, 1998). These studies are all examples of the validation of one widely used naturopathy supplement.

In contrast, a case report from the University of Washington Medical Center, Seattle, Washington, which is also the home city of Bastyr College, describes a bone marrow transplant recipient in whom hepatic zygomycosis developed after ingestion of multiple naturopathic medicines (Oliver, Van Voorhis, Boeckh, Mattson, & Bowden, 1996). *Mucor* was isolated from the patient's liver aspirate and from one of the naturopathic medicines. Arbitrary-primed polymerase chain reaction (PCR) analyses were performed on the *Mucor* isolates from the patient's liver aspirate and from his naturopathic medicine to see if they were genotypically related. *Mucor indicus* was the species identified in both the patient's liver aspirate and the naturopathic medicine. Arbitrary-primed PCR analysis revealed that these isolates were genotypically identical. The scientists concluded that this bone marrow transplant recipient acquired hepatic mucormycosis from ingestion of a naturopathic medicine containing *Mucor*.

SUMMARY

Naturopathy is a type of medical practice that uses natural remedies. It is based on ancient practices that have had a renaissance during the past 30 years. Naturopathic physicians work with patients to assess the underlying cause of the presenting malady and work to address the root cause, whether it be physical, psychological, mental, spiritual, or environmental in nature.

ASK YOURSELF

1. When did naturopathy begin in the United States?
2. Name at least 5 of the 6 principles on which the practice of naturopathy is based.
3. What is the duration and scope of a naturopathy doctor's (ND) education?
4. Do naturopaths have to be licensed to practice?
5. What conditions do NDs treat?
6. What does a typical treatment consist of?
7. How can I locate an ND?
8. Is there any research to support naturopathy treatments?

REFERENCES

Cassileth, B. R. (1999). *The alternative medicine handbook: The complete reference guide to alternative and complementary therapies.* New York: Norton.

Da Camara, C. C., & Dowless, G. V. (1998). Glucosamine sulfate for osteoarthritis. *Annals of Pharmacotherapy, 32,* 580–587.

Drovanti, A., Bignamini, A. A., Rovati, A. L. (1980). Therapeutic activity of oral glucosamine sulfate in osteoarthrosis: A placebo-controlled double-blind investigation. *Clinical Therapeutics, 3,* 260–272.

Lopez Vas, A. (1982). Double-blind clinical evaluation of the relative efficacy of ibuprofen and glucosamine sulphate in the management of osteoarthritis of the knee in out-patients. *Current Medical Research and Opinion, 8,* 145–149.

Oliver, M. R., Van Voorhis, W. C., Boeckh, M., Mattson, D., & Bowden, R. A. (1996). Hepatic mucormycosis in a bone marrow transplant recipient who ingested naturopathic medicine. *Clinical Infectious Diseases, 22*(3), 521–524.

Pujalte, J. M., Llavore, E. P., & Ylescupidez, F. R. (1980). Double-blind clinical evaluation of oral glucosamine sulphate in the basic treatment of osteoarthritis. *Current Medical Research and Opinion, 7,* 110–114.

Rovati, L. C. (1992). Clinical research in osteoarthritis: Design and results of short-term and long-term trials with disease modifying drugs. *International Journal of Tissue Reactions, 14,* 243–251.

RESOURCES

American Association of Naturopathic Physicians
601 Valley Street, Suite 105
Seattle, WA 98109
Phone: 206-298-0126 or 206-298-0129
Fax: 206-298-0125 Referral Line
E-mail: 74602.3715@compuserve.com
Web site: http://www.naturopathic.org

Provides a directory of naturopahic physicians and offers referrals to a nationwide network of accredited or licensed practitioners. On-line directory available at http://www.healthy.net/referrals.

American Naturopathic Medical Association
P.O. Box 96273
Las Vegas, NV 89193
Phone: 702-897-7053
Web site: http://www.anma.com.

Bastyr University College of Naturopathic Medicine
14500 Juanita Dr. N.E.
Kenmore, WA 98028-4966
Phone: 425-823-1300
Web site: http://www.bastyr.edu.

Internet

http://www.naturopathy.com

Mind-Body Therapies

Chapter Objectives

- Become familiar with a variety of the mind-body therapies used in some alternative and complementary therapy practices.
- Compare and contrast the quality and quantity of various mind-body therapies.
- Discover that some therapies are grounded in empirical evidence while others are based on an opinion or concept.

INTRODUCTION

The mental therapies gained recognition during the 1800s when psychiatrist Sigmund Freud and psychologist Carl Jung wrote about their patients and discoveries involving the complexities of the mind. Body-mind therapies explore the interactions between the body and the mind and the relationship this connection has to health. The term *body-mind* emerged when practitioners realized that the body affects the mind and visa versa. Healing within this modality emphasizes the importance of self-awareness and self-care, and illness and disease are often viewed as opportunities for personal growth (Fugh-Berman, 1997).

The therapies discussed in this chapter are not all inclusive but are representative of the vast array of mind-body treatments that currently exist and include:

- Psychotherapy
- Art therapy
- Music/sound therapies
- Imagery
- Hypnosis
- Meditation

PSYCHOTHERAPY

Psychotherapy is a general term for a range of practices in which the therapist uses verbal dialogue to help patients gain insight into their problems. Psychotherapists are also known as counselors, therapists, and/or mental health workers. Sigmund Freud, the founder of psychotherapy, said that the goal of therapy was to make the unconscious conscious.

Practitioners and Training Requirements

Psychotherapy practitioners range from university-educated doctors of philosophy to registered nurses with master's degrees to self-trained and/or certified mental health counselors. Anyone can call themselves a "psychotherapist," "counselor," or "therapist." In some states, that is, Colorado, anyone can legally practice psychotherapy, regardless of academic education or professional training. But in Colorado, for example, state law requires that all practicing psychotherapists pay a fee to be either licensed or listed in a state database kept by the Department of Regulatory Agencies (DORA). Each state has its own regulations.

Psychotherapists may hold a wide variety of master's and doctoral degrees. After graduating with one or more degrees, a person can qualify to become licensed by the state in that he or she resides. In addition, after completing certain postgraduate training programs or meeting specific criteria established by state or national professional organizations, therapists can obtain an ever-widening variety of certifications that may indicate additional achievement in a particular area of practice. However, there are also an increasing number of new experimental, nonaccredited training programs. It takes time to scrutinize and discriminate between the legitimately recognized universities and organizations and the more questionable ones.

Many other professionals may practice forms of psychotherapy:

- Pastoral counselors: master of divinity (MDiv), doctor of theology (ThD)
- Psychiatric nurses: registered nurse (RN), master's of science in nursing (MSN)
- Alcohol counselors: certified addiction counselors (CAC I, II, or III)
- Psychiatrists: medical doctors (MD), psychoanalysts (anyone trained or practicing Freudian or analytic styled psychodynamic approach), hypnotherapists (anyone trained or practicing hypnosis), sex therapists (anyone trained or practicing sex therapy)

TRAINING REQUIREMENTS

Licensed Psychotherapists

Having a license to practice psychotherapy indicates that the therapist has met minimum qualifications for academic knowledge as indicated by having a master's degree from an accredited graduate school, passed a qualifying exam, and completed two years approved supervised experience in the field. Generally, there are four kinds of licensed psychotherapists, but these terms may vary from state to state:

- Licensed psychologists
- Licensed clinical social workers (LCSW)
- Licensed marriage and family therapists (LMFT)
- Licensed professional counselors (LPC)

Patients can consider a prospective therapist's credentials along with the particular license they possess to determine the amount and kind of academic training and experience they have had. Doctors of philosophy (PhDs), doctors of psychology (PsyDs), or doctors of education (EdDs) have usually completed four or more years of graduate school and are eligible for licensing. However, only those who have been licensed can call themselves psychologists. Many doctors of philosophy from other related or unrelated academic fields still practice therapy without being licensed or clinically trained. Psychologists can also specialize in a wide variety of nonclinical practice areas, including statistical research, industrial psychology, and diagnostic testing and evaluations.

Licensed social workers, marriage and family therapists, and professional counselors usually have at least two years of graduate school and have earned a master's degree (some may have doctoral degrees). Licensed social workers often have other credentials: bachelor's of social work (BSW), master's of social work (MSW), Academy of Certified Social Workers (a two-year postgraduate national credential), board certified diplomate (BCD, a five-year postgraduate credential), or diplomate of clinical social work (DCSW, a five-year postgraduate credential). Social workers are also trained to specialize in a variety of areas in addition to clinical practice including community organization and development, and administrative management.

Licensed marriage and family therapists and professional counselors have other master's degrees: master of arts (MA), master of science (MS), or master of education (MEd). Marriage and family therapists have specialized training in the area of family systems while professional counselors may have a variety of more generalized training in the area of psychology and counseling.

Treatment

Psychotherapists treat a wide variety of problems, including:

- Anxiety and panic disorders
- Depression and mood disorders
- Addictions and recovery
- Incest issues
- Stress management

- Issues of the elderly
- Attention-deficit disorder
- Posttraumatic stress
- Couple and family therapy
- Adolescent and child problems
- Men's and women's issues
- Hypnosis
- Sex therapy
- Grief and bereavement
- Divorce and separation
- Chronic and terminal illness

The two psychotherapy treatment types are individual (one-on-one) or group psychotherapy. One-on-one therapy was most popular until the 1980s, when managed health care brought changes in allowable billing regulations. Since that time group therapy sessions are more common. Private practice treatment, often still using the one-on-one technique usually occurs in the therapist's office, while group sessions are held in a common room and used in many in-patient psychiatric facilities.

One of the primary differences between a psychotherapist and a psychiatrist (a medical doctor) is that the psychotherapist does not prescribe medications. Often, the two professionals will work together as a team, with the medical doctor prescribing psychotropic drugs and the psychotherapist doing the long-term individual and/or group counseling sessions

A number of different therapies exist under the umbrella term *psychotherapy*. A few are discussed here.

Body-Oriented Psychotherapy

Body-oriented psychotherapy seeks to enhance the psychotherapeutic process by incorporating a range of massage, bodywork, and movement techniques. Acknowledging the mind-body link, practitioners may use light touch, softer deep-tissue manipulation, breathing techniques, movement, exercise, or body awareness techniques to help address emotional issues.

Core Energetics

Core energetics is a form of body-oriented psychotherapy that aims to break down the client's defense mechanisms (such as rationalization, denial, and projection) in order to reach the "core" level of consciousness, or the spiritual self. By using bodywork and counseling techniques and offering spiritual guidance, the practitioner seeks to evoke cathartic reactions (dramatic, insightful breakthroughs) that open the way to the "core energy," enabling the client to become a more loving, creative, receptive, and vibrant person.

Gestalt Therapy

This psychotherapy aims to help the client achieve wholeness (*gestalt* is the German word for "whole") by becoming fully aware of his or her feelings, perceptions, and behavior. The emphasis is on the here and now of immediate experience rather than on the past. Gestalt therapy is often conducted in group settings, such as weekend workshops.

Pathwork

Pathwork is a therapy based on the work of Carl Jung and Jungian therapy. Jung's theory divides the psyche into three parts. The first is the ego, which Jung identifies with the conscious mind. Closely related is the personal unconscious, which includes anything that is not presently conscious but can be. The personal unconscious is like most people's understanding of the unconscious in that it includes both memories that are easily brought to mind and those that have been suppressed for some reason. But it does not include the instincts that Freud would have it include. The third part of the psyche that differentiates his theory from all others is the collective unconscious. This is the reservoir of our experiences as a species, a kind of knowledge we are all born with but one we can never be directly conscious of. It influences all of our experiences and behaviors, most especially the emotional ones, but we only know about it indirectly, by looking at those influences.

The contents of the collective unconscious are called archetypes. An archetype is an unlearned tendency to experience things in a certain way. The archetype has no form of its own but acts as an "organizing principle" on the things we see or do. Jung describes a number of archetypes and Jungian therapists work with patients to discover and understand their archetypes.

A personal growth process incorporating spirituality and psychology, pathwork encourages the individual to face and transform his or her "dark side" or shadow with the goal of promoting integration, inner peace, and greater consciousness. Through verbal dialogue, the practitioner assists the individual in removing physical, emotional, mental, and spiritual blocks often related to past traumas.

Advice to Patients

Initially, it may be confusing to your patient who seeks referral to a psychotherapist. There are so many different therapists and types of practice that you will want to help your patient narrow the field. First help them to focus on the specific type of assistance desired. Next suggest that they ask the prospective therapist the questions listed in Figure 9-1.

- How long is the wait for the first appointment?
- Is the office open during the evening and/or weekends?
- What is the fee for the initial visit?
- How long do the sessions last?
- Will the therapist accept the client's insurance? Who files the insurance claims?
- For how long does the patient's insurance cover therapy sessions?
- How does this therapist offer counseling sessions? Individual or group?
- Will the client return on a daily, weekly, or monthly basis?

Figure 9-1 Selected questions to ask a prospective psychotherapist

Lastly, explain to your patients that they should check the credentials and background of their potential therapist prior to engaging in complicated or long-term therapy.

Research

Most clinical research investigations validate the effectiveness of psychotherapy used either alone or in conjunction with medical therapy.

Patients with chronic forms of major depression are difficult to treat, and the relative efficacy of medications and psychotherapy is uncertain. One study randomly assigned adults with a chronic nonpsychotic major depressive disorder to 12 weeks of outpatient treatment with nefazodone (maximal dose 600 mg/day), the cognitive behavioral-analysis system of psychotherapy (16 to 20 sessions), or both (Keller, McCullough, Klein, Arnouv, Dunner, Gelenberg, Markowitz, Nemeroff, Russell, Thase, Trievedi, Zajecka, 2000). Results indicated that, of 681 patients, 662 attended at least one treatment session and were included in the analysis of response. The overall rate of response (both remission and satisfactory response) was 48% in both the nefazodone group and the psychotherapy group, as compared with 73% in the combined-treatment group. The conclusion was that although about half of patients with chronic forms of major depression have a response to short-term treatment with either nefazodone or a cognitive behavioral-analysis system of psychotherapy, the combination of the two is significantly more efficacious than either treatment alone.

Research suggests that cognitive-behavioral therapy (CBT) is the most effective psychotherapeutic treatment for bulimia nervosa. One exception is a study that suggested that interpersonal psychotherapy (IPT) might be as effective as CBT, although slower to achieve its effects (Apple, 1999). The present study is designed to repeat this important comparison. Two hundred-twenty patients meeting criteria for bulimia nervosa were allocated at random to 19 sessions of either CBT or IPT conducted over a 20-week period and evaluated for one year after treatment in a multisite study. Results found that CBT was significantly superior to IPT at the end of treatment in the percentage of participants recovered. This suggests that CBT should be considered the preferred psychotherapeutic treatment for bulimia nervosa (Agras, Walsh, Fairburn, Wilson, & Kraemer, 2000).

Pain is often poorly controlled in cancer patients. Chronic pain affects adult patients at all stages of cancer management, and optimal pain management may require attention to psychosocial variables and the inclusion of nonpharmacological techniques. Thomas and Weiss (2000) reviewed three nonpharmacological strategies that are effective in reducing pain caused by cancer—patient psychoeducation, supportive psychotherapy, and cognitive-behavioral interventions. Results validated that effective treatment of cancer pain begins with assessing the severity, characteristics, and impact of pain. Emotional distress (especially anxiety, depression, and beliefs about pain) emerged as predictive of patient pain levels. The conclusion was that patient psychoeducation empowers patients to actively participate in pain control strategies.

There is preliminary evidence that alexithymia may influence the course of coronary heart disease (CHD); however, this is the first study to explore attempts to modify alexithymic characteristics in cardiac patients (Beresnevaite, 2000). Twenty post-myocardial infarction (MI) patients (19 men and 1 woman) were placed in a treatment group that received weekly group psychotherapy for four months. Seventeen post-MI patients (16 men and 1 woman) were placed in a comparison group that received two educational sessions over a period of one month. The results indicate that group psychotherapy is able to decrease alexithymia and that for many patients this change can be maintained for at least two years. A reduction in the degree of alexithymia seems to influence favorably the clinical course of CHD.

ART THERAPY

Art therapy is a human service profession that combines psychotherapy and visual art in a creative process to further self-understanding. During treatment, the created art work becomes a reflection of the patient's personality, development, abilities, and conflicts. The American Art Therapy Association, Inc. (AATA) defines art therapy as ". . . a human service profession that utilizes art media, images, the creative art process and patient/client responses to the created products as reflections of an individual's development, abilities, personality, interests, concerns and conflicts." Art therapy is a rapidly growing field that had its beginnings in the treatment of severely emotionally disturbed and physically handi-

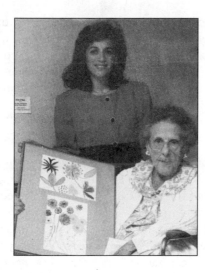

Figure 9-2 Art therapy can benefit patients of all ages.

capped children and adults through the use of art (see Figure 9-2). In recent years it has expanded to reach a broad range of populations, such as substance abusers, cancer patients, the mentally depressed, and survivors of trauma. Increasing numbers of health promotion practitioners include some form of art therapy in their practice. It may be as simple as having meaningful paintings on the office wall or as complex as working with clients to interpret their creations. Art therapy includes a range of modalities, including:

- Oil and acrylic painting on canvas, water color, or finger painting
- Basket or loom weaving
- Sculpture with wood, metal, marble, or other materials
- Wood carving or wood building
- Jewerly making
- Pottery making: design, clay work, or painting
- Music: sound, expression, writing, playing instruments, collecting or repairing instruments
- Glass blowing
- Journal writing and analysis
- Drama, theatre involvement, and screenplay writing

Practitioners

Art therapy practitioners range from the self-trained to university-educated professionals and may include a variety of other life experiences in their treatment. For example, a person who had studied dance before becoming a physical therapist may opt to include dance or some movement therapy into his or her practice. Another example is a psychiatrist who also does art work or sculpture may incorporate or even specialize in using expressive therapies coupled with mental healing. The professionally trained art therapist works in such settings as hospitals, community mental health centers, Child Life programs, shelters, prisons, nursing homes, and special schools.

TRAINING REQUIREMENTS

Art therapists generally have a bachelor's or a master of arts degree in art therapy. For example, the program at New York University's master's program began in the 1950s and in 1979 was one of the first of five programs to receive approval from the American Art Therapy Association.

Educational, professional, and ethical standards for art therapists are regulated by The American Art Therapy Association (AATA). The Art Therapy Credentials Board (ATCB), an independent organization, grants postgraduate supervised experience. Registered art therapists who pass the examination administered by the ATCB receives the Board Certified credential (ATR-BC).

Treatment

Art therapy is based on a knowledge of human developmental and psychological theories. This knowledge is implemented via assessment and treatment, including educational, psychodynamic, cognitive, transpersonal, and other therapeutic means of reconciling emotional conflicts, fostering self-awareness, developing social skills, managing behavior, solving problems, reducing anxiety, aiding reality orientation, and increasing self-esteem. Sometimes a therapy, such as painting, is done alone; at other times, the therapy is coupled or grouped, such as writing, directing, and acting in a screenplay. There are many art therapies, and some of them are detailed here.

EXPRESSIVE THERAPIES

Expressive therapies use the arts to promote physical health, mental health, and/or personal growth. Examples of expressive therapies include art therapy, dance therapy, drama therapy, music therapy, poetry therapy, and psychodrama.

JOURNALING

Recording thoughts in a journal may help relieve pain and, in some cases, even improve health. People who write daily about traumatic events may reduce their perception of stress from the focus event as they create a historical record that they can revisit in the future. The most common form of journaling is keeping a diary. People who keep a daily journal tend to report a deeper understanding of themselves and often become better able to achieve their goals, including health. Table 9-1 details the most effective forms of journaling.

TABLE 9-1	Health-Focused Journals
TYPE OF JOURNAL	**WHAT IT ACCOMPLISHES**
Gratitude journal	This is best performed at the end of the day, prior to going to bed. Its purpose is to help the writer better appreciate all there is to be grateful for. This is important, during times of crisis or ill health, when it is all too easy to see only the clouds and not the blue sky in which they are contained. Focusing on positive factors stimulates the immune system to operate more efficiently. People who are depressed, anxious, or generally pessimistic have less neuropeptide activity in their cells, whereas happy, optimistic, and confident people are found to have higher levels (Rybakowski & Twardowska, 1999; Caberlotto & Hurd, 1999). Suggest that each night your patient write down the things that occurred during the day that caused happiness, even things that otherwise might go unnoticed. Tell them to take time to really examine the day and make a list of all the people, things, and events that made them happy. As they do, they should reexperience that happiness as they write. Over time, this simple exercise may result in improved mood, self-esteem, and confidence levels while boosting the immune system.
Stream-of-consciousness morning journal	Whatever comes to mind is written down and then forgotten. Proponents of this method claim that it enables those who perform it to rid themselves of the "mental debris" lingering in their mind and thus to become better able to focus with more clarity on what they want to accomplish during the rest of the day. A variation of this exercise is to write for 15 minutes and then read over what was written, underlining all negative thoughts. When finished, each negative thought is rewritten as a positive thought.
Illness dialogue journal	Sickness often has an emotional component that may not be readily apparent. This form of journaling helps to bring the "hidden" meaning or message of the illness into consciousness in order to better understand the reasons behind the symptoms. Often, once these reasons are understood and accepted, the illness itself may swiftly disappear or a more appropriate way of treating it will be found. Recommend that your patient perform this exercise by asking the following question: "If this pain (or illness) could speak, what would it say?" Suggest that they write down the first impression. It is very important not to self-consciously edit as they listen for the response. They should be willing to write down whatever occurs, even if it seems ridiculous or is upsetting. After completion of the written response, have them read it over and ask the first question that surfaces. They should keep repeating this until no more questions occur or until discovery of an answer that can help. Usually this exercise needs repeating for at least a few days before one achieves resolution.

Research

In a study done to investigate the clinical effectiveness of a short course of drama therapy (an eclectic term encompassing all the arts therapies), a sample of 10 patients in a neuro-rehabilitation unit received five individual one-on-one sessions of therapy over a five-week period (McKenna, 1999). Semistructured interviews were carried out with each participant following the course. Qualitative analysis showed how this therapy helped psychological adjustment to severe disabilities resulting from neurotrauma. The four ways in which the participants were empowered and their self-esteem nutured were:

1. They were provided with a sense of personal space in an otherwise institutional setting.
2. They were allowed escapism and enjoyment.
3. Creativity and a sense of potency were awakened.
4. They were provided a metaphor to explore personal issues.

In another study, 26 patients aged 21–63 that were hospitalized for depression and 26 control individuals were asked to make a "funny" and a "sad" drawing (Miljkovitch & Miljkovitch, 1998). The drawings were scored using 22 variables describing their formal aspects and contents. Results showed that drawings of individuals with depression differ from those of control participants on a wide range of variables, sometimes very significantly. Prediction of participants' groups based on eight variables obtained by discriminate analysis was correct in 98% of cases. Results support the usefulness of asking for the two kinds of drawings and suggest that depression is better detected through formal aspects of drawings than through their contents.

MUSIC (SOUND) THERAPIES

Music is a universal language with many purposes and can be used in the health care setting to reduce stress and anxiety. The therapies that use music and/or sound can help clients attain therapeutic goals, which may be mental, physical, emotional, social, or spiritual.

Overview

Music therapy (MT) is a multisensorial technique as it may involve the hands, voice, emotions, mind, and spirit. Music is widely used to different ends in a variety of settings. Music therapy has two branches: active and passive. In active music therapy the utilization of instruments or of one's own voice is structured to correspond to all sensory organs so as to obtain suitable motor and emotional responses. For example, when following singing exercises, a patient with undiag-

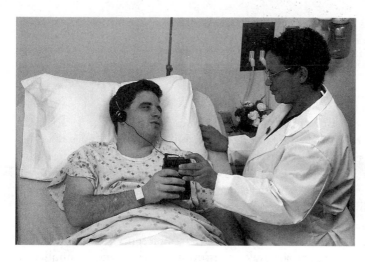

Figure 9-3 Music therapy helps patients relax.

nosable throat, larynx, or lung problems may have an insightful breakthrough as to the psychological meaning of their problems. In the passive branch, listening to specific music and/or sounds may be done in order to relax, stimulate, motivate, or soothe the body and mind (see Figure 9-3).

Music therapists assess emotional well-being, physical health, social functioning, communication abilities, and cognitive skills through musical responses. Therapists design music sessions for individuals and groups based on client needs using music improvisation, receptive music listening, song writing, lyric discussion, music and imagery, music performance, and learning through music. Individuals or groups participate in interdisciplinary treatment planning, ongoing evaluation, and follow-up. Most people can benefit from music therapy, but people with mental health needs, developmental and learning disabilities, and brain injuries, women in labor, cardiac patients, and patient's with Alzheimer's disease are especially noted.

HISTORY

The idea of music as a healing influence is as old as antiquity, when people sang and made music on crude instruments. The idea of formalizing music as a therapy came after musicians went to veterans' hospitals around the country to play for the thousands of veterans suffering both physical and emotional trauma from World Wars I and II. The patients' physical and emotional responses to music led hospital personnel and administrators to request the hiring of musicians by the hospitals. In time, the musicians realized that they would benefit by specialized training before entering the facility, and thus the demand was created for a college curriculum. The first music therapy degree program was founded at Michigan State University in 1944. The American Music Therapy Association (AMTA) was founded in 1998 as a union of the National Association for Music Therapy and the American Association for Music Therapy.

Practitioners

To become eligible for the national examination offered by the Certification Board for Music Therapists, music therapists must complete 1 of the 69 approved college music therapy curricula, including internship. Music therapists who successfully complete the independently administered examination hold the music therapist board-certified credential MT-BC. The National Music Therapy Registry (NMTR) serves qualified music therapy professionals who meet selected criteria. These individuals have met accepted educational and clinical training standards and are qualified to practice music therapy.

The AMTA is the professional association that represents over 5000 music therapists, corporate members, and related associations worldwide. Founded in 1998, its mission is the progressive development of the therapeutic use of music in rehabilitation, special education, and community settings. The AMTA sets the education and clinical training standards for music therapists.

Treatment

Music therapists work in psychiatric hospitals, rehabilitative facilities, medical hospitals, outpatient clinics, day care treatment centers, agencies serving developmentally disabled persons, community mental health centers, drug and alcohol programs, senior centers, nursing homes, hospice programs, correctional facilities, halfway houses, schools, and private practice.

Since music therapists serve a wide variety of persons with many different needs, there is no such thing as a typical session. Sessions are individually designed and music selected based on the individual client's treatment plan. Table 9-2 details four different locations where music therapy can occur and the music's potential effect on the patient.

Research

Findings from clinical research suggest that music may facilitate a reduction in the stress response, including decreased anxiety levels, decreased blood pressure and heart rate, and changes in plasma stress hormone levels. Findings from laboratory research using animal models provide beginning, although speculative, support for a physiological framework of the influence of music on the stress response (Watkins, 1997). Music therapy is useful in a wide range of clinical settings with patients experiencing health problems as diverse as hypertension/cardiovascular disease, migraine headaches, and gastrointestinal ulcers. In one study (Chlan, 1998) a single music therapy session was found to be effective for

TABLE 9-2	Practice Location and Music's Effect
PLACE OF PRACTICE	**EFFECT OF THE MUSIC**
Hospitals	• Alleviate pain in conjunction with anesthesia or pain medication • Elevate patients' mood and counteract depression • Promote movement for physical rehabilitation • Calm or sedate, often to induce sleep • Allay apprehension or fear • Promote relaxation
Nursing homes	• Increase or maintain patient's level of physical, mental, and social/emotional functioning
Psychiatric facilities	• Provide medium to explore personal feelings, make positive changes in mood and emotional states • Build a sense of control over life through successful experiences • Resolve conflicts leading to stronger family and peer relationships • Evoke thoughts, feelings, and memories helpful for change
In health promotion	• Use music for stress reduction via active music making, such as drumming and chanting, individually or in groups • Support and motivate for physical exercise

decreasing anxiety and promoting relaxation, as indicated by decreases in heart rate and respiratory rate over the intervention period with this sample of patients receiving ventilatory assistance.

IMAGERY

Imagery is a mind-body intervention aimed at easing stress and promoting a sense of peace and tranquility during a stressful or difficult time. It is also used to maximize potential or help one in transitions to higher levels of functioning (Dossey, Keegan, Cuzzetta, 2000). Imagery involves a process of incorporating the power of the mind to assist the body to heal, maintain, and improve health or relax by way of an inner communication involving all senses (Achteburg, Dossey, Kolkmeier, 1994; Shames, 1996).

Overview

Imagery provides an opportunity for people to directly focus on positive thoughts and images, thus allowing a sometimes necessary temporary mental escape from the mental content that causes the feeling of "overload" or the inability to cope with immediate problems. Clinical studies indicate that encouraging patients to listen to tapes or actual human voices that guide them through an imagery script during anesthesia induction and/or medical or surgical procedures decreases anxiety and stress levels significantly (Tusek, Church, Fazio, 1997; Tusek, Cwyner, Cosgrove, 1999). An effective imagery process can reduce the need for large doses of medication, thus reducing side effects and decreasing the recovery time frame.

HISTORY

Mental imagery has been recognized since the early 1900s. Roberto Assagioli, the Italian psychiatrist who introduced imagery into clinical practice in 1909, devised a theory of the wholeness of human consciousness and called it psychosynthesis. Since 1965, this practice has been used extensively in the healing professions, including nursing, medicine, and mental health. In the 1980s imagery was used and popularized in the treatment of cancer patients (Simonton, Matthews-Simonton, Sparks, 1980). In the 1990s the modality gained increased use as it was propagated, documented, and practiced by a number of well health care professionals. For example, Martin Rossmean, a physician and acupuncturist, and David Bressler, a health psychologist and acupuncturist, developed and ran the Academy of Guided Imagery in Mill Valley, California, and Bonney Schaub and Richard Schaub have an imagery-based practice on the U.S. East Coast and in Italy.

Practitioners

For the most part, practitioners who use the modality of imagery are health care professionals with an advanced degree: MD, PhD, MSN, or MSW. In addition to the professional degree, most practitioners become certified. There are several certification programs throughout the United States. One 150-hour certification program is offered by the Association for Guided Imagery in California. Guided imagery is one of several modalities the practitioner may offer clients.

Guided Imagery

Guided imagery involves using mental images to promote physical healing or changes in attitudes or behavior. Practitioners may lead clients through visualization exercises or offer instruction in using imagery as a self-help tool. Guided imagery is often used to alleviate stress and to treat stress-related conditions such as insomnia and high blood pressure. People with cancer, AIDS, chronic fatigue syndrome, and other disorders can use imagery to boost the immune system.

Treatment

The primary aim of guided imagery is to gently guide the person to a state where their mind is calm, silent, and still. It is a simple, low-cost, noninvasive tool that has been demonstrated to increase self-esteem, independence, and control that is often lost when a person is faced with emotional trauma or illness. The therapy may be done with individuals focusing on a specific problem or with a group using a universal healing theme.

A common guided imagery technique begins with a general relaxation process asking the person to slowly close their eyes and focus on their breathing. Clients are encouraged to relax, clear their mind, and surround themselves in images that are peaceful and calm. An example of the guided imagery process is shown in Figure 9-4.

- Assume a comfortable position in a quiet environment.
- Close your eyes and keep them closed until the exercise is completed.
- Breathe in deeply to a count of 4.
- Hold breath for a count of 4.
- Breathe out to a count of 4.
- Continue to breathe slowly and deeply.
- Think of your favorite place and prepare to take an imaginary journey there. Select a place in which you are relaxed and at peace.
- Picture in your mind's eye your favorite place. Look around you and see all the colors, the light and shadows, and the pleasant sights.
- Listen to all the sounds. Pay attention to what you hear.
- Feel all the physical sensations . . . the temperature . . . the textures . . . the movement of the air.
- As you take in a deep breath, smell the aromas of your favorite place.
- Taste the foods and drinks you usually consume in your favorite place. Savor each taste fully.
- Focus all your attention totally on your favorite place.
- Breathe in deeply to a count of 4.
- Hold breath for a count of 4.
- Breathe out to a count of 4.
- Resume your usual breathing pattern.
- Slowly open your eyes and stretch, if desired.

This procedure works best when all five senses are used. Like all other relaxation exercises, guided imagery becomes more effective with repetition.

Figure 9-4 Guided imagery exercise

Guided imagery is used to:

- Reduce stress and anxiety.
- Decrease pain.
- Decrease side effects.
- Decrease blood pressure.
- Decrease blood glucose levels (diabetes).
- Decrease allergy and respiratory symptoms.
- Decrease the severity of headaches.
- Enhance bone and wound healing.
- Enhance sleep.
- Enhance self-confidence.
- Assist in losses (job, divorce, death).
- Enhance quality of life.

A number of subsets of the modality are classified under the general umbrella term of imagery.

MINDFUL EATING

This imagery-related technique involves the attempt to bring awareness to the act of eating and to one's relationship with food. This is a useful skill when trying to lose or gain weight or gain an appreciation of food simply as nourishment. During mindful eating attention is focused on the origin and source of the food, the attention that was given to the food in preparation, how the food tastes and feels in the mouth, the aroma of the food, and the benefit of the digested food.

NEUROLINGUISTIC PROGRAMMING

This is a set of techniques whose goal is to alter limiting or restrictive patterns of thought, behavior, and language. In conversation, practitioners observe the client's language, eye movements, posture, breathing, and gestures in order to detect and then help change unconscious patterns linked to the client's emotional state.

The goal of this therapy is to reprogram the body's automatic mental and physical responses, replacing debilitating patterns with reactions that promise to combat illness. By teaching a client to substitute more positive thoughts and images for the previously negative thinking and imagery, neurolinguistic practitioners hope to remove the psychological roadblocks that obstruct the body's natural healing mechanisms.

Those who endorse neurolinguistic programming suggest that the brain begins to respond in kind to more positive images and behavior patterns, just as it did to negative ones. This, in turn, is said to stimulate the body's immune system, thus improving a person's chances of healing.

Rebirthing

Also known as conscious-connected breathing or vivation, rebirthing is an imagery-related technique in which the therapist guides clients through breathing exercises to help them reexperience past memories, including birth, and let go of emotional tensions long stored in the body.

Other studies were also supportive of the modality. For example, Schrock, Palmer, and Taylor (1999) looked at the effects of a six-week psychosocial intervention group on the survival of 21 breast cancer and 29 prostate cancer patients. Six 2-hour classes emphasized imagery and stress reduction techniques, along with covering attitudes, feelings, self-esteem, spirituality, nutrition, and exercise. The intervention group lived significantly longer than the matched controls, suggesting that short-term psychosocial interventions that encourage the expression of feeling, provide social support, and teach coping skills can influence survival.

Results from another study (Kolcaba & Fox, 1999) found guided imagery to be an effective intervention for increasing comfort and reducing anxiety in 53 women with early-stage breast cancer undergoing radiation therapy. The investigators designed and recorded imagery specifically for this study. Subjects were most likely to listen just before a treatment.

RESEARCH BOX: Effect of Imagery on Children's Pain and Anxiety during Cardiac Catheterization

Children who undergo cardiac catheterization present pain management challenges. In this experimental study, the investigator examined the effect of guided imagery on children's pain and anxiety during cardiac catheterization. Twenty-four children aged 9–17 years were randomly assigned to a control, presence, or imagery condition. Physiological, psychological, and behavioral data were used to rate children's pain and anxiety during cardiac catheterization. Children in the imagery condition displayed fewer distress behaviors during cardiac catheterization. Children in the presence condition reported the lowest levels of pain. Cortisol elevation over baseline was lowest in the control group, a result consistent with findings in previous studies.

Source: Pederson, C. (1995). Effect of imagery on children's pain and anxiety during cardiac catheterization. *Journal of Pediatric Nursing, 10*(6), 365–374.

HYPNOSIS

Hypnosis is a process or state of mind that can be manifest with suggestion or autosuggestion. It relates to altered brain wave patterns that are induced through deep relaxation.

Overview

Hypnosis is the process during which the subconscious mind can be engaged to work to bring about a desired goal such as smoking cessation or weight loss. This natural phenomenon usually contains all or some of the following characteristics:

- Focused concentration
- Increased physical and mental relaxation
- Heightened physiological and emotional suggestibility
- Heightened sensory awareness

The hypnotic state does not include:

- Loss of consciousness
- Weakening of will or control
- A process requiring a weak mind
- Disclosure of secrets
- A permanent state
- Any magic or potion that causes a change in behavior against one's will

Hypnosis can be used for a wide variety of conditions, disorders, and problems. Some common applications include stress management, smoking cessation, and weight control. Other uses involve improving study habits, learning and memory retrieval, self-esteem and confidence, sales motivation, and sleep habits.

Another area of emerging importance is the use of hypnosis for pain management. Some hypnosis subsets are called by different names, such as hypnotherapy and past life regression.

In 1995, the National Institutes of Health recommended that hypnosis be incorporated to a greater degree in the delivery of health care. In 1958, the American Medical Association (AMA) approved hypnosis for anesthesia.

Practitioners

Practitioners of hypnosis range from university-educated doctors of philosophy to self-trained entrepreneurs. The hypnotherapist may be a medical or mental health professional having a bachelor's degree or higher in psychology, counseling, social work, nursing, physical therapy, or related fields. He or she should be trained by a professional certified instructor (CI) of hypnotherapy and be certified by a national certifying organization, such as the National Guild of Hypnotists (NGH).

The NGH was established in 1951 by a group of hypnotists in Boston, Massachusetts. Within a short time, local chapters were formed and operated in many major cities throughout the United States and Canada. The NGH provides the service of testing and certifying hypnotherapists.

In most hypnosis training programs, a Level I curriculum provides a complete classical approach to hypnosis that enables the practitioner to immediately become a practicing hypnotherapist working with weight, smoking, and stress problems for both individuals and groups. Upon completion of Level II, the therapist is able to help clients deal with fears and anxieties, self-confidence and esteem issues, sports performance, career coaching, and sales performance.

To be certified, a hypnotherapist must attend and graduate from a recognized school of hypnosis or pass a test demonstrating his or her skills. In addition to remaining certified, the hypnotherapist must remain in good standing and continue to develop his or her skills by continuing his or her education in hypnotism.

Treatment

Hypnosis has proven effective in the relief of cancer pain, insomnia, tension headaches, chronic pain, certain dermatological conditions, alcoholism, allergies, myofascitis, and pain associated with childbirth. It has also been used successfully in weight reduction, smoking cessation, depression, confidence building, impotence, improving study habits, public speaking, stress reduction, trauma recovery, regression therapy, and controlling panic attacks.

The experience of hypnosis is similar to daydreaming or star gazing. A state of deep relaxation is achieved while remaining awake. It occurs through a series of therapist-guided suggestions and techniques. When the hypnotic state is achieved, the client is guided to explore deep-seated reasons for certain behaviors, and an attempt is made to finding an effective approach to behavior modification. There are a number of therapies that are classified under the umbrella term of hypnosis. An example is detailed next.

PAST-LIFE REGRESSION THERAPIES

Past-life regression therapy is based on the premise that many physical, mental, and emotional problems are rooted in the past—whether from childhood traumas or experiences in previous lifetimes. The practitioner of past-life regression therapy uses hypnosis (or altered states of consciousness) and relaxation techniques to access the source of these unresolved problems and helps clients analyze, integrate, and release past traumas that are interfering with their lives.

Advice to Patients

When advising a patient who wants to see a hypnotherapist, suggest that they choose a therapist with a focus on their issues and concerns. Furthermore, the therapist should be willing to answer your patient's questions about his or her experience and qualifications or about hypnosis in general. For patients who ask your opinion about the method and effectiveness of hypnosis, Table 9-3 can serve as a model for how to respond to the queries.

When advising your patient who wants to see a hypnotherapist, suggest that they choose a therapist with a focus on their issues and concerns. Furthermore, he or she should be willing to answer your patient's questions about his or her experience and qualifications, or about hypnosis in general. The hypnotherapist may be a medical or mental health professional (with a bachelor's degree or higher, in psychology, counseling, social work, nursing, physical therapy, or related field). He or she should have been trained by a professional Certified Instructor (CI) of hypnotherapy, and be certified by a national certifying organization, such as The National Guild of Hypnotists.

TABLE 9-3	**Typical Questions and Answers to Queries Patients Might Pose about Hypnosis**
TYPICAL QUESTION	**ANSWER**
What does hypnosis feel like?	Hypnosis feels a lot like daydreaming. You should be pleasantly relaxed, drowsy, and comfortable.
Will I be unconscious during the experience?	No. Even though you will feel very relaxed, you will actually be more acutely aware of everything that is happening. You will notice things that you may not have noticed before.
Do I have to concentrate?	The experience is much like being immersed in a good book or movie or not being aware of an injury while playing sports because your concentration is centered on the game. In times like these, you may not notice when someone talks to you.
Will I have a memory of what happened during the session?	Yes, events can be recalled, and you will feel a strong motivation to follow the plan of action decided upon by you and your therapist.
Will the hypnotic experience weaken my willpower?	No. In fact, quite the opposite occurs. Willpower is actually strengthened through the realization of the capacity of the subconscious mind to make up for the reduction in willpower caused by stress, anxiety, and tension in our everyday lives. With hypnosis, you can use this capacity to effect your desired change.

Research

Hypnosis has been around for a long time and a number of studies on its effectiveness exist, a few of which are discussed here.

STUDIES THAT SUPPORT USE OF HYPNOSIS

In one investigation, a MEDLINE search was conducted from January 1966 through December 1998 on key words related to hypnosis and skin disorders (Shenefelt, 2000). Findings included a wide spectrum of dermatological disorders that may be improved or cured using hypnosis as an alternative or complementary therapy. The conclusion of this investigation is that appropriately trained clinicians may successfully use hypnosis in selected patients as alternative or complementary therapy for many dermatological disorders.

A meta-analysis of 18 studies revealed a moderate to large hypnoanalgesic effect in most of the studies, supporting the efficacy of hypnotic techniques for pain management (Montgomery, DuHamel, & Redd, 2000). The results also indicated that hypnotic suggestion was equally effective in reducing both clinical and experimental pain.

Hypnosis has been used clinically to treat a variety of disorders that are refractive (do not respond) to pharmaceutical-based therapies, including asthma, but relatively little attention has been given recently to the use of clinical hypnosis as a standard treatment for asthma. Significant data suggest that hypnosis may be an effective treatment for asthma, but it is premature to conclude that hypnosis is unequivocally effective. Studies conducted to date have consistently demonstrated an effect of hypnosis with asthma. More and larger randomized, controlled studies are needed. Existing data suggest that hypnosis efficacy is enhanced in subjects who are susceptible to the treatment modality, with experienced investigators, when administered over several sessions, and when reinforced by patient autohypnosis. Children in particular appear to respond well to hypnosis as a tool for improving asthma symptoms (Hackman, Stern, & Gershwin, 2000).

Structured attention and self-hypnotic relaxation proved beneficial during invasive medical procedures. Hypnosis had more pronounced effects on pain and anxiety reduction and is superior to patient-controlled intravenous analgesia in that it also improves hemodynamic stability (Lang, Benotsch, Fick, Lutgendorf, Berbaum, Berbaum, Logan, & Spiegel, 2000).

STUDIES THAT DO NOT SUPPORT USE OF HYPNOSIS

Hypnosis in Smoking Cessation

Researchers reviewed 59 studies of hypnosis and smoking cessation to determine whether the research empirically supports hypnosis as a treatment (Green &

Lynn, 2000). Whereas hypnotic procedures generally yield higher rates of abstinence relative to wait-list and no-treatment conditions, hypnotic interventions are generally comparable to a variety of nonhypnotic treatments. The evidence for whether hypnosis yields outcomes superior to placebos is mixed. In essence, hypnosis cannot be considered a specific and efficacious treatment for smoking cessation. Furthermore, in many cases, it is impossible to rule out cognitive/ behavioral and educational interventions as the source of positive treatment gains associated with hypnotic treatments. Hypnosis cannot, as yet, be regarded as a well-established treatment for smoking cessation.

Hypnosis and Routine Endoscopy

A total of 124 subjects undergoing routine endoscopy were randomly assigned to one of three groups (Conlong & Rees, 1999). All three groups received lignocaine throat spray. The first group additionally received midazolam, the second received hypnosis, while the third only received lignocaine throat spray. Although hypnotized patients were deemed by an independent observer to be less agitated than the other two groups (p <0.03), they reported the gastroscopy to be significantly more uncomfortable (p <0.042) and scored higher in their memory for the procedure (p <0.001). They also took slightly longer to induce than the midazolam group. On the other hand, the midazolam group rated the procedure as significantly more comfortable although paradoxically were seen by an independent observer as being more agitated. They were also significantly more amnesic. The endoscopist encountered more procedural difficulties with this group, but this did not reach levels of significance. Hypnosis was not an effective alternative to intravenous sedation in gastroscopy.

MEDITATION

Although meditation assumes many forms and is used for many purposes, it is essentially a tool that helps facilitate a sense of being centered, a feeling of the body being rooted in itself in its place on earth. Meditation is a naturally occurring rest state—resting in the body while remaining awake and alert. Meditation is innate, and the body already knows how to do it. The human body has an instinctive ability to shift into profound rest states in order to heal, energize, integrate, tune itself up, and assimilate learning.

Meditation can take many forms. For example, it can be a directed or nondirected practice, a visualization, the repetition of a mantra (a set of meaningful repetitive words), the counting of breaths, the naming of breath activity (i.e., in through the nose, out through the mouth), utter silence, mindful watching of mental activity, prayer, contemplation, or total immersion in a movement exercise such as hatha yoga, tai chi, or Sufi dancing. Extensive research over the past

20 years has demonstrated meditation's powerful healing effect on a wide range of conditions, from asthma to high blood pressure. Many meditate simply to reduce stress and improve their overall sense of well-being.

History

Hunters, singers, dancers, drummers, and hermits probably discovered meditation independently, each in their own way. People tend to encounter meditative states whenever they throw themselves with total intensity into life's callings. The knowledge of how to cultivate meditative states is a kind of craft knowledge. Meditation did not come from India or Tibet, but rather those are the places where it was widely practiced before it was written down. Since the 1980s meditation has become increasingly popular in the United States, with schools, institutes, and programs offered nationwide.

Practitioners

Meditation practitioners are people who have studied meditation and use it in their personal lives. Meditation teachers, on the other hand, are skilled, long-term meditators who have mastered the skill and want to guide others in the process. Teachers may be self-taught masters or professionals who know the modality and choose to incorporate it into their practice. For example, a professional incorporating meditation is Dean Orinish, a physician and well-known researcher who has documented the positive effects of lifestyle changes, particularly in heart health. The primary therapies he uses are diet, exercise, and meditation. Herbert Benson, a medical doctor at the Harvard Clinic in Boston, has worked with health care professionals to incorporate the practice of meditation in their practices.

Meditation Practice

Meditation is paradoxical in that a person is resting yet wide awake inside. It is very similar to taking a nap without falling asleep. If done properly, one can actually awaken to a heightened awareness of the details of everyday life. Even a few minutes of meditation may help a person move through the world more relaxed and alert. In essence, meditation gives one's attention a chance to explore its full range, both inward and outward. It is a conversation between the inner and outer life. Generally, a meditation master or teacher will lead a group or class of students or meditators who range from novices to experienced people. The group will "sit" together for a stated duration of time and through a verbal guiding process the teacher will instruct the student in focusing and quieting the mind (see Figure 9-5). There are several different forms to this practice.

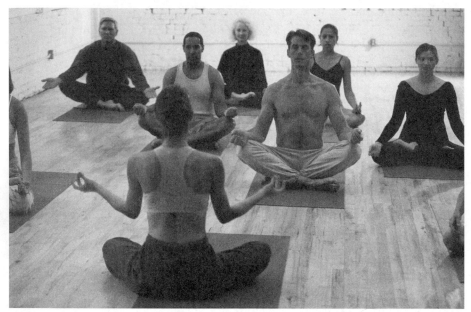

Figure 9-5 A meditation teacher leading a class. (Photo courtesy of Photodisc.)

Mindfulness

Best described as moment-to-moment awareness, mindfulness is often viewed as the heart of meditation. One can develop mindfulness by cultivating attention to objects in one's field of awareness, such as the flowing of one's breath, body sensations, sounds, thoughts, feelings, perceptions, impulses, and one's relationship to the world.

This method involves the cultivation of mindfulness through the practice of specific methods (formal meditation practice) and through moment-to-moment, nonjudgmental awareness of all aspects of daily life (informal meditation practice).

Focusing

This self-help tool is based on the premise that information about one's life issues can be accessed through a "felt sense" in the body. This skill can be used either alone or in partnership with someone else to resolve day-to-day issues (such as decision making), to negotiate profound changes (such as recovery from abuse), and to foster spiritual development.

Relaxation Response

Relaxation response is an integrated psychophysiological response originating in the hypothalamus that leads to a generalized decrease in arousal of the central nervous system. It is the direct opposite of the stress response. This hypometabolic state is the foundation of many interventions. Relaxation interventions have been taught for centuries. They include many theoretic and philosophic traditions and an array of specific strategies. The possible outcomes using relaxation response strategies are numerous and enable the patient to use the body's own innate mechanisms for health and healing. The relaxation response is used for reducing hypertension, insomnia, anxiety, pain, and medication use across multiple populations, diagnostic categories, and settings.

The response occurs through the repetition of a word or short phrase, and the gentle return to this repetition whenever distracting thoughts occur, in order to trigger a series of physiological changes (slowed breathing, heart rate, blood pressure, etc.) that reduce stress. The relaxation response has proven to be beneficial in treating stress-related conditions such as muscle tension pains, insomnia, and hypertension.

Research

Increased peripheral vasoconstriction has been implicated as playing an important role in the early development of essential hypertension. Some studies have demonstrated that transcendental meditation (TM) reduces high blood pressure, but the hemodynamic adjustments behind these blood pressure reductions have not been elucidated. The aim of one study was to provide a preliminary investigation of the acute effects of TM on temperature, pulse, and respiration (TPR) (Barnes, Treiber, Turner, Davis, & Strong, 1999). Subjects were 32 healthy adults divided into a TM group of long-term TM practitioners and a control group. Hemodynamic functioning was assessed immediately before and during three conditions: 20 minutes of rest with eyes open (all subjects), 20 minutes of TM (TM group), and 20 minutes of eyes-closed relaxation (control group). During eyes-open rest, the TM group had decreases in systolic blood pressure (SBP) and TPR, compared with increases in the control group (SBP: −2.5 vs. +2.4 mm Hg, p <0.01; TPR: −0.7 vs. +0.5 mm Hg/liter per minute, p <0.004). During TM, there was a greater decrease in SBP due to a concomitantly greater decrease in TPR compared with the control group during eyes-closed relaxation (SBP: −3.0 vs. +2.1 mm Hg, p <0.04; TPR: −1.0 vs. +0.3 mm Hg/liter per minute, p <0.03). The TPR decreased significantly during TM. Decreases in vasoconstrictive tone during TM may be the hemodynamic mechanism responsible for reduction of high blood pressure over time. The results of this study provide a preliminary contribution to the understanding of the underlying hemodynamic mechanisms responsible for the beneficial influence of TM on cardiovascular risk factors.

A classic investigation examined the extent to which advanced meditative practices might alter body metabolism and the electroencephalogram (EEG) in three Tibetan Buddhist monks living in the Rumtek monastery in Sikkim, India (Benson, Malhotra, Goldman, Jacobs, & Hopkins, 1990). Researchers found that during the practice of several different meditative practices, resting metabolism (VO2) could be both raised (up to 61%) and lowered (down to 64%). The reduction from rest is the largest ever reported. On the EEG, marked asymmetry in alpha and beta activity between the hemispheres and increased beta activity were present. From these three case reports, conclusions were that advanced meditative

RESEARCH BOX: Effects of Relaxation Response Training on Menopausal Symptoms

The specific aim of this study was to investigate the efficacy of elicitation of the relaxation response for the treatment of menopausal hot flashes and concurrent psychological symptoms. The volunteer sample consisted of 33 women between the ages of 44 and 66 years who were in general good health, with a minimum of 6 months without a menstrual period, experiencing at least five hot flashes per 24 hours, and not using hormone replacement therapy. The setting was an outpatient clinic in a tertiary care teaching hospital. The interventions used were relaxation response training and an attention control group and a daily symptom diary measuring both the frequency and intensity of hot flashes, the Spielberger State-Trait Anxiety Inventory (STAI) and the Profile of Mood Scale (POMS) were the measures used. This was a randomized, controlled, prospective study. Subjects were randomly assigned to one of three groups (relaxation response, reading, or control) for the 10-week study. In the first 3 weeks baseline measurements were taken of the frequency and intensity of hot flash symptoms, and these and the preintervention psychological scores were compared with the final 3 weeks measurement of frequency and intensity and the postintervention psychological scores for symptomatic improvement. The relaxation response group demonstrated significant reductions in hot flash intensity ($p < 0.05$), tension-anxiety ($p < 0.05$), and depression ($p < 0.05$). The reading group demonstrated significant reductions in trait-anxiety ($p < 0.05$) and confusion-bewilderment ($p < 0.05$). There were no significant changes for the control group. Daily elicitation of the relaxation response led to significant reductions in hot flash intensity and the concurrent psychological symptoms of tension-anxiety and depression.

Source: Irvin, J. H., Domar, A. D., Clark, C., Zuttermeister, P. C., & Friedman, R. (1996). The effects of relaxation response training on menopausal symptoms. *Journal of Pyschosomatic and Obstetrics and Gynaecology, 17*(4), 202–207.

practices may yield different alterations in metabolism (there are also forms of meditation that increase metabolism) and that the decreases in metabolism can be striking.

SUMMARY

Mind-body therapies explore the interactions between the body and the mind, and the relationship this connection has to health. the focus of this chapter was on psychotherapy, art therapy, music/sound therapies, imagery, hpnosis, and meditation. Practioners in the field range from the self-trained person to those who have post-graduate education. Research is proliferating in the mind-body arena as numerous studies document the effectiveness of these mosalities.

ASK YOURSELF

1. Describe which of the therapies is most appealing to you and why. Do any of the therapies make you feel uncomfortable? Which ones would you recommend or not recommend to your patients? Why or why not?
2. Which one or more of your patients or clients might benefit from a referral to a mind-body therapist? Elaborate on why.

REFERENCES

Achteberg, J., Dossey, B., & Kolkmeier, L. (1995). *Rituals of healing: Using imagery for health and wellness*. New York: Bantam Doubleday Dell.

Agras, W. S., Walsh, T., Fairburn, C. G., Wilson, G. T., & Kraemer, H. C. (2000). A multicenter comparison of cognitive-behavioral therapy and interpersonal psychotherapy for bulimia nervosa. *Archives of General Psychiatry, 57*(5), 459–466.

Barnes, V. A., Treiber, F. A., Turner, J. R., Davis, H., & Strong, W. B. (1999). Acute effects of transcendental meditation on hemodynamic functioning in middle-aged adults. *Psychosomatic Medicine, 61*(4), 525–531.

Benson, H., Malhotra, M. S., Goldman, R. F., Jacobs, G. D., & Hopkins, P. J. (1990). Three case reports of the metabolic and electroencephalographic changes during advanced Buddhist meditation techniques. *Behavioral Medicine, 16*(2), 90–95.

Beresnevaite, M. (2000). Exploring the benefits of group psychotherapy in reducing alexithymia in coronary heart disease patients: A preliminary study. *Psychotherapy and Psychosomatics, 69*(3), 117–122.

Caberlotto, L., & Hurd, Y. L. (1999). Reduced neuropeptide Y mRNA expression in the prefrontal cortex of subjects with bipolar disorder. *Neuroreport, 10*(8), 1747–1750.

Chlan, L. (1998). Effectiveness of a music therapy intervention on relaxation and anxiety for patients receiving ventilatory assistance. *Heart Lung, 27*(3), 169–176.

Conlong P., & Rees, W. (1999). The use of hypnosis in gastroscopy: A comparison with intravenous sedation. *Postgraduate Medical Journal, 75*(882), 223–225.

Dossey, B., Keegan, L., & Guzzetta, C. (2000). *Holistic nursing: A handbook for practice.* Gaithersburg, MD: Aspen.

Fugh-Berman, A. (1997). *Alternative medicine: What works.* Baltimore, MD: Lippincott Williams & Wilkins Healthcare.

Green, J. P., & Lynn, S. J. (2000). Hypnosis and suggestion-based approaches to smoking cessation: An examination of the evidence. *International Journal of Clinical and Experimental Hypnosis, 48*(2), 195–224.

Hackman, R. M., Stern, J. S., Gershwin, M. E. (2000). Hypnosis and asthma: A critical review. *Journal of Asthma, 37*(1), 1–15.

Irvin, J. H., Domar, A. D., Clark, C., Zuttermeister, P. C., & Friedman, R. (1996). The effects of relaxation response training on menopausal symptoms. *Journal of Psychosomatic Obstetrics Gynaecology, 17*(4), 202–207.

Keller, M. B., McCullough, J. P., Klein, D. M., Arnouv, B., Dunner, D. L., Gelenberg, A. J., Markowitz, J. C., Nemeroff, C. B., Russell J. M., Thase, M. E., Trievedi, M. H., Zajecka, J. (2000). A comparison of nefazodone, the cognitive behavioral-analysis system of psychotherapy, and their combination for the treatment of chronic depression. *New England Journal of Medicine, 342*(20), 1462–1470.

Kolcaba, K., & Fox, C. (1999). The effects of guided imagery on comfort of women with early stage breast cancer undergoing radiation therapy. *Oncology Nursing Forum, 26*(1), 67–72.

Lang, E. V., Benotsch, E. G., Fick, L. J., Lutgendorf, S., Berbaum, M. L., Berbaum, K. S., Logan, H., & Spiegel, D. (2000). Adjunctive non-pharmacological analgesia for invasive medical procedures: A randomised trial. *Lancet, 355*(9214), 1486–1490.

McKenna, P., & Haste, E. (1999). Clinical effectiveness of dramatherapy in the recovery from neuro-trauma. *Disability and Rehabilitation, 21*(4), 162–174.

Miljkovitch de Heredia, R. M., & Miljkovitch, I. (1998). Drawings of depressed inpatients: Intentional and unintentional expression of emotional states. *Journal of Clinical Psychology, 54*(8), 1029–1042.

Montgomery, G. H., DuHamel, K. N., & Redd, W. H. (2000). A meta-analysis of hypnotically induced analgesia: How effective is hypnosis? *International Journal of Clinical and Experimental Hypnosis, 48*(2), 138–153.

Rybakowski, J. K., & Twardowska, K. (1998). The dexamethasone/corticotropin-releasing hormone test in depression in bipolar and unipolar affective illness. *Journal of Psychiatric Research, 33*(5), 363–370.

Schrock, D., Palmer, R., & Taylor, B. (1999). Effects of a psychosocial intervention on survival among patients with stage 1 breast and prostate cancer: A matched case-control study. *Alternative Therapies in Health and Medicine, 5*(3), 49–55.

Shames, K. H. (1996). *Creative imagery in nursing.* Albany, NY: Delmar Thomson Learning.

Shenefelt, P. D. (2000). Hypnosis in dermatology. *Archives of Dermatology, 136*(3), 393–399.

Simonton, O., Matthews-Simonton, S., & Sparks, T. F. (1980). Psychological intervention in the treatment of cancer. *Psychosomatics, 21*, 226–227.

Thomas, E. M., & Weiss, S.M. (2000). Nonpharmacological interventions with chronic cancer pain in adults. *Cancer Control, 7*(2), 157–164.

Tusek, D., Church, J.M., & Fazio, V. W. (1997). Guided imagery as a coping strategy for perioperative patients. *Association of Operating Room Nurses Journal, 66*(4), 644–649.

Tusek, D. F., Cwynar, R., & Cosgrove, D. M. (1999). Effect of guided imagery on length of stay, pain and anxiety in cardiac surgery patients. *Journal of Cardiovascular Management, 22*(1), 109–127.

Watkins, G. R. (1997). Music therapy: Proposed physiological mechanisms and clinical implications. *Clinical Nurse Specialist, 11*(2), 43–50.

RESOURCES

Organizations

Center for Mind-Body Medicine
5225 Connecticut Ave, NW, Suite 414
Washington, DC 20015
Phone: 202-966-7338
Fax: 202-966-2589
E-mail: center@cmbm.org
Web site: www.cmbm.org

Center for Mindfulness Stress Reduction Clinic
University of Massachusetts Medical Center
Worcester, MA
Phone: 508-856-2656

Mind/Body Medical Institute Division of Behavioral Medicine
Beth Israel Deaconess Medical Center
Boston, MA
Phone: 617-632-9530

Associations

American Art Therapy Association, Inc.
1202 Allanson Road
Mundelein, IL 60060-3808
Phone: 888-290-0878 or 847-949-6064
Fax: 847-566-4580
E-mail: arttherapy@ntr.net

American Music Therapy Association
8455 Colesville Road, Suite 1000
Silver Spring, MD 20910
Phone: 301-589-3300
Fax: 301-589-5175
E-mail: info@musictherapy.org

Journals

Advances: The Journal of Mind-Body Health, John E. Fetzer Institute, Kalamazoo, MI
Alternative Therapies in Health and Medicine, Innovision Communications, Aliso Viejo, CA
Brain, Behavior, and Immunity, Academic Press, San Diego, CA
Mind-Body Medicine, Decker Periodicals, Hamilton, Ontario

CHAPTER 10

Posture and Mobility

Chapter Objectives

- Discover the range of modalities related to posture and mobility.
- Find that some modalities have research to validate effectiveness.
- Become familiar with a variety of the posture and mobility therapies used in some alternative and complementary therapy practices.
- Compare and contrast the quality and quantity of various therapies.
- Find that some therapies are grounded in empirical evidence while others are based on opinion, life experience, or concept.

INTRODUCTION

The posture and mobility classification of modalities has to do with how individuals hold and move their bodies. To the untrained eye, posture goes unnoticed, but a skilled observer can recognize and treat body postures that can contribute to unhealthy conditions. In many instances, clients seek therapy only after poor posture has become a chronic state and a remedy is sought for the consequence. The enlightened individual may seek postural integration to prevent the onset of related deleterious conditions.

Some therapies described in this chapter are widely recognized and offer certification or other training, while others are used by individuals in loosely organized groups. These therapies are not all inclusive but are representative of the vast array of posture and mobility modalities that currently exist. Some are techniques while others are a recognized therapy complete with its own body of literature. However, both are reported as there are practitioners and consumers of both. The therapies in this chapter are:

- ■ Movement therapies
  - Alexander technique
  - Aston Patterning
  - Body-mind centering
  - Dance/movement therapies

- • Feldenkrais method
- • Gyrotonics
- • Pilates method
- • Rosen method
- ■ Tai chi
  - • Qigong
- ■ Yoga
  - • Kripalu yoga
  - • Phoenix rising

MOVEMENT THERAPIES

The posture and movement of most children and young adults are supple, erect, and graceful. But as we grow older most people's posture deteriorates, often quite seriously. This happens as we become busy, focused on work, and unconsciously tense in reaction to life's worries and concerns. Our shoulders may become hunched and our necks stiff, and we may sit either slumped or holding ourselves in a rigid upright position.

Humans have a series of reflexes throughout the body that support us against the force of gravity and naturally coordinate our movements. Inappropriate muscular tension creates an interference with these reflexes, and the result is that many of us move in ways that are awkward and inefficient. This can give rise to a wide range of common ailments such as arthritis, neck and back pain, migraine, and sciatica. Many of our postural problems can be traced to overtensed neck muscles that interfere with the free movement of the head in relationship to the spine. Other tensions and tightly held muscle groups, over time, result in an unbalanced body that has lost the suppleness and easy movement of youth.

Most movement therapies deal with posture, muscle groups, and how to increase mental awareness of the body. The individual therapies involve different types and kinds of training, exercise, and/or motion of both large and small muscle groups. Therapies within this grouping appeal to a large variety of people who are interested in improving their movement and/or coordination skills, including people with neuromotor difficulties (i.e., cerebral palsy and strokes), chronic pain, and injuries as well as musicians, actors, dancers, athletes, and martial artists.

Many of the movement therapy modalities evolved from the experience of one person who found benefit in a particular form of posture, coordination, and breathing. Some therapies have associations and certification programs while others are still too new to have developed an organization or certification program.

A number of the therapies use the term reeducation to describe what they do or how they work. Reeducation is a term that refers to unlearning old patterns that usually involves muscle groups and substituting the behavior with newly acquired and practiced ways, that is, becoming conscious of postural stance and making a concerted effort to correct posture to effect a change in the voice. The goal is to break through unconscious habits to address harmful postural and mental sets, that is, being mentally unconscious of one's slumping postural stance. Also, some of the therapies use the term *mind-body technique* or *strategy*. This is because the focus is to alert the mind to become increasingly conscious of the body and its movements and behavior.

Practitioners

Movement therapy is an emerging field and, as such, many of the modalities are not structured into organizations. In some instances practitioners are self-trained, and in others they are professionally educated with certification in a specific movement therapy. Most therapies have their own associations and certification programs; however, there are also aptly skilled, but noncertified practitioners of the modality.

Alexander Technique

The Alexander technique (AT) is an educational discipline of psychophysical reeducation. Alexander technique teachers and physical therapists work with people who have both posture and movement dysfunctions. Physical therapists treat their patients within a medical model while AT practitioners regard themselves as teachers and work within an educational model. The two fields have many intertwining interests and concerns.

The AT involves a process of unlearning the acquired habits that interfere with innate balance, poise, and clarity, that is, slumping and rolling the shoulders forward when typing at a computer keyboard. This mind-body movement therapy was developed by F. Matthias Alexander (1869–1956), an Australian orator and actor who created the method after concluding that bad posture was responsible for his own chronic voice loss. He developed the method through the use of trial and error both with himself and with students/clients. Practitioners of the AT use gentle hands-on guidance and verbal instruction to teach simple, efficient ways of moving as a means to improve balance, posture, and coordination and relieve tension and pain. The client learns methods of increasing mental awareness of what is happening in the physical body and how to alter the body stance.

The AT has been successful in reducing musculoskeletal tension, thereby providing relief from chronic pain, as well as improving overall physical and mental health. It has long been popular among performers: vocalists, instrumentalists, actors, dancers, and athletes.

The Society of Teachers of the Alexander Technique (STAT), established in 1958, is the largest regulatory body of AT practitioners. Practitioners of this modality consider themselves to be teachers rather than therapists; therefore, often the client is referred to as the student.

Aston Patterning

Judith Aston, a student of Ida Rolf, was looking for an alternative to the painful force used in Rolfing, a deep, forceful massage technique, and conceived of this gentle movement education modality now known as Aston Patterning. The goal is to increase efficiency in movement and push the body to peak performance. The practitioner combines soft tissue bodywork and reeducation of everyday movements. Aston Patterning is a comprehensive, integrated system of three-dimensional deep-tissue release and movement education. It is based on the recognition of the relationships between body-mind and spirit to well-being. It combines massage and deep-tissue work, movement education, and ergonomics.

Body-Mind Centering

Body-mind centering is a movement-reeducation approach that explores how the body's systems (skeletal, muscular, nervous, etc.) contribute to movement and self-awareness. The approach also emphasizes movement patterns that develop during infancy and childhood. For example, a child who was frequently punished at the dinner table may grow up and unconsciously slump during eating. This occurs as a result of learned behavior during childhood that served to protect the child from persecution. Body-mind centering incorporates guided movement, exercise, imagery, and hands-on work. It can be used to help people of all ages resolve movement problems and facilitate the dialogue between the mind and body. For example, sometimes people unconsciously drum their fingers on a table or swing their crossed leg when nervous. The person who is working on body-mind centering seeks to alter those movement patterns. The more mentally aware individuals become of the body movement patterns and their relationship to psychological triggers, the better able they will be to alter the pattern.

Dance/Movement Therapies

Dance/movement therapy is the psychotherapeutic use of movement as a process that furthers the emotional, cognitive, social, and physical integration of the individual. This modality uses expressive movement as a therapeutic tool for both personal expression and psychological or emotional healing.

Dance/movement therapists work with individuals who have social, emotional, cognitive, and/or physical problems and are employed in psychiatric hospitals, clinics, day care, community mental health centers, developmental centers, correctional facilities, special schools, and rehabilitation facilities. Practitioners work with people who are familiar with dancing and choose this method of expression to work on their healing. They work with people of all ages in both groups and individually. They also serve as consultants and engage in research.

The American Dance Therapy Association (ADTA) was founded in 1966, and works to establish and maintain high standards of professional education and competence in the field of dance/movement therapy. The ADTA stimulates communication among dance/movement therapists and members of allied professions through publication of the *ADTA Newsletter,* the *American Journal of Dance Therapy,* monographs, bibliographies, and conference proceedings.

The ADTA distinguishes between dance/movement therapists prepared to work in professional settings within a team under supervision and those prepared for the responsibilities of working independently in private practice or providing supervision. They use the following credentials to differentiate levels of training:

- Dance therapist registered (DTR) therapists have a master's degree and are fully qualified to work in a professional treatment system.

- Academy of Dance Therapists registered (ADTR) therapists have met additional requirements and are fully qualified to teach, provide supervision, and engage in private practice.

Feldenkrais Method

The Feldenkrais method was developed by Moshe Feldenkrais (1904–1984), an engineer and physicist, the first European black-belt in Judo, and a student of Gurdjieff's work. The Feldenkrais method stresses gaining "awareness through movement" using movement to restore a person's natural ability to function optimally. His teachings contend that our thoughts, feelings, actions, sensations, and emotions are all related to our self-image. Therefore, Feldenkrais has a wide range of applications to behavior, whether for purposes of physical and emotional health, artistic expression, sports performance, or the enjoyment of everyday life. This method supports improving self-knowledge as well as the efficacy and quality of our actions.

The Feldenkrais method combines movement training, gentle touch, and verbal dialogue to help people move more freely and efficiently. Feldenkrais seeks to retrain the body's movements, muscle by muscle, using a system of gentle, seemingly innocuous floor exercises as well as individual, hands-on bodywork sessions termed "functional integration." In individual hands-on functional integration sessions, the practitioner uses touch to address the client's breathing and body alignment and in a series of classes of slow, nonaerobic motions helps promote "awareness through movement"; students learn improved ways in which their bodies can move. The Feldenkrais method is frequently used to treat stress and tension, to prevent recurring injury, and to help athletes and others improve their balance and coordination.

A number of Feldenkrais professional training programs throughout the country offer participants extensive practical experience and in-depth training in both *awareness through movement* (ATM) and *functional integration* (FI). Training programs also provide a thorough exploration of the theory underlying the Feldenkrais method through lectures, discussions, study groups, and assigned readings. By exploring the neurological, biological, and psychological aspects of the Feldenkrais method students gain the knowledge and skills necessary to become qualified practitioners.

Gyrotonics

This exercise system emphasizes circular motions similar to those used in swimming, tai chi, and yoga. Juliu Horvath, a Hungarian raised in Romania, began his professional career as a ballet dancer. Soon after defecting to the United States in the late 1960s, he learned that he could successfully combine the benefits of swimming, gymnastics, yoga, and dance into one system in which all the major muscle groups work interdependently and in an integrated manner. He designed his first machine, the Tower Handle Unit, to develop the inner strength necessary to perform his moving yoga. Over the years, Juliu added other machines to this system. Although originally designed for dancers who benefit from the broader range of motion that these machines provide, the Gyrotonic Expansion System works for anyone wishing to gain strength, flexibility, and coordination. The fundamentals of the Gyrotonic Expansion System (the Juliu Horvath Method) consists of a totally new exercise system using Gyrokinetics as the basis for exercising the muscles while mobilizing and articulating the joints. The Gyrotonic system uses key principles of gymnastics, swimming, ballet, and yoga through which major muscle groups are worked interdependently and in an integrated manner. The uniqueness of the system is that it stretches and strengthens at the same time with minimal effort while it increases the range of motion and develops coordination. The Gyrotonic Expansion System emphasizes multiple joint articulation and strengthening the surrounding ligaments and each attachment.

Pilates Method

The exercises derived from the program first developed by Joseph H. Pilates work the deeper muscles to achieve efficient and graceful movement, improve alignment and breathing, and increase body awareness. The exercises deliver simultaneous stretching and strengthening in a nonimpact, balanced system of body-mind control that works as well for the seasoned athlete as it does for the injured and sedentary individual. Pilates is a full-body, exercise system that emphasizes body alignment and correct breathing. With the help of an instructor, clients perform strength, flexibility, and range-of motion exercises on specially designed equipment. The Pilates method may be performed by people of any age or fitness level in order to improve flexibility, and range of motion, and people in physical therapy may use the method to aid in their recovery.

Several certification programs on both coasts have been created to meet growing demands. The structure of several certification programs is weekend introduction programs and concentration studies of 10 weeks.

Rosen Method

Developed by former physical therapist Marion Rosen, the Rosen method combines gentle touch and verbal communication to evoke relaxation and self-awareness. Because it can bring up buried feelings and memories, it is used as a tool for personal growth as well as pain relief. Combining breathwork, massage, relaxation techniques, and psychoanalysis, this unique body-mind form of therapy operates on the premise that the body is an "autobiography of traumas" that can be read and purged through light to deep hands-on bodywork, breathwork, and verbal dialogue to help process the insights. Rosen focuses on allowing the body to give up chronic muscle tension, thus helping the body return to its natural function and shape. Emphasis is placed on increasing awareness of tension and feelings. The results of Rosen method bodywork and movement frequently include a lessening of pain and tension and an increase in vitality. Many individuals experience a new sense of clarity about their life direction and goals. They are better able to make decisions that improve the quality of their life and can more easily align with their purpose. The Rosen method purports to:

- Relax muscle tension and chronic muscular holding
- Increase flexibility and vitality
- Deepen physical and emotional awareness
- Invite personal growth
- Complement other therapeutic modes and psychospiritual disciplines

Rosen method bodywork came out of Marion Rosen's 50 years of experience as a physical therapist and health educator. Her unique approach to bodywork and movement earned her recognition as a leader and originator in the field of body-oriented therapies. In the 1930s, Rosen studied breath and relaxation in Munich, Germany, with Lucy Heyer, who had been trained by Elsa Gindler, a renowned innovator of body therapies. Licensed in physical therapy, both in Stockholm and at the Mayo Clinic, Rosen developed the Rosen method over the course of many years in private practice. Rosen's purpose is to realize a vision of health and well-being by making the benefits of the Rosen method widely available to the general public. The Rosen Method Professional Association (RMPA) is the main source for Rosen method bodywork referrals (see the resources at the end of the chapter).

Advice to Patients

Most American adults could benefit from one of the movement therapies; this group of therapies will likely proliferate during the coming decade. Many older adults are too sedentary with consequent muscle and joint stiffness and a loss of flexibility. Thus, if your patient seems stiff, aching, and out of shape, you may want to recommend one of the above therapies. Suggest they look for postings of classes at their local cultural activity center, community college, art center, and food market or in the telephone book or newspaper.

Also, your patient should be aware that acute traumatic injuries are common with ballet dancers (Macintyre, 2000). Consequently, dance therapy or other strenuous therapy is more suitable for a young adult, while an older adult may be better suited to a less active therapy.

Advise your patient to ask the therapist about where they trained and if they have certification. If your patient is in poor physical condition, suggest that they begin the therapy slowly and not to exceed their limits. You may need to remind them that it took time to get to the shape they are currently in and so it will take time to undo the effects.

Research

Very little research exists on the movement therapies compared to the other more recognized movement modalities such as tai chi or yoga; however, there are some studies. One study was done to determine whether arthrosis begins at an unusually early age in professional dancers, there is a correlation between hypermobility and osteoarthrosis in dancers, and osteoarthrosis is a contributing factor to retirement from a professional career in this population (Teitz & Kilcoyne, 1998). Changes of arthrosis were found in 34 of 56 joints in 14 dancers and in 3 of 36 joints in 36 nondancers. Hip calcifications were found in 10 hips in 7 dancers and in 1 nondancer's hip. The prevalence of arthrosis in knees, ankles, and first metatarsophalangeal joints in young dancers was increased when compared to that of nondancers in the same age group. Since some professional dancers move on to become dance therapists, it is significant that they be aware of these data.

TAI CHI

Tai chi (pronounced tie-chee) is an extensive series of flowing, graceful movements used for health, meditation, and self-defense. Tai chi practice is based on a sequence of movements called "a form." The tai chi form takes around 8 minutes to do and is generally done daily. The aim of tai chi is to cultivate and circulate

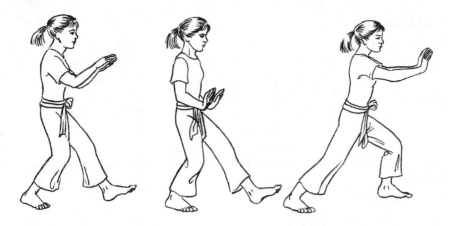

Figure 10-1 A common tai chi movement known as "grasp the bird's tail"

the body's vital energy. The movements are natural and are likened to a floating cloud or running stream. The arms move in a relaxed, circular fashion. Each step is taken very slowly, while the other foot remains firmly rooted to the ground. The body weight shifts gently from one side to the other during the form. Figure 10-1 shows an example of a tai chi movement.

Breathing is central to the form and is centered in the abdomen. This exercise system combines slow, graceful movement with calm, regular breathing. It has many styles and uses throughout the world and is becoming increasingly popular as a means of maintaining good health and feelings of relaxation and calm.

History

Tai chi has its origins in China around the twelfth century. However, Chinese cave paintings and references in ancient medical texts from earlier dates indicate that exercise systems similar in style to what we know as tai chi were practiced much earlier than that, perhaps even as early as 3000 B.C. Like the many other systems of self-care practiced by the Chinese, such as acupuncture or divination, tai chi probably has its real origins in the days before recorded history.

Today, tai chi has spread worldwide and is no longer an activity confined to Chinese parks and village halls. Most American towns offer tai chi classes in sports or adult learning centers, university or college campus, or cultural activity centers. Tai chi is also incorporated as a teaching media in numerous arts and therapy organizations. It is used in drama schools, in acupuncture colleges, on board cruise ships, and in senior citizen centers.

Practitioners

Tai chi teachers are generally mature students who have studied with a tai chi or qigong master for many years. More often than not, teachers do not have a professional or academic degree, rather it is their presence and reputation that attracts students. Although there are associations for tai chi practitioners, this practice is more loosely organized than other alternative therapies and gains its status from a history of personal testimonial and observational success. New students are attracted to tai chi because of its recognizable benefits.

The Practice

Tai when translated from the Chinese into English means "big," or "great," while *chi* means something like "ultimate energy" or "great system." Tai chi, therefore, is all about generating and feeling energy through movement, the ultimate energy that powers the universe—everything from the greatest star down to the smallest of microscopic creatures.

The yin and the yang are the two great polarities of Oriental philosophy and science—celebrated in areas as diverse as Oriental medicine, literature, and painting. The yin is *cool, negative, evening, winter, and autumn*; while the yang is *warm, positive, morning, summer, and spring*. The earliest references to the yang and yin in the literature is the ancient Chinese "Book of Changes," the *I Ching*. The yin and the yang are two halves of one great whole—hence the term *tai chi*.

Many people use tai chi as a guide toward understanding the principles of Taoism, the ancient Chinese philosophy of "the Way" or "the Path" through life that remains still to this day at the heart of Oriental philosophy and culture. Taoism is built on moderation, humility, and integrity. It celebrates the forces of nature and recognizes the interplay of yin and yang in all things, and in many respects it is a very modern way of looking at the world. People who practice tai chi regularly often arrive at an understanding of their own individual tao, or path, which subsequently helps them connect to the greater Tao of nature.

One of the more popular forms uses a sequence of 108 movements. Tai chi is the most widely recognized and practiced whole-body qigong exercise. Both of these practices are based on the ancient Chinese principle that the body has channels, called meridians, which can be used to cultivate, stimulate, and balance the body's vital energy, the qi. It is believed that we can learn to balance this energy and eventually increase the flow of qi in order to enhance well-being and vitality by dissolving any energy blocks within our body.

The cultivation of qi may take many forms. It is the awareness of, or tuning in to, qi that separates these practices from other exercises. Qigong and tai chi both promote the integration of mind, body, and spirit with the intent of achieving an inner harmony or state of balance with the energy of life. Both approaches are used not only for healing but also for prevention (see Figure 10-2).

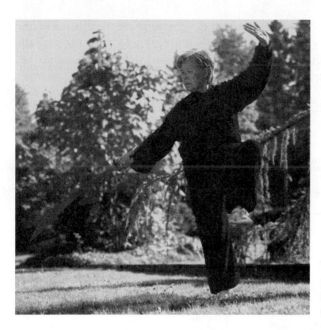

Figure 10-2 A woman performing tai chi chuan, a variation of tai chi. (Photo courtesy of Photodisc.)

Qigong

Also referred to as chi-kung, this is an ancient Chinese exercise system that aims to stimulate and balance the flow of qi (chi), or vital energy, along the acupuncture meridians, or energy pathways. Qigong is a variant of tai chi that has been used by the Chinese people for over 7000 years as a means to promote self-healing and inner harmony. For 20 years (from the 1960s to the 1980s), the practice of qigong was suppressed by the Communist Party. Eventually, interest in qigong and tai chi was renewed, and today more than 70 million Chinese people practice qigong tai chi on a daily basis. Qigong is used to reduce stress, improve blood circulation, enhance immune function, and treat a variety of health conditions.

The word *qi* (pronounced chee) signifies "life energy, vital energy, breath of life, force, power, air." The word *gong* means work and force, or power. *Qigong* is literally translated as "working with the energy of life" (see Figure 10-3). It refers to

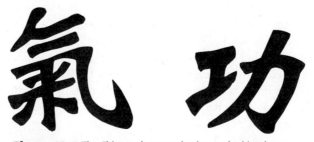

Figure 10-3 The Chinese characters for the words *chi* and *gong*.

the art and science of regulating internal energy to improve health, calm the mind, and condition the body. Qigong is actually a program for working with life energy that includes breathing and relaxation exercises, massage, visualization, meditation, and other natural methods.

Advice to Patients

Suggest your patients enroll in a tai chi or qigong program to take advantage of many benefits, including lowering blood pressure, stress management, increased concentration, weight control, and many other long-term advantages. Like yoga, the patient will have to stay with the practice for months in order to reap the advantages. Generally patients who are attracted to yoga will also like tai chi and find this gentle art/exercise form greatly beneficial to improving health and stamina and helping to minimize the deleterious effects of long-term chronic illnesses.

RESEARCH BOX: Effects of Tai Chi on Blood Pressure

This randomized clinical trial study compared the effects on blood pressure of a 12-week moderate-intensity aerobic exercise program and a tai chi program of light activity. Sixty-two sedentary older adults (45% black, 79% women, aged 60 years or more) with systolic blood pressure 130–159 mm Hg and diastolic blood pressure < 95 mm Hg (not on antihypertensive medication) were randomized to a 12-week aerobic exercise program or a light-intensity tai chi program. The goal of each condition was to exercise four days per week, 30 minutes per day. Blood pressure was measured during three screening visits and every two weeks during the intervention. Estimated maximal oxygen uptake and measures of physical activity level were determined at baseline and at the end of the intervention period. Results showed mean (SD) baseline systolic and diastolic blood pressures of 139.9 (SD 9.3) mm hg and 76.0 (SD 7.3) mm hg, respectively. For systolic blood pressure, adjusted mean [standard error (SE)] changes during the 12-week intervention period were –8.4 (SE 1.6) mm hg and –7.0 (SE 1.6) mm hg in the aerobic exercise and tai chi groups, respectively (each within-group $p < 0.001$; between-group $p = 0.56$). For diastolic blood pressure, corresponding changes were –3.2 (SE 1.0) mm Hg in the aerobic exercise group and –2.4 (SE 1.0) mm Hg in the tai chi group (each within-group $p < 0.001$; between-group $p = 0.54$). Body weight did not change in either group. Estimated maximal aerobic capacity tended to increase in aerobic exercise ($p = 0.06$) but not in tai chi ($p = 0.24$). The conclusions of this study are that programs of moderate-intensity aerobic exercise and light-intensity tai chi exercise may have similar effects on blood pressure in previously sedentary older individuals. If additional trials confirm these results, promoting light-intensity activity could have substantial public health benefits as a means to reduce blood pressure in older aged persons.

Source: Young, D. R., Appel, L. J., Jee, S., and Miller, E. R., III. (1999). The effects of aerobic exercise and T'ai Chi on blood pressure in older people: Results of a randomized trial. *Journal of the American Geriatric Society, 47*(3), 277–284.

Balance Control, Flexibility, and Cardiorespiratory Fitness among Older Tai Chi Practitioners

Tai chi chuan (TTC) exercise has beneficial effects on the components of physical condition and can produce a substantial reduction in the risk of multiple falls. Previous studies have shown that short-term TCC exercise did not improve the scores in the single-leg stance test with eyes closed and the sit and reach test. There has apparently been no research into the effects of TCC on total-body rotation flexibility and heart rate responses at rest and after a 3-minute step test.

In this cross-sectional study, 28 male TCC practitioners with an average age of 67.5 years and 13.2 years of TCC exercise experience were recruited to form the TCC group. Another 30 sedentary men aged 66.2 were selected to serve as the control group. Measurements included resting heart rate, left and right single-leg stance with eyes closed, modified sit and reach test, total-body rotation test (left and right), and a 3-minute step test. Compared with the sedentary group, the TCC group had significantly better scores in resting heart rate, 3-minute step test heart rate, modified sit and reach, total-body rotation test on both right and left sides ($p < 0.01$), and both right and left leg standing with eyes closed ($p < 0.05$). According to the American Fitness Standards, the TCC group attained the 90th percentile rank for sit and reach and total-body rotation test, right and left. From these results we can conclude that long-term regular TCC exercise has favorable effects on the promotion of balance control, flexibility, and cardiovascular fitness in older adults.

Source: Hong, Y., Li, J. X., & Robinson, P. D. (2000). Balance control, flexibility, and cardiorespiratory fitness among older Tai Chi practitioners. *British Journal of Sports Medicine, 34*(1), 29–34.

(Continued on next page)

Effect of Tai Chi on Cardiorespiratory Function in Patients with Coronary Artery Bypass Surgery

This study prospectively evaluated the training effect of a one-year TCC program for low-risk patients with coronary artery bypass surgery (CABS) after a postoperative outpatient (phase II) cardiac rehabilitation program. Twenty patients with mean age of 56.5 ± 7.4 years completed this study. The TCC group included 9 men who practiced classical yang TCC with an exercise intensity of 48%–57% heart rate range (HRR). The control group included 11 men whom were recommended to do a home-based self-adjusted exercise program with similar intensity of phase II cardiac rehabilitation. Graded exercise tests were performed before and after one year of training for all subjects. Mean attendance of the TCC group was 3.8 ± 1.5 times weekly, in contrast to 1.7 ± 1.1 times for the control group. During the follow-up examination, the TCC group increased 10.3% in VO2 peak (from 26.2 ± 4.4 to 28.9 ± 5.0 ml • kg −1 • min −1, p <0.01) and increased 11.9% in peak work rate, (from 135 ± 26 to 151 ± 28 W, p <0.01). However, the control group showed slight decrease in VO2 peak, from 26.0 ± 3.9 to 25.6 ± 4.6 ml • kg −1 • min −1, and in peak work rate, from 131 ± 23 to 128 ± 32 W. At the ventilatory threshold, the TCC group also showed significant increase in VO2 and work rate (p <0.05). The control group did not significantly change in these variables. The conclusion of this study demonstrates that a one-year TCC program for low-risk patients with CABS can favorably enhance cardiorespiratory function.

Source: Lan, C., Chen, S. Y., Lai, J. S., & Wong, M. K. (1999). The effect of Tai Chi on cardiorespiratory function in patients with coronary artery bypass surgery. *Medicine and Science in Sports and Exercise, 31*(5), 634–638.

Tai Chi Practice Reduces Movement Force Variability for Seniors

The purpose of this study was to examine whether tai chi practice can reduce the inconsistency of arm movement force output in older adults. Twenty seniors took part in the eight-week-long exercise intervention program (12 in tai chi practice, mean (M) = 79.3 years, Standard Deviation (SD) = 2.4; and 8 in a locomotor activity group, walking or jogging, M = 79.5 years, SD = 1.9). Linear and curvilinear manual aiming movements were tested at the beginning (pretest), during the fourth week (retest), and at the end of the exercise program (posttest). The measure of vertical pressure on the surface of a tablet served as the dependent variable. The findings suggest that tai chi participants significantly reduce more pressure variability than the participants in locomotor activity group after eight weeks of practice. Additionally, seniors produced higher pressure variability in the curvilinear task than in the linear task. Evidence from this study proposes that tai chi practice may serve as a better real-world exercise for reducing force variability in older adults' manual performance.

Source: Yan, J. H. (1999). Tai chi practice reduces movement force variability for seniors. *Journal of Gerontology. Series A, Biological Sciences and Medical Sciences, 54*(12), M629–634.

Effect of Tai Chi and Chronic Back Pain

Researchers at the University of California at San Diego have also shown that tai chi can help younger adults with low back pain. In their report, about 50 volunteers between the ages of 18 and 65 with daily back pain were divided in half. Those in the tai chi group were taught 11 movements over a six-week period and asked to practice the technique at home at least once a week. They saw a significant reduction in their pain and a slight improvement in their mood.

Source: Bhatti, T. I., Gillin, J. C., et al. (1998, Apr. 4). T'ai Chi Chuan as a treatment for chronic low back pain: A randomized, controlled study. In *Proceedings of the Third Annual Alternative Therapies Symposium* (p. 216).

YOGA

Yoga is one of the oldest systems of physical and spiritual healing as it dates back 5000 years. Yoga is from the Sanskrit word *yug,* meaning union (with the Divine). There are various types of yoga, but all of them have the same goal—unification with the Divine. Classical yoga includes a variety of techniques that help students achieve their personal goals while also presenting new opportunities for expanding these goals. The techniques of yoga seek to bring into balance all the disparate aspects of the body, mind, and personality so that the student ends up with energy, strength, and clarity of purpose supported by the whole being.

There are several forms of yoga. The best known and most widely practiced are listed in Table 10-1.

In the West, many only know yoga as hatha yoga, which is mainly physical exercise and postures (asanas). Actually asanas are only a single step in the eight-step

TABLE 10-1	Common Forms of Yoga
Hatha yoga	Focuses mainly on body postures and breath control techniques.
Raja yoga	Focuses on the mind using meditation.
Ashtanga yoga	Combines hatha and raja.
Kundalini yoga	Concentrates on awakening the subtle energy referred to as a coiled snake located at the base of the spine.
Tantric yoga	Uses sexual energy as means of awakening the dormant kundalini in order to heighten awareness.

path and are to be used as a stepping stone for the higher paths. This is because in classical yoga, simply working on the beauty and welfare of an impermanent object (the body) is considered a waste of time and effort. What is important is to enhance the whole body, mind, and spirit.

The practice of Yoga involves activation of body chakras. Chakras are psychic centers or trigger points of awareness and prana (life force) situated in specific areas of the body. These centers have been known for thousands of years by yogis, rishis, and sages by psychic introspection. From knowledge of these chakras, the great yogic science of kundalini yoga developed, which is concerned with awakening the energy that flows through the chakras.

At a subtle level, the seven major chakras correspond to the endocrine glands of the physical body, as well as major nerve plexes, thereby creating a nerve-hormone-chakra complex. You can image such a point as being formed by a needle and thread sewing the mental, spiritual, and physical bodies together. Chakras are the intersection of mind and body energies. Each chakra has certain characteristic colors and mantras associated with it. A mantra is a word or phrase that has psychic and spiritual properties when repeated during meditation practice.

Practitioners

Yoga teachers are generally mature students who have studied with a yoga master for many years. More often than not, teachers do not have a professional or academic degree; rather it is their presence and reputation that attracts students. Although there are associations for yoga practitioners, this practice is more loosely organized than other alternative therapies and gains its status from a history of personal testimonial and observational success. New students are attracted to yoga because of its recognizable benefits.

For the most part, yoga is still loosely organized in terms of national associations, conventions, and certification programs. There are, however, a number of associations in the country. The American Yoga Association, organized in 1968, under the direction of Alice Christensen, founder and president, is an example of one of the several associations in the country.

Techniques of Yoga

Basic yoga, in its simplest form, consists of three basic techniques as described in Table 10-2. More advanced forms are used when the student or class is deemed ready by the yoga teacher.

TABLE 11-2	Basic Yoga Techniques
TECHNIQUE	**EFFECT**
Exercise	Yoga exercises are designed to efficiently improve muscle tone, limberness, and circulation. Yoga also strengthens the nervous system, which builds concentration, poise, and a more stable emotional nature. Students quickly learn to recognize and reduce physical tension in an enjoyable and relaxing daily routine.
Breathing	Various yoga breathing techniques help to speed recovery from stress reactions, relieve insomnia, and improve concentration and stamina.
Meditation	The student learns a total-body relaxation technique followed by meditation, which is simply learning how to quiet the mind so that it rests from daily stresses. Regular meditation practice teaches one how to relax at will and also stimulates the intuitive, creative, and problem-solving capacities that we all have but often do not use.

There are many variations on the theme as certain teachers have developed the practice in their own specific way.

Phoenix Rising Yoga Therapy

This form of yoga therapy is designed to help clients achieve greater spiritual balance in their lives. A therapy session combines hands-on support in performing yoga postures with therapeutic dialogue techniques.

Kripalu Yoga

Kripalu yoga uses classical hatha yoga postures and breathing techniques to help students enter a state of "meditation in motion" (see Figure 10-4). Kripalu yoga teachers offer guidance in these yoga techniques and provide an atmosphere in which sensations, thoughts, and emotions can be experienced in a safe and

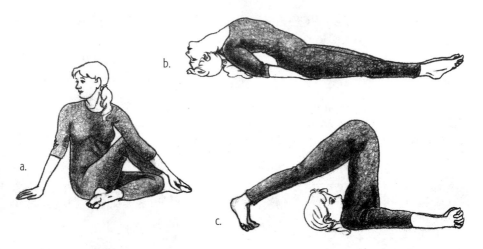

Figure 10-4 Examples of different yoga postures: (a) spinal twist, (b) the fish, and (c) the plough

relaxed atmosphere. The principles of kripalu yoga are the foundations for phoenix rising yoga therapy and kripalu bodywork.

Advice to Patients

When you refer patients for yoga therapy, you will want to explain that the best results come from long-term involvement with a skilled and patient teacher. At first their muscles may be sore with the multiple postures and stretching techniques. In addition, it may take months to years to comprehend and appreciate many of the subtleties and benefits of this modality.

Occasionally, an injury occurs. Vertebral artery dissection has been reported following minor head and neck trauma. Such activities as rapid head turning, which may occur in yoga and other vigorous exercise, have been implicated (DeBehnke & Brady, 1994). Consequently, as with the other modalities, it is important to advise your patients to not try to do too much too soon, but rather gradually work into the technique.

Research

Yoga has been valued for centuries as an enhancement of health. Other less well-known conditions may also be helped with yoga. Carpal tunnel syndrome is a common complication of repetitive activities and causes significant morbidity. One study was done to determine the effectiveness of a yoga-based regimen for relieving symptoms of carpal tunnel syndrome on 42 employed or retired individuals with carpal tunnel syndrome (median age 52 years; range 24–77 years) (Garfinkel, Singhal, Katz, Allan, Reshetar, & Schumacher, 1998). Researchers

RESEARCH BOX: Lipid Profiles Following Yoga Interventions

The effect of yogic lifestyle on the lipid status was studied in angina patients and normal subjects with risk factors of coronary artery disease. The parameters included body weight, estimation of serum cholesterol, triglycerides, high- and low-density lipoproteins (HDL, LDL), and the cholesterol-HDL ratio. A baseline evaluation was done and then the angina patients and risk factor subjects were randomly assigned as control ($n = 41$) and intervention (yoga) groups ($n = 52$). Lifestyle advice was given to both groups. An integrated course of yoga training was given for four days followed by practice at home. Serial evaluation of both the groups was done at 4, 10, and 14 weeks. Dyslipidemia was a constant feature in all cases. An inconsistent pattern of change was observed in the control group of angina ($n = 18$) and risk factor subjects ($n = 23$). The subjects practicing yoga showed a regular decrease in all lipid parameters except HDL. The effect started at 4 weeks and lasted for 14 weeks. Thus, the effect of yogic lifestyle on some of the modifiable risk factors could probably explain the preventive and therapeutic beneficial effect observed in coronary artery disease.

Source: Mahajan, A. S., Reddy, K. S., & Sachdeva, U. (1999). Lipid profile of coronary risk subjects following yogic lifestyle intervention. *Indian Heart Journal, 51*(1), 37–40.

were looking for changes from baseline to eight weeks in grip strength, pain intensity, sleep disturbance, Phalen sign, and Tinel sign and in median nerve motor and sensory conduction time. Subjects in the yoga groups had significant improvement in grip strength and pain reduction, but no significant differences were found in sleep disturbance, Tinel sign, and median nerve motor and sensory conduction time. In this preliminary study, a yoga-based regimen was more effective than wrist splinting or no treatment in relieving some symptoms of carpal tunnel syndrome.

SUMMARY

With the exception of tai chi and yoga, many of the movement therapies are still young and in the process of development. As our sedentary population ages and people become stiffer and less flexible, these therapies should become increasingly useful and popular. The posture and mobility therapies detailed in this chapter serve to awaken interest and open doors. If one or more of these therapies appeal to you, then begin an in-depth exploration of its tradition, practice, training methods, and documented effectiveness. Some of the therapies in the chapter are ripe for research investigation as health care professionals continue to compile data to support or challenge the use of alternative and complementary therapies.

ASK YOURSELF

1. Which five or more posture and mobility therapies may be used in an alternative or complementary care practice?
2. Which one or more therapies have research to support their effectiveness?
3. What type of person might be best served by deciding to begin a posture or mobility therapy?
4. How might you suggest to one of your patients that he or she would benefit from a movement or posture therapist?

REFERENCES

DeBehnke, D. J., & Brady, W. (1994). Vertebral artery dissection due to minor neck trauma. *Journal of Emergency Medicine, 12*(1), 27–31.

Garfinkel, M. S., Singhal, A., Katz, W. A., Allan, D. A., Reshetar, R., Schumacher, H. R., Jr. (1998). Yoga-based intervention for carpal tunnel syndrome: A randomized trial. *Journal of the American Medical Association, 280*(18), 1601–1603.

Hong, Y., Li, J. X., & Robinson, P. D. (2000). Balance control, flexibility, and cardiorespiratory fitness among older Tai Chi practitioners. *British Journal of Sports Medicine, 34*(1), 29–34.

Macintyre, J., & Joy, E. (2000). Foot and ankle injuries in dance. *Clinical Sports Medicine, 19*(2), 351–368.

Teitz, C. C., & Kilcoyne, R. F. Premature osteoarthrosis in professional dancers. *Clinical Sports Medicine, 8*(4), 255–259.

RESOURCES

American Dance Therapy Association National Office
Phone: 410-997-4040
Fax: 410-997-4048
Internet: www.adta.org

North American Society of Teachers of the Alexander Technique
3010 Hennepin Ave. S., Suite 10
Minneapolis, MN 55408
Phone: 800-473-0620 or 612-824-5066

Rosen Method Professional Association
Phone: 800-893-2622

The main source for Rosen method referrals.

International Kundalini Yoga Teachers Association (IKYTA)
Executive Director of IKYTA
Route 2, Box 4, Shady Lane
Espanola, NM 87532
Phone: 505-753-0423
Fax: 505-753-5982

American Yoga Association
P.O. Box 19986
Sarasota, FL 34276
Phone: 941-927-4977
Fax: 941-921-9844

Touch Therapies and Bodywork

Chapter Objectives

*   Discover the range of modalities related to touch therapies and bodywork.
*   Become familiar with a variety of the touch and bodywork therapies used in some alternative and complementary therapy practices.
*   Compare and contrast the quality and quantity of various therapies.

INTRODUCTION

Touch therapies are as old as healing itself. People instinctually knead, rub, or touch an area that is sore, tired, or overused. Hands-on touch modalities such as massage, acupressure, and shiatsu are currently used by more than 30,000 nurses in hospitals each year, and the procedures are documented as legitimate medical techniques. The American Massage Therapy Association (AMTA) represents more than 40,000 massage therapists in 30 countries.

Teams of health care practitioners combine medical skills with hands-on touch and energy techniques in most major cities of the United States. The world's first Touch Research Institute is at the University of Miami's Medical School. Its purpose is to further explore and document the benefits of touch therapy. Documented studies show that with hands-on work there is an array of effects:

*   ■ It benefits hospital patients (Smith, Stallings, Mariner, & Burnall, 1999).
*   ■ Bulimic adolescents benefit (Field, Schanberg, Kuhn, Fierro, Henteleff, Mueller, Yando, Shaw, & Burman, 1998).
*   ■ Circulation and breathing improve postsurgically (Morhenn, 2000).
*   ■ Premature infants have enhanced growth rate (Feldman & Eidelman, 1998; Hayes, 1998).

Bodywork is a general umbrella term that includes an array of techniques including massage, deep-tissue manipulation, movement awareness, and energy balancing, all of which are employed to improve the structure, harmony, and balance of the body and its functioning. Bodywork helps reduce pain, soothe injured muscles, stimulate blood and lymphatic circulation, and promote deep relaxation. Practitioners use hands-on techniques to manipulate the bones, muscles, and other tissues.

THE MODALITIES

Some of the therapies described in this chapter are widely recognized and offer certification or other training, while individuals in loosely organized groups use others. Although some of the therapies discussed in this chapter may seem esoteric to some, it is important that health care providers be aware of their existence in order to offer their patients the best possible advice. The therapies discussed in this chapter are:

(a) Massage

- Bonnie Prudden myotherapy
- Breema bodywork
- Craniosacral therapy
- Deep-tissue bodywork
- Gyrotonics
- Hellerwork
- Infant massage
- Kripalu bodywork
- Myofascial release
- Naprapathy
- Neuromuscular therapy
- Ohashiatsu
- Orthobionomy
- Rolfing
- Rubenfeld synergy method
- Soma neuromuscular integration
- Structural integration
- Swedish massage
- Trager bodywork

(b) Acupressure

- Integrative acupressure
- Jin Shin Do bodymind acupressure
- Jin Shin Jyutsu
- Reflexology
- Shiatsu
- Trigger point/myotherapy

MASSAGE THERAPY

Massage therapy is a general term for a range of therapeutic approaches with roots in both Eastern and Western cultures. It involves the practice of kneading or otherwise manipulating muscles or other soft tissue with the intent of improving a person's well-being or health.

Overview

Massage has a long history in most cultures, and its universal goal is to help promote relaxation, relief from sore and injured muscles, and an overall sense of well-being and improved health. Swedish massage is the most common form encountered in this country. Created by Per Henrik Ling in the 1800s, Swedish massage combines ancient Oriental techniques with modern principles of anatomy and physiology to relieve tension from chronically contracted muscles. Benefits include increased blood circulation to muscles and organs and the flushing out of waste and by-products such as lactic acid, allowing oxygen in the blood to nourish and rehabilitate, benefits that stem largely from the fact that massage stimulates sensory receptors in the soft tissues and increases lymphatic flow. Several specialized forms of massage therapy have developed in recent years, most notably sports massage, pregnancy massage, infant massage, and Thai and Lomi Lomi massage.

There are numerous indications that massage therapy is gaining acceptance and growing. Of the types of alternative care explored in a recent study, people say they would be most likely to use massage therapy (80%), vitamin therapy (80%), herbal therapy (75%), and chiropractic (73%) (Landmark report, 1997). Consumers spent between $4 and $6 billion annually on visits to massage therapists, approximately 27% of the $21.2 billion spent on unconventional health care in 1997. Collectively, they visited massage therapists 114 million times each year, yielding about 18% of the 629 million annual visits to alternative health care providers (Eisenberg, Davis, Ettner, Appel, Wilkey, Van Rompay, & Kessler, 1998). Of primary care physicians and family practitioners, 54% say they would encourage their patients to pursue massage therapy as a complement to medical treatment (Blumberg, Grant, Hendrick, Kamps, & Dewan, 1995).

HISTORY

Massage has both Western and Eastern origins. The first written records date back 3000 years to Chinese and Ayurvedic records (see Figure 11-1). During the height of the Greek civilization, the art of bathing and massage emerged as therapeutic treatments for both illness and relaxation (Dossey, Keegan, Guzzetta, 2000; Hover-Kramer, Mentgen, Scandrett-Hibdon, 1996). When the Greek civilization fell and the Romans acquired the sites, bath houses and therapeutic massage were expanded and improved. Therapeutic baths followed by massage

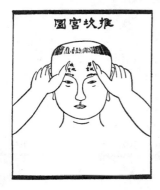

Figure 11-1 The practice of massage has both Eastern and Western origins. This illustration is from the Chinese work *Synopsis of the Technique of Remedial Massage,* 1889. (Courtesy of New York Public Library picture collection.)

became an accepted and sought-after therapy and recreation. Modern Western massage had its renaissance in the late 1800s, when Per Henrik Ling, a Swedish athlete, reintroduced massage, calling it Swedish massage, a method that combined hands-on techniques with active movements.

The practice of massage therapy has grown exponentially during the past few decades. Therapeutic backrubs were a part of general nursing care from the inception of hospital nursing in the United States in the late 1800s until the 1970s, when the practice was gradually discontinued as part of hospital care (see Figure 11-2). The skill was deleted from many curriculums at that time because it was not thought to be a scientifically validated intervention. When research studies began to validate its effectiveness in the 1980s and 1990s, it was reintroduced. Many nurses began entrepreneurial or independent practices during those decades and added the practice of massage to their repertoire. Most of these nurses had learned the technique in school and then took additional continuing education courses. Some nurses even took the massage therapy curriculum and became licensed in that as well as in nursing. As the therapy became more popular, massage therapy schools developed and attracted both nurses and nonnurses alike.

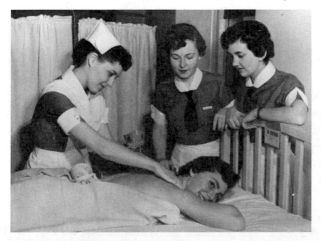

Figure 11-2 Therapeutic backrubs were a part of general nursing care from the inception of hospital nursing until about the 1970s, when the practice was gradually discontinued. (Courtesy of the Center for the Study of the History of Nursing, School of Nursing, University of Pennsylvania.)

Practitioners

The number of massage therapists is estimated to be between 150,000 and 190,000 working as part- and full-time practitioners, including students, while the AMTA's membership has increased threefold in the 1990s to over 36,000 members (AMTA, 1999).

There are many different kinds of massage training, some more in-depth than others. A well-trained massage therapist has graduated from a school with between 500 and 1000 hours of training, not including continuing education, training in specialties, or hours of experience.

REGULATION

The AMTA was founded in 1943 to develop guidelines for the ethical practice of massage, such as a Practice Standards document and a Code of Ethics. Such standards help to ensure a safe and nurturing environment for all who seek the benefits of massage.

The AMTA initiated the creation of the National Certification Board for Therapeutic Massage and Bodywork (NCBTMB), which is formally recognized by the National Commission of Certifying Agencies. The National Certification Exam has become the standard for licensure used by at least 16 of the 26 states that regulate massage to measure a competent and qualified practitioner.

The designation Nationally Certified in Therapeutic Massage and Bodywork indicates that the therapist has met certain basic standards in knowledge and training or experience and subscribes to a code of ethics. More than 29,000 massage therapists now have national certification from the NCBTMB. Therapists who have passed the National Certification Exam can be found through the NCBTMB. Some therapists may not have certification but may have membership in a recognized professional organization, such as the Associated Bodywork and Massage Professionals (ABMP), AMTA, or International Massage Association (IMA).

Treatment

Massage therapy is generally done in half-hour or one-hour sessions. Some therapists may do 90-minute sessions (or more). During the massage, only the part of the body being worked on is uncovered. Those parts of the body generally considered private are not uncovered or worked on. Patients interested in massage therapy should have an opportunity to discuss any particular preferences about parts of their body to be exposed and worked on prior to the massage session. If uncomfortable with any aspect of the massage, the patient should inform the therapist immediately. As patients get to know their therapist over repeated sessions, some of their preferences and levels of comfort may very well change, at which time they may renegotiate any aspect of their treatment with the therapist.

A host of various massage techniques abound. Swedish massage is probably the most commonly practiced form of massage in Western countries (see Figure 11-3). It integrates ancient Eastern techniques with modern principles of anatomy and physiology. Practitioners rub, knead, pummel, brush, and tap the muscles. The most common strokes are a combination of stroking (effleurage), friction, vibration, percussion, kneading (petrissage), stetching, compression, or passive and active joint movements within the normal physiological range of motion. Figure 11-4 presents a classification of massage movements.

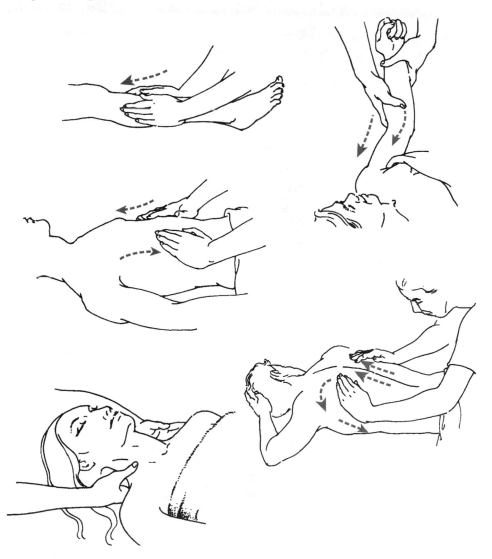

Figure 11-3 Effleurage, or stroking movements, is a commonly used massage technique.

1. Touch
   a. Superficial
   b. Deep
2. Gliding or effleurage movements
   a. Aura stroking
   b. Superficial
   c. Deep
3. Kneading movements
   a. Kneading or petrissage
   b. Fulling
   c. Skin rolling
4. Friction
   a. Circular friction
   b. Transverse or cross-fiber friction
   c. Compression
   d. Rolling
   e. Chucking
   f. Wringing
   g. Vibration
      • Manual
      • Mechanical
5. Percussion movements
   a. Hacking
   b. Cupping
   c. Slapping
   d. Tapping
   e. Beating
6. Joint movements
   a. Passive joint movements
   b. Active joint movements
      • Active assistive movements
      • Active resistive movements

Figure 11-4 Classification of massage movements

Numerous beneficial physiological effects come from massage therapy. Table 11-1 lists some of these effects.

TABLE 11-1 Physiological Benefits of Massage	
BODY SYSTEM	**PHYSIOLOGICAL EFFECT**
Circulation of the blood and lymph	Increases in the blood and lymph circulation are the most widely recognized and frequently described positive physiological effects of the stimulation received in massage therapy. Removal of waste material by increased blood flow and increase in oxygen delivery and other nutrients to cells result from massage.
Skeletal muscle	Benefits such conditions as muscle spasm, muscle hypertonicity, overuse injury, and tension headaches.
Fibrosis and contracture	Helps to stretch contracted muscles to begin reapportioning them back to their normal shape.
Pain control	Massage may act directly on the source of pain to alleviate nociceptive stimulation, or act centrally to alter the processing of nociceptive input, or affect conduction of pain impulses in the peripheral nerves.
Respiratory function	Chest percussion in combination with postural drainage and massage and manipulation of the respiratory musculature are known benefits in chronic obstructive pulmonary disease (COPD).

The numerous more common forms of massage therapy practiced throughout the United States are discussed in the following pages.

Infant Massage

This intervention is often referred to as touching and caressing, tender in caring (TAC-TIC) therapy. This therapy is used with a variety of infants, including healthy preterm babies and high-risk ventilated premature neonates (Fugh-Berman, 1997).

Trained instructors teach infant massage to new parents. Infant massage practices are designed to enhance the bonding between parent and baby. As preventive therapy, infant massage can help strengthen and regulate a baby's respiratory, circulatory, and gastrointestinal functions.

Bodywork

As discussed previously, bodywork differs from massage in that bodywork is a general umbrella term that includes an array of techniques including massage, deep-tissue manipulation, movement awareness, and energy balancing, all of which are employed to improve the structure, harmony, and balance of the body and its functioning. As with massage, bodywork practitioners employ a variety of treatment methods, some of which are discussed here.

BONNIE PRUDDEN MYOTHERAPY

Developed by a fitness expert in Reiki (see Chapter 13), this bodywork method is designed to relax muscle spasms, improve circulation, and alleviate pain. Using this technique, the practitioner uses elbows, knuckles, or fingers to apply pressure for several seconds to trigger points—highly irritable spots on muscle tissue that may radiate pain to other areas. Clients also perform specific exercises for the freed muscles.

BREEMA BODYWORK

Breema bodywork is an ancient, nondiagnostic health improvement method that uses a series of gentle, rhythmic movements to release tension and promote health, vitality, and inner harmony. Treatments are designed to create structural, physiological, emotional, and energetic balance in both the practitioner and the recipient. Breema bodywork is done fully clothed, with the recipient lying or sitting on a carpeted floor.

CRANIOSACRAL THERAPY

Craniosacral therapy is a manual therapeutic procedure for remedying distortions in the structure and function of the brain and spinal cord, the bones of the skull, the sacrum, and interconnected membranes. It is used to treat chronic pain, migraine headaches, temporolmandibular joint (TMJ) problems, ear infections, stroke recovery, spinal cord injuries, cerebral palsy, and a range of other conditions.

This bodywork modality was developed by osteopaths and chiropractors to work with the craniosacral mechanism—brain, spinal cord, skull, sacrum, and related membranes. Cerebrospinal fluid (CSF) pathways surround the brain and spinal cord and can be inhibited by trauma. Through hands-on manipulation, the practitioner holds or kneads the hollow at the craniosacral area and thus releases connective muscle tissue. Gentle touch on head, neck, and spine to loosen joints and fascia (connective tissue) frees trapped energy, which in turn helps restore the body's ability to heal itself.

DEEP-TISSUE BODYWORK

This is a general term for a range of therapies that seek to improve the function of the body's connective tissues and/or muscles. This form of neuromuscular reprogramming and therapy combines massage techniques with muscle testing to help people learn how to use their muscles with greater strength and less effort. Among the conditions deep-tissue bodywork treats are whiplash, lower back and neck pain, and degenerative diseases such as multiple sclerosis. Conscious bodywork is used to treat persistent joint and muscle pain and restrictions of movement caused by injury.

ROLFING

This technique uses deep manipulation of the fascia (connective tissue) to restore the body's natural alignment, which may have become rigid through injury, emotional trauma, or inefficient movement habits. The process, developed by biochemist Ida P. Rolf in the 1920s, has roots in yoga, the Alexander technique, and osteopathic medicine. Rolf viewed the body as a tower of children's building blocks, claiming that if one block slips out of alignment, the structure becomes unstable. Rolfing focuses on restructuring the musculoskeletal system by working on patterns of tension held in deep tissue. The practitioner uses deep manipulation of the fascia (connective tissue) in specific areas, which vary depending upon where and how the client's weight is carried, to restore the body's natural alignment and balance. While the client works to rebalance the body, emotional pain and memories are often released, allowing for the possibility of change in the client's attitude and behavior. Today, Rolfing is not considered as harsh as it once was. Rolfing takes place over a series of ten 1-hour sessions, each session focusing on a different part of the body.

HELLERWORK

Developed by former aerospace engineer (and one-time Rolf Institute president) Joseph Heller, this technique combines deep-tissue muscle therapy and movement reeducation with dialogue about the emotional issues that may underlie a physical posture. Heller studied Rolfing under Ida Rolf and developed Hellerwork as a more gentle form of deep-tissue muscle therapy—manipulation of the fascia (connective tissue)—than Rolfing. Stressing the mind-body connection, Hellerwork is used in a series of sessions to treat chronic pain or to help "well" people learn to live more comfortably in their bodies. Hellerwork stresses the importance of the body-mind connection through its emphasis on movement reeducation and its belief that we hold emotions and memories in the body. Through deep-tissue therapy, these emotions and memories are triggered, and the Hellerworker then engages the client in dialogue about what has been triggered in order for the client to gain insight and possible resolution of the issue or memory. The proper Hellerwork series involves eleven 60–90-minute sessions, each session focusing on a different part of the body. Hellerwork is also increasingly used as an adjunct in psychotherapy.

MYOFASCIAL RELEASE

Myofascial release is a hands-on deep-tissue bodywork technique akin to Rolfing or Hellerwork, as it is similarly focused on loosening the fascia (connective tissue) in order to restore structural alignment in the body as well as promote a balanced relationship between all parts of the body. The primary distinction between this technique and Rolfing or Hellerwork, however, lies in the fact that the latter two involve 10 or 11 sessions, while this modality is locally applied; it is not part of a prescribed treatment series.

This hands-on technique seeks to free the body from the grip of tight fascia, or connective tissue, thus restoring normal alignment and function and reducing pain. Using their hands, therapists apply mild, sustained pressure to gently stretch and soften the fascia. Myofascial release is used to treat neck and back pain, headaches, recurring sports injuries, and scoliosis, among other conditions.

KRIPALU BODYWORK

Based on the principles of Kripalu yoga, this bodywork method seeks to promote a deep state of relaxation and help recipients reconnect with the healing wisdom of their bodies. Along with specific massage strokes, Kripalu bodyworkers use verbal and nonverbal means to guide recipients into a meditative state in which physical and mental tension may be accessed and released.

NAPRAPATHY

Developed in the early 1900s, this system of manually applied movements (both passive and active) is designed to bring motion, consequently releasing tension from abnormally tense and rigid ligaments, muscles, and articulations of the human body. Naprapathy's philosophy is based upon a belief that all biological processes are aimed at survival and perpetuation of the species and that these processes are responsible for the rehabilitation of the human organism. Naprapathy's procedures help the body to maintain a favorable internal environment by releasing points of tension and by employing rational dietary and hygienic measures. The word *naprapathy* is a combination of the Czech word *napravit,* meaning "to correct," and the Greek *pathos,* meaning "suffering."

NEUROMUSCULAR THERAPY

This general term incorporates a range of bodywork practices that have a therapeutic (not simply relaxing) intent. Practitioners stress client education and follow-up. Among the conditions they address are chronic back pain, headaches, tension, and emotional illnesses. Neuromuscular therapy emphasizes the role of the brain, spine, and nerves in muscular pain. One goal is to relieve tender, congested spots in muscle tissue and compressed nerves that may radiate pain to other areas of the body.

OHASHIATSU

This is a system of physical techniques, exercise, and meditation used to relieve tension and fatigue and to induce a state of harmony and peace. The practitioner first assesses a person's state by feeling the *hara* (the area below the navel). Then, using continuous and flowing movements, the practitioner presses and stretches the body's energy channels, working in unison with the person's breathing.

ORTHO-BIONOMY

Developed by a British osteopath, ortho-bionomy involves the use of noninvasive, gentle touch along with dialogue and instruction in common movements such as walking, sitting, standing, and reaching. Practitioners may also sometimes work with the energy field surrounding the person. The goal of the work is the client's enhanced well-being and empowerment, rather than just physical healing.

RUBENFELD SYNERGY METHOD

The Rubenfeld synergy method uses gentle touch, movement, verbal exchange, and imagination to help access memories and emotions locked in the body. Developed by healer Ilana Rubenfeld, it integrates elements of the Alexander technique, the Feldenkrais method, gestalt therapy, and hypnotherapy. Because it combines bodywork and psychotherapy, this technique may be used for specific physical or emotional problems or for personal growth.

SOMA NEUROMUSCULAR INTEGRATION

This bodywork method seeks to improve posture, joint function, and body alignment through deep manipulation of the muscular and connective tissue, balancing and aligning the physical structure of the body and thereby integrating the nervous system into a healthier functioning body. The 10-session process, which incorporates movement training, also seeks to promote greater access to the functioning of each hemisphere of the brain. People with conditions such as chronic back pain, arthritis, asthma, scoliosis, and headaches have sought relief through this method.

Soma works with body psychology (somography), the balancing of brain hemispheres, and movement reeducation (awareness about how we move and how to move with optimum efficiency). Soma involves a series of ten 1-hour sessions. Soma is also used as an adjunct to psychotherapy.

STRUCTURAL INTEGRATION

A systematic approach to relieving patterns of stress and impaired functioning, structural integration seeks to correct misalignments in the body created by gravity and physical and psychological trauma. As in Rolfing, the practitioner uses his or her hands, arms, and elbows in a series of 10 sessions to apply pressure to the fascia, or connective tissue, while the client participates through directed breathing.

TRAGER BODYWORK

Developed by Milton Trager, a medical doctor and a former acrobat and boxer, this movement education approach seeks to address the mental roots of muscle tension. Trager began this technique as a result of studying "effortless movement" and the neuromuscular workings of the body. He observed that psychological "holdings" in the body as a result of physical or emotional traumas, poor posture, or stress could be released by gently rocking the trunk of the body and lulling the client into a "hookup" (a peaceful, meditative state transferred between practitioner and client). Trager theorized that given a choice between old, painful holdings and new, freer movements, the unconscious will automatically choose the latter.

By gently rocking, cradling, and moving the client's body, the practitioner encourages the client to see that physically restrictive patterns can be changed. Trager bodywork is meant to promote relaxation and increase mobility and mental clarity. It is used by athletes for performance enhancement as well as by people with musculoskeletal and back problems. Trager is unusual among bodywork modalities in that it does not use forceful manipulation.

Advice to Patients

Sometimes people are afraid of trying something as different as massage or may be shy and reluctant to expose themselves. Reassure patients that touch practitioners are trained and skilled in their modality and that the modesty and dignity of their body will be respected. Massage rooms should be warm, clean, and comfortable. Anything less than that should not be tolerated. The safest way to determine if your patient will like the therapist and their environment is to go to the setting before scheduling the treatment and meet with the therapist.

Advise your patient to fully disclose accurate health information to the therapist and state what particular problems or concerns are bothering him or her. Also have them tell the therapist if there are certain things that they do or do not like, such as the type of music used or the lighting.

RESEARCH BOX: Effects of Massage on Sleep

Critically ill patients are deprived of sleep and its potential healing qualities, although many receive medications to promote sleep. Prior to this study, no one had adequately evaluated holistic nonpharmacological techniques designed to promote sleep in critical care practice. This study was done to determine the effects of (1) a back massage and (2) combined muscle relaxation, mental imagery, and a music audiotape on the sleep of older men with a cardiovascular illness who were hospitalized in a critical care unit. Sixty-nine subjects were randomly assigned to a 6-minute back massage ($n = 24$); a teaching session on relaxation and a 7.5-minute audiotape at bedtime consisting of muscle relaxation, mental imagery, and relaxing background music ($n = 28$); or the usual nursing care (controls, $n = 17$). Polysomnography was used to measure one night of sleep for each patient. Sleep efficiency index was the primary variable of interest. One-way analysis of variance was used to test for the difference in the index among the three groups. Descriptive statistics showed improved quality of sleep among the back-massage group. Initial analysis showed a significant difference among the three groups in sleep efficiency index. Post hoc testing with the Duncan procedure indicated a significant difference between the back-massage group and the control group; patients in the back-massage group slept more than 1 hour longer than patients in the control group. However, the variance was significantly different among the three groups, and reanalysis of data with only 17 subjects in each group revealed no difference among groups ($p = 0.06$). The conclusion was that back massage is useful for promoting sleep in critically ill older men.

Source: Richards, K. C. (1998). Effect of a back massage and relaxation intervention on sleep in critically ill patients. *American Journal of Critical Care, 7*(4), 288–299.

Effects of Massage on Neonates

Twenty-eight neonates born to HIV-positive mothers were randomly assigned to a massage therapy or control group. The treatment infants were given three 15-minute massages daily for 10 days. The massage group showed superior performance on almost every Brazelton newborn cluster score and had a greater daily weight gain at the end of the treatment period, unlike the control group, who showed declining performance.

Source: Scafidi, F., & Field, T. (1996). Massage therapy improves behavior in neonates born to HIV-positive mothers. *Journal of Pediatric Psychology, 21*(6), 889–897.

ACUPRESSURE

Acupressure is natural hands-on healing art over 5000 years old. It is a natural response to hold the place on your body that is aching, wounded, or tense. The impulse that makes you double over and press your stomach in response to abdominal cramps is an example of the instinctive practice of acupressure. It may well be the most ancient form of physical therapy.

Overview

Acupressure is based on the same Taoist principles as acupuncture. This ancient Chinese technique involves the use of finger pressure (rather than needles) along the body's energy meridians in order to regulate the flow of chi (life energy or life force). Acupressure focuses on manipulating soft tissues at specific points along the body to treat ailments such as arthritis, tension and stress, aches and pains, and menstrual cramps. The system is also used for general preventive health care. The flow of the breath is an important part of the healing process, as is balancing body-mind-spirit and stimulating self-healing.

Practitioners

Most acupressure practitioners are health care providers who have chosen to augment their practice with acupressure therapy. Many, however, have chosen one or two of the modalities and taken certification programs. Generally, the programs are taught in sections of weekend or multiweek segments with clinical practice hours requirements. Some of the modalities have their own individual certificate or certification program, others are affiliated with the American Oriental Bodywork Therapy Association (AOBTA).

The AOBTA is a national not-for-profit professional association of practitioners of bodywork therapies of Asia. All forms recognized by the AOBTA have their roots in China. Over the centuries China, Japan, Thailand, Korea, and more recently, North America and Europe have changed and evolved these forms into separate and distinct modalities. The AOBTA recognizes 12 forms of bodywork:

Acupressure

AMMA therapy

Chi nei tsang

Five element shiatsu

Integrative eclectic shiatsu

Japanese shiatsu

Jin Shin Do bodymind acupressure

Macrobiotic shiatsu

Shiatsu anma therapy

Traditional Thai massage

Tuina

Zen shiatsu

The AOBTA was formed in 1989 with the coming together of a number of associations that represented individual disciplines of Asian bodywork therapy. The AOBTA currently has 1400 active members in the United States and abroad. Qualification for membership varies with the type and level of membership sought. The AOBTA requires documentation of training that conforms to its curriculum requirements for certified practitioner (minimum of 500 hours) and associate (minimum of 150 hours). All training must either be taken with an AOBTA certified instructor or be reviewed and approved by an AOBTA certified instructor with the use of an AOBTA national transcript.

There are four AOBTA practitioner levels of membership: (1) certified practitioner, (2) certified instructor, (3) associate, and (4) student certified practitioner. Acceptance into the AOBTA as a certified practitioner may be granted to:

■ Graduates of a school or program of a participating member of AOBTA council of schools and programs (COSP)

■ Nationally certified practitioners who hold a current "Diplomate, OBT (NCCAOM)"

■ Graduates of a 500-hour program taught by an AOBTA certified instructor with training documented on a 500-hour AOBTA transcript form

■ Graduates of at least 500 hours of training and coursework with apprenticeship program(s) and/or school(s), with training documented on a 500-hour AOBTA transcript form, proving fulfillment of educational requirements

Treatment

Acupressure is a way of accessing and releasing blocked or congested energy centers in the body. These energy centers, or acupoints, lie on energy pathways called meridians. When acupoints or meridians become blocked or congested, pain or discomfort on a physical level may manifest. By using deep but gentle finger pressure on specific acupoints, the acupressure practitioner unblocks the energy, allowing the body and mind to relax, easing physical discomfort, and creating an opportunity to explore thought patterns, memories, and belief systems. This therapy should result in less discomfort and stress. Acupressure is purported to:

Reduce stress

Transform emotional blocks

Maintain good health

Acupressure can be used for a wide variety of conditions, including:

Minor aches and pains

Headaches

Digestive problems

Insomnia

The World Health Organization (WHO) recognizes the ability of acupuncture and traditional Oriental medicines to treat over 43 common disorders, including:

- Gastrointestinal disorders, such as food allergies, peptic ulcer, chronic diarrhea, constipation, indigestion, gastrointestinal weakness, anorexia, and gastritis

- Urogenital disorders, including stress incontinence, urinary tract infections, and sexual dysfunction

- Gynecological disorders, such as irregular, heavy, or painful menstruation; infertility in women and men; and premenstrual syndrome (PMS)

- Respiratory disorders, such as emphysema, sinusitis, asthma, allergies, and bronchitis

- Disorders of the bones, muscles, joints, and nervous system, such as arthritis, migraine headaches, neuralgia, insomnia, dizziness, and low back, neck, and shoulder pain

- Emotional and psychological disorders, including depression and anxiety

- Addictions, such as alcohol, nicotine, and drugs

- Eye, ear, nose, and throat disorders

- Supportive therapy for other chronic and painful debilitating disorders

The focus of acupressure is to alter the flow of qi (life essence or energy) in the body meridians. Gentle manipulation and pressure on specific points located on these meridians allow blocked energy to be released. A number of different modalities have arisen from the basic acupressure form.

INTEGRATIVE ACUPRESSURE

Integrative acupressure is a variation of traditional acupressure that combines structural soft tissue balancing and body realignment with a repatterning of the flow of lymph fluids through the body. It reeducates the mind's patterns and enhances the immune system's natural healing ability.

JIN SHIN DO BODYMIND ACUPRESSURE

Developed by a psychotherapist, Jin Shin Do, this technique combines acupressure, Taoist yogic breathing methods, and Reichian segmental theory (which addresses how emotional tension affects the body). Jin Shin Do seeks to release physical and emotional tension known as "armoring" through gentle, prolonged point holding along one or more of the 12 longitudinal, body energy meridians for 1–5 minutes. The technique aims to promote a pleasant trance state in which the participant can address the emotional factors that may underlie various physical conditions. Frequently, client and practitioner enter a meditative state together in order to balance body and mind energies.

JIN SHIN JYUTSU

This Asian system is designed to harmonize the flow of energy through the body. It holds that tension, fatigue, and illness can trap energy in the body's 26 "safety energy locks." Practitioners use their hands to restore balance and reduce stress. Jin shin jyutsu is not a form of massage, however, as it does not involve the physical manipulation of muscles.

REFLEXOLOGY

An ancient Egyptian practice, reflexology is based on the idea that specific points on the feet and hands correspond to specific organs, glands, and other parts of the body. With fingers and thumbs, the practitioner applies pressure to these points to treat a wide range of stress-related ailments (see Figure 11-5).

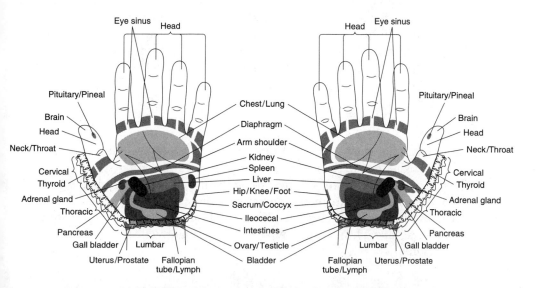

Figure 11-5 Pressure points of the hand used in reflexology

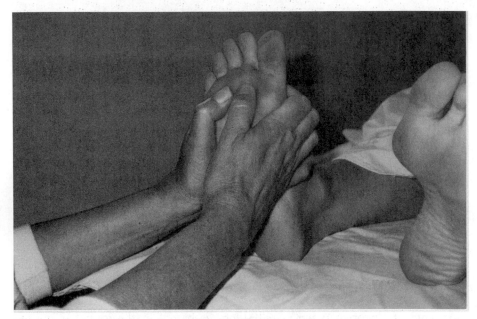

Figure 11-6 A reflexologist applies pressure to specific points in the feet.

When pressure is applied to these areas with fingers and thumbs, the corresponding organ or gland is positively affected (see Figure 11-6). Practitioners of reflexology maintain that restoring the body's energy flow will rid the body of certain disorders. Ten energy channels are believed to begin and end in the toes and extend to the fingers and the top of the head. Each channel relates to a body zone and to the organs in that zone. Reflexology claims to treat a wide range of symptoms: sinus congestion, kidney disorders, PMS, headaches, and asthma. Reflexologists stress that they act merely as mediators; it is the patient's body that heals itself.

SHIATSU

Used in Japan far more than 1000 years, this acupressure technique manipulates muscle tissue by stretching it rhythmically and by tapping specific body points with varying degrees of firmness using the fingertips. Shiatsu is the most common form of acupressure therapy used in the United States. The Shiatsu therapist believes that holding pressure for 3–5 seconds on specific body points stimulates chi (vital energy). Shiatsu is reported to be highly effective in relieving muscle tension.

TRIGGER POINT/MYOTHERAPY

Practitioners of this technique apply pressure to specific points on the body to relieve tension. Trigger points are tender, congested spots in muscle tissue that may radiate pain to other areas. Though the technique is similar to shiatsu or acupressure, it uses Western anatomy and physiology as its basis.

Advice to Patients

Explain to your patients that an acupressure session usually begins with the therapist doing a preliminary assessment of physical, emotional, and energetic states by asking about their history and current problems. Occasionally a therapist will do further assessments such as checking the tension or sensitivity of the back or leg muscles. The appropriate acupoints are then held with gentle, deep finger pressure in a way that encourages the tension to release. As patients become mindful of the tension, they will notice how the initial sensation quickly changes to a deepening sense of warmth, with relaxation lasting for days after the session. Acupressure sessions last from 10 to 60 minutes, so patients may wish to allow some quiet time after the session to fully appreciate the experience. The effects of an acupressure session will vary from person to person and by the condition being addressed.

SUMMARY

The touch, massage, and bodywork therapies detailed in this chapter serve to awaken interest and open doors. If one or more of them appeal to you, then explore their tradition, practice, training methods, and documented effectiveness. Many of these modalities are ripe for research investigation as health care professionals continue to compile data to support the use of alternative and complementary therapies.

ASK YOURSELF

1. Which five or more touch and/or bodywork therapies may be used in an alternative or complementary care practice?
2. Which of the therapies are most appealing to your patient and why?
3. Which therapies have research to support their effectiveness?
4. What type of person might seek touch therapy?

REFERENCES

American Massage Therapy Association (AMTA). (1999, January). Market analysis exhibit.

Blumberg, D. L., Grant, W. D., Hendricks, S. R., Kamp, C. A., & Dewan, M. J. (1995). The physician and unconventional medicine, *Alternative Therapies in Health and Medicine, 1*(3), 31–35.

Dossey, B., Keegan, L., & Guzzetta, C. (2000). *Holistic nursing: A handbook for practice.* Gaithersburg, MD: Aspen.

Eisenberg, D. M., Davis, R. B., Ettner, S. L., Appel, S., Wilkey, S., VanRompay, M., Kessler, R. C., (1998). Trends in alternative medicine use in the United States, 1990–1997. *Journal of the American Medical Association, 280*(18), 1569–1575.

Feldman, R., & Eidelman, A. I. (1998). Intervention programs for premature infants. How and do they affect development? *Clinics in Perinatolgy, 25*(3), 613–626.

Field, T., Schanberg, S., Kuhn, C., Fierro, K., Henteleff, T., Mueller, C., Yando, R., Shaw, S., & Burman, I. (1998). *Adolescence, 33*(131), 555–563.

Fugh-Berman, A. (1997). *Alternative medicine: What works.* Baltimore, MD: Lippincott Williams & Wilkins Healthcare.

Hover-Kramer, D., Mentgen, J., & Scandrett-Hibdon, S. (1996). *Healing touch.* Albany, NY: Delmar Thomson Learning.

Hayes, J. A. (1998). TAC-TIC therapy: A non-pharmacological stroking intervention for premature infants. *Complementary Therapies in Nursing and Midwifery, 4*(1), 25–27.

The Landmark report on public perceptions of alternative care, November 1997. Sacramento, CA.

Morhenn, V. B. (2000). Firm stroking of human skin leads to vasodilatation possibly due to the release of substance P. *Journal of Dermatological Science, 22*(2), 138–144.

Smith, M. C., Stallings, M. A., Mariner, S., & Burrall, M. (1999). Benefits of massage therapy for hospitalized patients: A descriptive and qualitative evaluation. *Alternative Therapies in Health and Medicine, 5*(4), 64–71.

RESOURCES

Associations and Organizations

Acupressure Institute
1533 Shattuck Ave.
Berkeley, CA 94709
Phone: 510-845-1059

American Academy of Osteopathy
3500 DePauw Blvd., Suite 1080
Indianapolis, IN 46268-1136
Phone: 317-879-1881

American Academy of Reflexology
606 E Magnolia Blvd., Suite B
Burbank, CA 91501-2618
Phone: 818-841-7741

American Massage Therapy Association
820 Davis St., Suite 100
Evanston, IL 60201-4444
Phone: 847-864-0123
Fax: 847-864-5196
E-mail: intoinet.amta@massage.org
Web address: http://www.amtamassage.org

AMTA's web site at www.amtamassage.org provides information about the benefits of massage therapy, recent research on its efficacy, and a means to locate qualified massage therapists.

American Oriental Bodywork Therapy Association
1010 Haddonfield-Berlin Road, Suite 408
Voorhees, NJ 08043
Phone: 856-782-1616
Fax: 856-782-1653
Web address: AOBTA@prodigy.net

American Osteopathic Association
142 E Ontario St.
Chicago, IL 60611
Phone: 800-621-1773
Web address: http://www.am-osteo-assn.org

Associated Bodywork & Massage Professionals
1271 Sugarbush Drive
Evergreen, CO 80439-7347
Phone: 800-458-2267 or 303-674-8478

Cranial Academy
8606 Allisonville Road, Suite 130
Indianapolis, IN 46250
Phone: 317-594-0411

Feldenkrais Guild
524 Ellsworth St., Box 489
Albany, OR 97321-0143
Phone: 800-775-2118
Fax: 541-926-0572
E-mail: feldngld@peak.org
Web address: http://www.feldenkrais.com

Gyrotonic Expansion System, international home base
560 W. 43rd St., Suite 40E
New York, NY 10036
Phone: 212-594-5025
Fax: 212-594-5026
Web address: www.gyrotonic.com

International Institute of Reflexology
P. O. Box 12462
St. Petersburg, FL 33733-2642
Phone: 727-343-4811
E-mail: ftreflex@concentric.net

Jin Shin Do Foundation for Bodymind Acupressure
1084G San Miguel Canyon Road
Watsonville, CA 95076
Phone: 408-763-7702
Fax: 408-763-1551

Jin Shin Jyutsu
8719 E. San Alberto Dr.
Scottsdale, AZ 85258
Phone: 602-998-9331
Fax: 602-998-9335

National Certification Board for Therapeutic Massage and Bodywork
8201 Greensboro Dr., Suite 300
McLean, VA 22102
Phone: 800-296-0664 or 703-610-9015
Fax: 703-610-9005
Web address: http://www.ncbtmb.com

North American Society of Teachers of the Alexander Technique
3010 Hennepin Ave. S., Suite 10
Minneapolis, MN 55408
Phone: 800-473-0620 or 612-824-5066

Rolf Institute of Structural Integration
205 Canyon Blvd.
Boulder, CO 80302
Phone: 800-530-8875
E-mail: rolfinst@aol.com
Web address: http://www.rolf.org

TRAGER Institute
21 Locust Ave.
Mill Valley, CA 94941
Phone: 415-388-2688
E-mail: admin@trager.com

Chiropractic

David Wells, DC, LAC

Chapter Objectives

- Gain a general understanding of the practice of chiropractic and its place in the modern health care system.
- Learn about the nature of chiropractic practice.
- Discover the roots of chiropractic.
- Understand what typically occurs in the chiropractic setting.

INTRODUCTION

Of all the complementary and alternative practices, chiropractic is the best established in this country. It is used by approximately 7% of the general population and is included in most insurance reimbursements.

Chiropractic is a manual therapy based on the concept that manipulation of joints to remove nerve interference allows the body's natural recuperative powers to restore and maintain health. It differs from massage techniques in that it is based on moving bones to restore nerve function as opposed to manipulating soft tissues. It differs from osteopathy, another manual manipulation technique, because osteopathy is focused on restoring blood flow, not nerve function. In addition to eschewing drugs and surgery, chiropractic is also distinct from allopathic medicine in that chiropractic holds that the susceptibility to disease and dysfunction is related to nerve interference rather than biochemical disorders or infectious disease.

Overview

Chiropractic is the art and science of promoting and restoring health through manual manipulation of the spine and extremities to correct impingement on the nervous system. The word *chiropractic* is made up of Greek and Latin roots. *Chiro* is Greek for "hand." *Practic* is Latin for "to do" or "perform." Taken together, chiropractic means "performed by hand." The corrective thrust performed is called an "adjustment," as its purpose is to adjust the position of the bone. The misalignment of one or more bones in a joint is called a "subluxation." The term derives from *sub,* meaning "below" or "less than," and *luxation,* meaning "dislocation of a joint." Thus, subluxation is a partial dislocation of a joint.

History

The origins of joint manipulation are lost in the prehistoric past. Many cultures around the world have a long tradition of joint manipulation to improve flexibility and reduce pain. The ancient Chinese have a system of joint manipulation combined with massage called tui na (literally "push-pull"). In the Pacific islands, deep-tissue massage and joint manipulation is called lomi lomi. In merry old England, practitioners of the art were referred to as bonesetters. Even Hippocrates, the ancient Greek "father of medicine" is reported to have said, "First and foremost, look to the spine for the cause of disease." Hippocrates is said to have treated sciatica by manipulating the spine of patients who were hung by their feet over a wall for traction.

On September 18, 1895, in Davenport, Iowa, a healer named Daniel David Palmer noticed an irregularity in the alignment of the upper thoracic spine while examining a partially deaf janitor named Harvey Lillard. To correct that misalignment, Palmer performed a rapid forceful thrust on the vertebra, resulting in a popping sound. To their mutual surprise, Harvey Lillard reported that he could, "hear the wagons on the street." This so astonished Palmer that he devoted the rest of his life to developing and promoting this healing art he named chiropractic. Three years later he opened the Palmer College of Chiropractic in Davenport. In 1910, he wrote *The chiropractic adjuster: A textbook of the science, art and philosophy of chiropractic for students and practitioners.*

The theoretical basis on which Palmer built the profession of chiropractic is as follows:

- The innate wisdom of the body is the source of all healing.
- That wisdom (often called "innate" by chiropractors) is not only information but also the energy of life itself (in this way, chiropractic is similar to other forms of vitalism).
- That wisdom flows from the brain down through the spinal nerves to every organ, muscle, and tissue in the body.
- The body in turn communicates its needs back to the brain through the nervous system.
- Vertebra and other bones, if subluxated, can impinge on the free flow of information and life force flowing through the nervous system.
- The chiropractor needs only remove the pressure on the nerves by correcting the subluxation, and the body will heal itself.

PRACTITIONERS

With over 60,000 practicing in the United States, doctors of chiropractic make up the second largest primary care profession after allopathic medical doctors. Chiropractors are licensed in all 50 states and U.S. protectorates and in over 30 other countries around the world. Because of their education and licensing status, chiropractors are referred to as doctors of chiropractic (DC).

Training Requirements

To earn a doctor of chiropractic degree, a minimum of six years of college (two undergraduate and four chiropractic) are required. Of the 16 accredited chiropractic colleges in the United States, 4 require a bachelor's degree prior to matriculation. Chiropractors are *not* required to pass an entrance exam comparable to the MCAT required of medical students.

All chiropractic colleges include clinical internship and most offer postgraduate externship programs. At 4822 hours, chiropractic education is the equivalent of standard preclinical medical training of 4667 hours. Chiropractic education includes substantially more hours in basic medical sciences such as anatomy and physiology than does medical training and fewer hours in public health. The chief difference between chiropractic education compared with medical education is that chiropractic clinics, not hospitals, are the venue for hands-on training and patient contact. Medical doctors have three years of on-the-job training through internship and residency (3467 hours) compared with 1405 clinic hours for chiropractors.

Postdoctoral training is also available in several specialties through chiropractic colleges and specialty councils. High standards of chiropractic education are maintained with the help of oversight from the Council on Chiropractic Education (CCE) and its Commission on Accreditation. The CCE has been recognized by the United States Department of Education since 1974 as the accrediting body for chiropractic schools and colleges.

Postgraduate specialty board certifications are available, including specialties in orthopedics, clinical neurology, nutrition, pediatrics, family practice, sports medicine, radiology, industrial consulting, rehabilitation, and applied chiropractic sciences. These specialty certifications may be earned by taking one- to three-year training courses followed by rigorous examinations. Specialty certification is maintained by meeting continuing education requirements. Doctors of chiropractic possessing specialty certifications are referred to as diplomates in the particular specialty.

Chiropractic education has been limited by its exclusion from the medical mainstream. Access to public funding of research and education and access to hospitals have been nearly absent during chiropractic's 100 plus years of history. This can be expected to change in the coming years for two reasons:

1. Until 1980, the American Medical Association (AMA) Code of Ethics expressly forbade any professional association with chiropractors. The AMA had also lobbied legislatures and hospitals to exclude chiropractic. Following a 12-year lawsuit that finally resolved in 1987 at the level of the Supreme Court, the AMA was forced to drop its policy to "contain and eliminate the profession of chiropractic."
2. The National Institutes of Health, Office of Alternative Medicine, has increased funding to study the effectiveness of chiropractic. This research funding will help chiropractic colleges by providing an additional (small) source of revenue.

Licensure

After completion of studies, state licensure must be obtained to practice chiropractic. The National Board of Chiropractic Examiners (NBCE) was established in 1963 to promote consistency and reciprocity between state licensing boards. The NBCE exams consist of four parts, each part composed of two days of rigorous testing. Although 49 states require Part I, 48 require Part II, 45 require Part II, and 21 require Part IV of the national boards, all but 10 states administer additional examinations. The NBCE also offers a separate examination in techniques of physical therapy for those states that include these modalities in their scope of practice.

In addition to setting educational and licensing requirements, the state licensing boards of chiropractic provide ongoing consumer protection though disciplinary actions made in response to consumer complaints. Participation in continuing education is required for license renewal in 47 of the 50 states, with the median number of required hours being 12 per year.

While the scope of practice varies somewhat from state to state, it always includes manual manipulation of the spine and extremities, spinal analysis and X-ray. Most states include soft tissue massage, the application of hot, cold, therapeutic exercise and modalities such as ultrasound, diathermy, traction, and electrical stimulation, and dispensing of nutritional advice and nutritional supplements. Chiropractors may not prescribe drugs in any state. In a number of states, chiropractors may sign birth and death certificates and perform acupuncture, pelvic and rectal exams, and venipuncture for diagnostic purposes. In Oregon, chiropractors may perform minor surgery: proctology and obstetrical procedures. Five states (Michigan, Mississippi, New Jersey, South Carolina, Tennessee, and Washington) limit chiropractors to examination by spinal analysis and X-ray and treatment to manual manipulation of the spine for subluxations.

Doctors of chiropractic are not generally prohibited from treating specific health conditions by law; however, purporting to treat, for example, heart disease, cancer, and pneumonia through chiropractic adjustments is not considered to be within the community standard of practice and may subject the chiropractor to licensing sanctions or charges of malpractice.

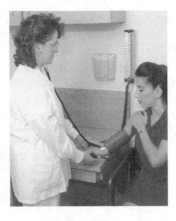

Figure 12-1 A first visit to a chiropractor has many similarities to a first visit to a general practitioner.

TREATMENT

A first visit to a doctor of chiropractic has many similarities to a first visit to a general practitioner in private medical practice. The patient will usually fill out an extensive medical history form, then the doctor or an assistant will take and record vital signs (height, weight, blood pressure, pulse and respiration rate, and temperature if indicated) (see Figure 12-1). The examination itself will generally include a full or regional orthopedic and neurological examination and a standard physical exam (e.g., auscultation; percussion; eyes, ears, nose, and throat; and abdominal palpation). At this point the chiropractic exam becomes more specifically oriented to the search for subluxations of the spine and extremities. Chiropractors are very well trained in the art of palpation, both static and motion palpation (see Figure 12-2). The doctor of chiropractic will palpate the area of complaint and related

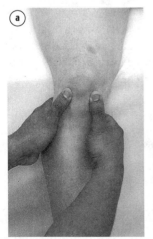
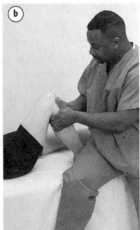
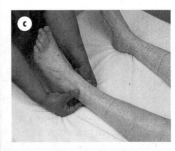

Figure 12-2 Chiropractors are well trained in palpation to identify misalignments or evaluate tissue tone: (a) palpation of the tibiofemoral joint; (b) palpation of the ankle; (c) testing the cruciate ligaments of the knee.

areas of the spine to identify misalignments that could be restricting nerves or full joint motion. The chiropractor will also palpate soft tissues to evaluate tissue tone that may support or impede recovery and may also contribute to nerve entrapment of joint dysfunction. Another aspect of chiropractic evaluation is careful evaluation of posture and movement to determine habits, weakness, or abnormal muscle tension that may be contributing to the symptomology.

After the physical examination, the doctor of chiropractic may decide that an X-ray of the area of complaint and/or related area of the spine is needed. A note of caution here is that many chiropractors believe they need to take an X-ray to determine the exact position of a subluxation rather than to rule out pathology. Overutilization of X-rays is a frequent complaint against chiropractors. If an X-ray is recommended, inquire about the medical necessity. While the dosage of X-ray received from a spinal X-ray is lower than the amount of exposure that occurs in an hour of daytime flight in a jet airliner (the solar radiation is less shielded at high altitude), there is no safe amount of X-ray. Furthermore, the cost of the X-ray may not be justified by clinical necessity. Following the exam and X-ray or other laboratory test, if indicated (chiropractors in most states may order blood tests, magnetic resonance imaging, etc.), the doctor of chiropractic will explain the results of the examination and propose a treatment plan. Assuming the patient agrees, treatment will then commence.

The centerpiece of chiropractic treatment is the adjustment (see Figure 12-3). There are almost as many ways to perform an adjustment as there are chiropractors. Most commonly, the chiropractor will position the joint at end-range, then apply a rapid, forceful, high-velocity thrust to the bone in question to move it just slightly beyond the normal physiological range. This motion may produce a popping sound and generally produces immediate relief of localized or referred pain and muscle spasm. The popping, if it occurs, is not the result of bone moving against bone; it is the result of air popping out of solution to accommodate the rapidly expanding joint space.

Adjustments may also be performed using manual pressure on the bones or through the use of a mechanical aid such as an Activator instrument. As mentioned

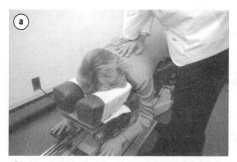 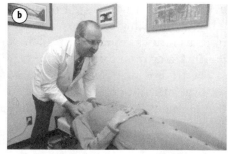

Figure 12-3 The centerpiece of chiropractic treatment is adjustment: adjusting (a) the back and (b) the neck. (Photos copyright of the American Chiropractic Association. Used with permission.)

before, there are many techniques for moving bones and many schools of thought within the chiropractic profession. Because chiropractic is taught by private colleges without government or drug company funding, and because chiropractors do not generally have hospital privileges (with all the attendant oversight and professional contact), chiropractic practice has diverged into many schools of thought. Some of these philosophies and practices are outside of the mainstream of chiropractic care. Caution should be exercised selecting a practitioner who conforms to the generally recognized practice norms. In addition to the adjustment, chiropractors often utilize physical modalities such as heat, cold, diathermy, ultrasound, electrical stimulation, massage, therapeutic exercise, and stretching to promote soft tissue rehabilitation. Many chiropractors also recommend nutritional supplements or dietary advice. Some recommend herbal products or homeopathics. The reason for this is that the profession of chiropractic became the refuge for all other forms of natural healing that were suppressed by the medical profession as it rose to dominance in the early part of the twentieth century. Homeopaths, herbalists, naturopaths, nutritionists, and others from the Natural Hygiene movement, the Eclectic School, and so on, became chiropractors as that was the only nonallopathic profession (besides osteopathy) to obtain licensure to practice.

Chiropractic generally requires several treatments to correct a musculoskeletal problem. This is because the tissues supporting the joint take time to heal. For sprains, about six to eight weeks are needed for the body to repair muscle and connective tissue. Chiropractic adjustments during this time of tissue healing reinforce the correct position and full range of motion of the joints until the muscle and connective tissue tone can take over the job. If the patient depends passively on care and does not work to strengthen and rebuild muscle tone, dependency on chiropractic adjustments can result.

ADVICE TO PATIENTS

A few years ago the *Los Angeles Times* ran a front page story entitled "Chiropractic Manipulation Causes Stroke." The article stated that the "chiropractic manipulation" was performed by a medical doctor who had taken a weekend seminar on spinal adjusting. However, many people who did not read the article, only the title, avoided chiropractic care. This kind of misrepresentation frequently keeps patients away from chiropractors.

The truth is that chiropractic is actually quite safe, especially compared with medical interventions. As the article above illustrates, the greatest risk from spinal manipulation is that a rapid forceful movement of the neck could break loose a blood clot in a person with arteriosclerosis (hardening of the arteries). To protect against that possibility, chiropractors are taught to take a thorough history to screen high-risk patients. Risk factors include age over 65, diabetes, obesity, long-term use of birth control pills, and alcoholism. If a patient has risk factors, the chiropractor makes a clinical judgment as to whether or not to perform vascular screening tests. These are simple, in-office procedures such as asking the patient to turn the head to one side and lean back while reporting any dizziness or other unusual symptoms. During the maneuver, the chiropractor will watch the patient's eyes to see if the eyes jerk rapidly back and forth. If that is the case, forceful cervical manipulation is contraindicated. The chiropractor may then use an Activator or other soft techniques.

The other adverse effect that scares some people away from chiropractic is the possibility of injury to the discs in the lower back. Again, chiropractors are taught to carefully screen patients to determine which type of adjustment is best for that individual. Adverse events are extremely rare, as the following article by a researcher at the RAND think tank suggests: "for cervical manipulation the estimated risk for serious complications is 6.39 per 10,000,000 manipulations and for lumbar manipulation the estimate is 1 serious complication per 100,000,000 manipulations" (Coulter, 1998).

The most common risk associated with referring a patient to a chiropractor is the tendency of some chiropractors to overtreat. Some chiropractors have a near-religious fervor about their mission of detecting and correcting spinal subluxations that leads them to believe that all persons should receive frequent, regular spinal adjustments to prevent disease and maintain health. While there may be truth in this belief, overtreatment may also result in laxity of ligaments and possibly microtears in the muscle fibers around the joints. Overtreatment will certainly result in higher costs and time away from work or other activities. Chiropractic as a profession is currently undergoing a paradigm shift away from passive care (the doctor performing treatment to the patient) toward a model of active care. Active care means teaching the patient correct posture, stretching, and exercise to correct and prevent future problems. Most insurers and the worker's compensation systems are promoting active patient involvement as the best way to minimize costs and maximize health. This is consistent with chiropractic's philosophy of healing from within.

Cautions

There are a number of chiropractors who purport to treat non-neuromusculoskeletal conditions such as asthma, allergy, and childhood ear infections. There is little to no research to support the efficacy of chiropractic for these conditions. Furthermore, caution should be exercised if a chiropractor advocates treatment several times a week for months at a time. Most acute neuromusculoskeletal conditions resolve with or without treatment in four to six weeks. A small percentage of conditions will never improve or will obtain only temporary symptomatic relief from chiropractic care. The greatest benefit for most people with neuromusculoskeletal complaints is to begin a program of stretching and rehabilitative exercise. Advise patients that if a chiropractor does not recommend such a program with two weeks of initiating care, they might consider seeking a second opinion.

A further caution is that some chiropractors insist on taking X-rays of every patient. According to medical and chiropractic radiologists, only a small percentage of patients require X-rays.

RESEARCH

The chiropractic's mechanism of action is in need of further research. Evidence suggests that the chiropractic adjustment does indeed reduce pressure on spinal nerve roots, increase circulation of blood and lymph in the area of the joint, release muscle spasm, and facilitate optimal joint motion.

In contrast to allopathic medicine, throughout the history of chiropractic, almost all research has been self-funded by the chiropractic profession. This has been changing in recent years as the government and insurers are taking an increased interest in manipulative therapies. There are currently 14 chiropractic peer-reviewed journals. More research is being done now than at any other time in the history of chiropractic. We can expect to see more definitive results in the near future.

The proposed mechanisms of action for the effectiveness of a chiropractic adjustment are twofold:

1. Reduction of compressive forces on neural tissues
2. Stimulus-induced reflex effects

As to the former, the adjustment is hypothesized to relieve compression on the nerve root. One study in support of the first hypothesis was performed in 1976 at the University of Colorado by Chung Ha Suh. His experiment found that as little as 2 mm Hg pressure on a spinal nerve root could reduce function by 60% within minutes. The stimulus reflex effects are hypothesized to occur from rapid stretching of soft tissue in an adjustment producing activity in joint and muscular mechanoreceptors. The impulses from these mechanoreceptors are proposed to induce inibitory effects on the nervous system, that is, pain relief. While further studies are needed to fully understand chiropractic's mechanism of action, large-scale outcome studies have already proved chiropractic's value in treating musculoskeletal disorders, as the following studies will demonstrate.

U.S. Government Endorses Effectiveness

The U.S. Agency for Health Care Policy and Research (AHCPR) Report (1994) was the result of literature review and the consensus of a multidisciplinary panel of independent experts. The panel concluded that relief of acute lower back pain in adults can be achieved most safely and effectively with spinal manipulation: "Chiropractic is the most effective treatment for acute lower back pain."

Further evidence of government support was demonstrated in 1972, when Congress amended the Medicare Act to include chiropractic services.

Cost-effectiveness: *The Manga Report, 1993*

This study, performed at the University of Ottawa, overwhelmingly supported the safety, scientific validity, patient satisfaction, and cost-effectiveness of chiropractic: "Evidence from Canada and other countries suggests potential savings of hundreds of millions annually. . . . The literature clearly and consistently shows that the major savings from chiropractic management come from fewer and lower costs of auxiliary services, fewer hospitalizations, and a highly significant reduction in chronic problems, as well as in levels and duration of disability."

Journal of Manipulative and Physiological Therapeutics, 1993

This two-year study of 395,641 patients with neuromusculoskeletal conditions revealed that patients receiving chiropractic care incurred significantly lower health care costs than did patients treated solely by medical or osteopathic physicians.

Chiropractors Best Qualified to Perform Manual Manipulation

THE NEW ZEALAND COMMISSION REPORT, 1980

This 377-page report to the New Zealand House of Representatives was, in the words of the commission that produced it, "probably the most comprehensive and detailed independent examination of chiropractic ever undertaken in any country." The commission, composed primarily of medical doctors who were initially skeptical of chiropractic, concluded that:

Spinal manual therapy in the hands of a registered chiropractor is safe.

Spinal manual therapy can be effective in relieving musculoskeletal symptoms such as back pain and other symptoms known to respond to such therapy, such as migraine.

Chiropractors are the only health practitioners who are necessarily equipped by their education and training to carry out spinal manual therapy.

HIGH PATIENT SATISFACTION, 1991

A 1991 Gallup poll revealed that 90% of chiropractic patients felt their treatment was effective and nearly 75% felt most of their expectations had been met during their chiropractic visits.

FLORIDA WORKER'S COMPENSATION STUDY, 1988

"Analysis of 10,652 worker's compensation cases revealed that a claimant with a back-related injury, when initially treated by a chiropractor versus a medical doctor, is less likely to become temporarily disabled or if disabled, remain disabled for a shorter period of time; and claimants treated by medical doctors were hospitalized at a much higher rate than claimants treated by chiropractors."

UTAH WORKER'S COMPENSATION STUDY, 1991

This study, published in the 1991 *Journal of Occupational Medicine*, indicated that costs were significantly higher for medical claims than for chiropractic claims for the same diagnostic codes. Furthermore, the number of days lost from work was nearly 10 times higher for those who received medical care instead of chiropractic care.

EFFECTIVE FOR MIGRAINE HEADACHES, 1978

A study published in the *ACA Journal of Chiropractic* indicated that 47.6% of patients with recurring headaches, including migraines, were either cured or experienced reduced headache symptomatology after receiving chiropractic manipulation.

EFFECTIVE ON PATIENTS DISABLED BY BACK PAIN, 1985

In a University of Saskatchewan study of 283 patients "who had not responded to previous conservative or operative treatment" and who were initially classified as totally disabled, "81% . . . became symptom-free or achieved a state of mild intermittent pain with no work restrictions" after daily spinal manipulations were administered.

SUMMARY

Chiropractic is the best established form of complementary and alternative health care in the United States and provides effective treatment for acute and chronic neuromusculoskeletal conditions. In seeking a chiropractor, advise your patients to look for one who involves them in a program of stretching, exercise, and other forms of self-care. Also advise them to beware of the chiropractor who insists on X-raying every patient or who pressure patients to sign up for extended treatment plans.

ASK YOURSELF

1. What type of patient might seek chiropractic therapy?
2. What does the scope of practice for a chiropractor generally include?
3. What advice or precautions can you offer patients seeking chiropractic treatment?

REFERENCES

Anderson, R. (1992). Spinal manipulation before chiropractic. In S. Halderman (Ed.), *Principles and practice of chiropractic.* Norwalk CT: Appleton and Lange.

Bigos, S., Bowyer, O., Braen, G., (1994). *Acute low back problems in adults: Clinical practice guideline No. 14. AHCPR Publication No. 95–0642.* Rockville, MD: Agency for Health Care Policy and Research, U.S. Department of Health and Human Services, Public Health Service.

Blunt, K. L., Gatterman, M. I., & Bereznick, D. E. (1995). Kinesiology: An essential approach toward understanding chiropractic subluxation. In M. I. Gatterman (Ed.), *Foundations of chiropractic: Subluxation.* St. Louis, MO: Mosby.

Coulter, I. (1988). Efficacy and risks of chiropractic manipulation: What does the evidence suggest? *Integrative Medicine, 1*(2).

Coulter, I., Adams, A., Coggan, P., Wildes, M., & Gonyea, M. (1998). A comparative study of chiropractic and medical education. *Integrative Medicine 1;* 61–66.

Council on Chiropractic Education. (1996). *Biennial report* (Feb. 94–Jan. 96). Scottsdale, AZ: Author.

Eisenberg, D. M., Kessler, R. C., Foster, C., et al. (1993). Unconventional medicine in the United States. *New England Journal of Medicine 328*(4), 246–252

Federation of Chiropractic Licensing Boards. (1997). *Official Directory of the Federation of Chiropractic Licensing Boards: 1997–1998.* Greeeley, CO: Author.

Getzendaner, S. (US District Judge). (1987, August 27). *Memorandum, Opinion, and Order. Wilk, et al., v American Medical Association, et al.* Northern District of Illinois, Eastern Division.

Gillette, R. G. (1995). Spinal cord mechanisms of referred pain and neuroplasticity. In M. I. Gatterman (Ed.), *Foundations of chiropractic: Subluxation.* St. Louis, MO: Mosby.

Hu, J. W., Yu, X. M., Vernon, H., & Sessle, B. J. (1993). Excitatory effects on neck and jaw muscle activity of inflammatory irritant applied to cervical paraspinal tissues. *Pain, 55,* 243–250.

Lamm, L. C., Wegner, E., & Collord, D. (1995). Chiropractic scope of practice: What the law allows—update 1993. *Journal of Manipulative and Physiological Therapeutics, 18,* 16–20.

Lantz, C. A. (1995). The vertebral subluxation complex. In M. I. Gatterman (Ed.), *Foundations of chiropractic: Subluxation.* St Louis, MO: Mosby.

Le Bars, D., Villanueva, I., Bouchassira, D., & Miller, J. C. (1992). Diffuse noxious inhibitory controls (DNIC) in animals and in man. *Patologicheskaia Fiziologiia Eksperimentalnaia Terapiia, 4,* 55–65.

Lomax, E. (1997). Manipulative therapy; an historical perspective. In A. A. Buerger & J. S. Tobis (Eds.), *Approaches to the validation of manipulation therapy.* Springfield, IL: Charles C. Thomas.

Palmer, D. D. (1910). *The chiropractic adjuster: A textbook of the science, art and philosophy of chiropractic for students and practitioners.* Portland, OR: Portland Printing House.

Pressman, A. H., & Nickles, S. L. (1984). Neurological and nutritional considerations of pain control. *Journal of Manipulative and Physiological Therapeutics, 2,* 38–42.

Suh, C. H., Sharpless, S. K., Macgregor, R. J., Luttges, M. W. (1974). *Researching the fundamentals of chiropractic.* Unpublished manuscript, University of Colorado at Boulder.

Triano, J. J. (1992). Studies on the biomechanical effects of a spinal adjustment. *Journal of Manipulative and Physiological Therapeutics, 15,* 71–75.

Triano, J. J. (2000). The mechanics of spinal manipulation. In W. Herzog (Ed.), *Clinical biomechanics of the spine.* St Louis, MO: Mosby.

Wolinsky, H., & Brune, T. (1994). *The serpent and the staff: The unhealthy politics of the American Medical Association.* New York: Jeremy P. Tarcher/Putnam.

RESOURCES

American Chiropractic Association
1701 Clarendon Blvd.
Arlington, VA 22209
Phone: 703-276-8800
Web site: http://wuw.amerchiro.org.

International Chiropractors Association
1110 North Glebe Rd., Suite l000
Arlington, VA 22201
Phone: 800-423-4690
Web site: http://www.chiropractic.org.

Energetic Therapies

Chapter Objectives

- Discover the range of modalities related to energetic therapies.
- Become familiar with a variety of the energetic therapies used in some alternative and complementary therapy practices.
- Compare and contrast the quality and quantity of various therapies.

INTRODUCTION

Energy therapies work to change or alter the flow of body energies. Most of the modalities involve hand movement or magnetic treatment in the nonphysical but theorized energetic realm surrounding the physical body.

OVERVIEW

Energy therapies work with the flow of the body's life force, which is known by several names: chi in China, ki in Japan, prana in India, aura in the West, and the biofield or bioenergetic field within certain Western healing modalities. Various cultures throughout the world recognize the presence of a vital energy or life force that vivifies the human body (see Figure 13-1). Most advocates of energy work believe this life force is a vital essence found in all matter, animate and inanimate. By manipulating and regulating this life energy, a healer can gently improve a patient's health.

Energetic therapies are perhaps the most controversial of the alternative and complementary therapies in that there is only limited scientific evidence that such an area actually exists around the human species. Other dimensions of the energetic realm are biological biofeedback therapies, in which actual physiological feedback is obtained from measurement tools (Dossey, Keegan & Puzzetta, 2000). The recipient is offered this feedback data along with specific interventions in which to alter the patterned response.

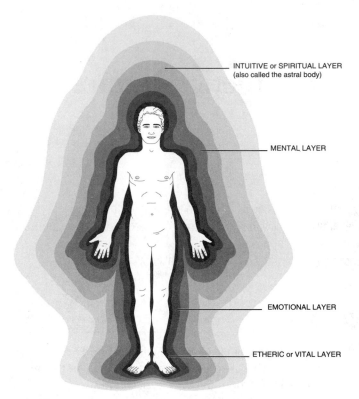

INTUITIVE or SPIRITUAL LAYER
(also called the astral body)

MENTAL LAYER

EMOTIONAL LAYER

ETHERIC or VITAL LAYER

Figure 13-1 Energy therapies are based on the recognition of the presence of a vital energy field that surrounds the body. This illustration identifies four major layers of this field.

History

Energetic healing has its roots in Chinese and Indian antiquity but had its renaissance in the West during the 1800s in esoteric schools of thought. The most popular of the therapies and the one most used by nurses, therapeutic touch, began in New York in the 1970s with Delores Krieger, a professor at New York University, who developed the technique with the aid of her lay healer friend, Dora Kunz. During the last quarter of the twentieth century, permutations of therapeutic touch evolved. Other energetic modalities, such as Reiki, are based on principles similar to healing touch. These are discussed later in this chapter.

PRACTITIONERS

Practitioners of the energetic therapies range from self-trained to professionals with university degrees and certification. Some of the modalities, such as Reiki, therapeutic touch, and healing touch, have definitive certification programs and their own body of professional literature. Other modalities are taught by master teachers to enrolled or interested students.

THE THERAPIES

Practitioners of these therapies look for weaknesses in the energy field in and around the client's body and seek to restore its proper circulation and balance. Energy channeled through the practitioner is directed to strengthen the body's natural defenses and help the client's physical, mental, emotional, and/or spiritual state. Sessions may or may not involve the physical laying-on of hands. The modalities in this chapter are:

Barbara Brennan healing science

Bioenergetics

Biofeedback

Biological terrain assessment

Healing touch

Magnet therapy

Neurofeedback

Polarity therapy

Reiki

Robert Jaffe advanced healing energy

SHEN therapy

Spiritual healing

Therapeutic touch

Barbara Brennan Healing Science

Developed by physicist, teacher, and healer Barbara Brennan, who devoted more than 25 years to researching the human energy field. This spiritual healing system seeks to reorganize and revitalize the client's energy field. Using hands-on techniques and other approaches, the healer works to clear the client's field of unhealthy and blocked energies, charge depleted areas, repair distorted patterns, and balance the entire field. The goal is to promote health on physical, emotional, mental, and spiritual levels.

Bioenergetics

Bioenergetics holds that repressed emotions and desires affect the body and psyche by creating chronic muscle tension and diminished vitality and energy.

Through physical exercises, breathing techniques, psychotherapy, and other forms of emotional release, the therapist attempts to loosen this "character armor" and restore natural well-being.

Biofeedback

A technique used especially for stress-related conditions such as asthma, migraines, insomnia, and high blood pressure, biofeedback is a way of monitoring minute metabolic changes in one's own body (e.g., temperature changes, heart rate, and muscle tension) with the aid of sensitive machines. By consciously visualizing, relaxing, or imagining while observing light, sound, or metered feedback, the client learns to make subtle adjustments to move toward a more balanced internal state.

Biofeedback is a tool for empowering the mind by training it to take control of certain conscious and autonomic processes. Electronic equipment is used to read brain wave patterns, muscle tension, or electrical skin resistance; the individual then tries through various means to control the mind and thereby raise or lower the response on the biofeedback machine. Through repeated practice, a patient can train him or herself to control physical conditions and psychological states. Biofeedback works well for high blood pressure, insomnia, headaches, and other tension-causing conditions. It is also an excellent tool for teaching relaxation.

Biological Terrain Assessment (BTA 1000)

This new health-monitoring technology, based on the biochemistry of the body, uses a technological device to measure three bodily fluids—blood, saliva, and urine—for specific data. The device is not diagnostic for any particular pathology or disease state; rather, the test imparts analytical data about the lymph system, the blood, and the kidney blood filtration system. These include oxygen transport, nutrient delivery, waste removal, mineral retention, cellular absorption, and multiple metabolic chemical interactions. The practitioner administering testing then recommends a variety of therapies and nutritional alternatives based on the information provided.

Healing Touch

Healing touch uses hands-on and energy-based techniques to balance and align the human energy field, accelerate wound healing, relieve pain, promote relaxation, prevent illness, and ease the dying process. Janet Mentgen developed this approach in the 1970s primarily for use by nurses, but it expanded into use by other health care providers who receive training in the method. Healing touch utilizes the techniques of therapeutic touch as well as the elements of Barbara Brennan healing science and other eclectic philosophies and modalities.

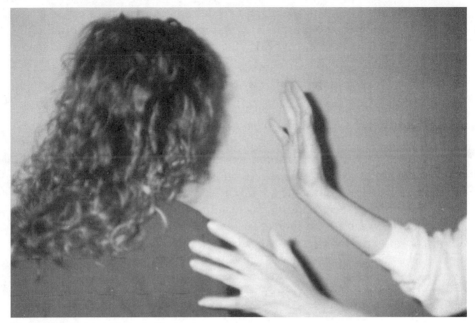

Figure 13-2 Administering healing touch

Body, mind, emotion, and spirit are touched through this therapeutic process, and each individual is empowered to participate fully in his or her healing journey. Healing touch is a different and often complementary mode of facilitating the healing process, but it functions from an energy perspective rather than from only a physical one. The healing touch practitioner uses light touch or works with his or her hands near the client's body in an effort to restore balance to the client's energy system, realign the energy flow, and reactivate the mind-body-spirit connection to eliminate blockages to self-healing (see Figure 13-2).

HEALING TOUCH CERTIFICATION PROGRAM

The three-level Healing Touch (energy healing) Certification Program is designed for health care professionals as well as for interested lay people:

- Level I is for beginners from all backgrounds. It covers the theory and scientific aspects of energy healing, and 10 techniques can be practiced immediately after completing the class. This 15–20-hour course is held over a weekend.

- Level IIA guides the student through a full healing sequence in an hour that includes back, neck, and other advanced techniques. This 15–20-hour course is held over a weekend.

■ Level IIB focuses on the adaptation of Barbara Brennan's work and provides more advanced techniques that increase the power and duration of the results of the work. This 15–20-hour course is held over a weekend.

■ Level IIIA and Level IIIB are the practitioner level courses. They are residential and held from Thursday evening through Sunday noon.

The competency of the practitioner is gained through practice and continued study as well as participation in, for example, community practice groups and retreats. Beginners are encouraged to practice on themselves, family, and friends. The number of years a person has been actively practicing therapeutic touch is the best indicator of competence. Year-long programs for the purpose of developing expertise are available from some advanced teachers. A variety of workshops enhance the practice of therapeutic touch, including imagery and intuitive training.

Courses are available from individual teachers and through some community colleges. Each of the three introductory levels involves 8–10 hours of theory and supervised practice. The three levels can be taken over a six-month period; some workshops may be held over an extended period. Healing touch teachers suggest that students of therapeutic touch repeat course work with a variety of healing touch teachers, since all bring their own experience into their teaching.

Magnet Therapy

Magnet therapy (also known as magnetic field therapy or biomagnetic therapy) involves the use of magnets, magnetic devices, or magnetic fields to treat a variety of physical and emotional conditions, including circulatory problems, certain forms of arthritis, chronic pain, sleep disorders, and stress. The theory that magnets can heal is not new. In ancient times, mineral-rich lodestones were thought to have therapeutic powers. In the eighteenth century, Frenchman Franz Anton Mesmer wrote himself into the history books by "mesmerizing" people—and curing them—using magnets. Today, electronic magnetic resonance imaging is used in most hospitals for taking detailed images of the inner workings of the body.

This controversial form of therapy is usually used to relieve pain, primarily muscle and joint pain, but occasionally headaches, carpal tunnel syndrome, and other types of pain as well. Among its many applications are muscle strains; sprains of the spine, neck or limbs; hip and joint pain; arthritis; phantom limb pain; fibromyalgia; osteoarthritis; persistent rotator cuff tendinitis; and chronic pelvic pain. In addition, magnetic fields are sometimes used to speed the healing of bone fractures, and some proponents even advocate magnets to relieve stress, combat infections, and prevent seizures.

The studies that have been conducted on the efficacy of magnets have typically yielded quite contradictory results. Proponents announce favorable findings, only to find themselves debunked in subsequent trials. They usually respond that the follow-up studies failed to properly employ the precise magnetic devices responsible for initial success.

TREATMENTS

For pain management, small magnetic discs are usually taped to the body over the areas that radiate the pain, known as the pain trigger points. Magnets used for this type of therapy typically generate a field measured at 350–500 gauss, or about 10 times the strength of a typical refrigerator magnet.

To relieve stress and insomnia, some practitioners advocate magnetic blankets and beds. These devices produce a much stronger field in order to compensate for the loss of potency caused by their greater distance from the skin. For example, in such conditions, a 4000-gauss magnet is needed to deliver 1200 gauss to the patient.

Although all magnets have two poles—positive (south) and negative (north)—they vary drastically in size and strength. If using a magnet for pain relief, it is best to purchase a therapeutic magnet from a reputable, medical vendor who will allow you to use it on a trial basis. Magnets delivering between 300 and 500 gauss are considered safe for home use.

Depending on the nature and severity of the condition, the following recommendations should be followed:

Treatment time. The magnet may be left in place for as little as 3 minutes or as long as several days.

Treatment frequency. Often the magnet is applied several times per day for several days or weeks at a time. Many people use this therapy at the first sign of a recurrence of pain.

RATIONALES FOR MAGNETIC FIELD THERAPY

The leading theories of how and why magnetic field therapy works are as follows:

- *Pain relief.* Some advocates ascribe the therapy's purported benefits to its affect on the nervous system, which depends on electrical charges to deliver its signals. Others say that magnets exert a pull on charged particles within bodily fluids, thereby promoting the flow of blood to the damaged joints or muscles, boosting levels of oxygen and nutrients, and ultimately relieving pain. It remains to be seen whether either theory is valid. One fact, however, is certain: Magnets will not cure the underlying cause of muscle or joint pain, and once the devices are removed, the pain may return.

- *Stress.* Some proponents say that a negative magnetic field applied to the top of the head has a calming, sleep-inducing effect. Since stress is a factor in a wide range of ailments, they say the therapy can be beneficial as an adjunct in virtually any circumstance. (The treatments cannot, however, be relied on to remedy the problem.)

■ *Infections.* A few advocates of magnetic therapy go so far as to say that negative magnetic fields can destroy bacterial, fungal, and viral infections. However, there is no definitive proof of such an effect, and mainstream physicians warn against any attempt to substitute magnets for traditional antibiotics.

■ *Central nervous system disorders.* Some magnetic therapy practitioners have reported that placing small ceramic neodymium or iron oxide magnets upon patients' heads can relieve seizures, panic attacks, and hallucinations without disturbing mental alertness. There have been no formal clinical trials, however, to validate this contention.

Because magnetic therapy is a noninvasive, drug-free form of treatment, physicians who prescribe it claim it is one of the safest long-term remedies available, more effective than aspirin or other over-the-counter medications. Fans of this therapy even argue that treatment outcomes are more predictable than most traditional approaches.

Practitioners of this therapy recommend a number of additional precautions:

■ Never use a magnetic bed for more than 8 hours.

■ Wait at least 60 minutes after meals before applying magnets to the abdomen. Earlier application is said to interfere with normal contractions in the digestive tract.

■ Remember that the magnetic devices will stick to other metal products, possibly causing injury. Be cautious, for example, when removing a pan from the stove while wearing a device on your wrist.

■ Be careful to keep the devices away from anyone wearing a pacemaker or defibrillator.

Many magnet therapy advocates believe magnets either fight pain or stimulate circulation or both. Since popular wisdom holds that one key to managing pain is managing the way the nervous system handles the messages it receives, magnets may interfere with the transmission of impulses, making the recipient feel as if their pain is gone. Another basic belief is that better circulation means less pain and swelling and faster healing. Within these two schools of thought are two more theories about how magnets work:

1. *Molecular changes.* At the most basic level—within the molecules that make up the cells in your body—magnets might cause changes in ions, electrically charged particles that are responsible for nerve impulses and

muscle contractions. Altering the movement or electronic state of these molecules may affect the transmission of nerve signals—such as the kind that scream "pain"—across the synapses that separate the cells.

2. *Cellular changes.* Magnets might also create a change in the cells' action, such as altering the way a nerve cell handles a message of pain or how a muscle cell responds to a signal from the nervous system. Cellular change also would include the theory that magnets may stimulate circulation of blood because they attract iron that is contained in the hemoglobin, though that theory is fairly outdated. In one author's opinion (Livingston, 1996), one way a magnet works, if it works at all, is to change the way chemical messages are carried from one nerve to the next. He postulates that it would be easier for a magnet to influence a tiny molecule than the cell as a whole, whether it is a blood cell, a nerve cell, or a muscle cell.

Magnets are becoming more popular for treating injuries in professional football. Ryan Vermillion, director of rehabilitation for the Miami Dolphins, calls magnets an adjunct to his entire rehabilitation program and has used them for four years, treating everything from bumps and bruises to postsurgery pain in most of his players. Treatments may be applied by a practitioner, self-applied, or applied as part of a self-care program. One of the advantages of magnet therapy is that it does not have any known side effects.

A common criticism of magnet therapy is that the magnets used to treat pain carry only a tiny force. Magnet strength is measured in gauss, a unit related to the amount of iron a magnet can lift. The magnets used in commercial pain-relieving products (and employed in the studies discussed here) typically measure between 300 and 1000 gauss. (For comparison, a refrigerator magnet is generally about 50 gauss.)

David Ramey, an equine veterinarian in Glendale, California, who has studied magnetic products for both horses and people, says that the typical therapeutic pads he has measured carry a magnetic field that can be measured only millimeters away from its surface; if you go more than a centimeter away, there is no force at all. Thus, any effect that an external magnet could have on your body must be very superficial.

Although health care providers await positive results from clinical trials, consumers are buying magnetic products, apparently swayed by strong marketing and personal testimonials. Magnets are for sale everywhere: in health food stores, in the back of golf and tennis magazines, in celebrity endorsements, and, oddly, in places such as arts and crafts shows. Mail-order companies have been offering magnets to cure everything from headaches to osteoporosis for years. However, it has been only recently that health care professionals have acknowledged that magnets might have something to offer.

For anyone thinking about using magnets, consider the following before purchase:

- Carefully read the literature on the magnet you buy to determine how to best use it. Manufacturers and researchers are miles away from agreeing on how best to apply magnets—directly on the sore spot, for example, or over a so-called trigger point that could be in another part of the body entirely. It is important to keep in mind, however, that the effects of magnet therapy are still being studied.

- Make sure the therapeutic magnet you buy comes with a money-back guarantee if you are not satisfied. Magnets are not cheap: Small ones run about $25, and magnet-filled mattress pads sell for several hundred dollars.

- Buy a magnet that is at least 400 gauss—refrigerator magnets are not strong enough. Put it directly on the place that hurts, wear it as much as you can, and wait for results (Lawrence, 1998).

- Therapeutic magnets come in a wide range of shapes and sizes and can be purchased in a variety of products. The North America Academy for Magnetic Therapy (NAAMT) recommends magnets between 200 and 1000 gauss.

Neurofeedback

Neurofeedback (electroencephalogram biofeedback) is a process in which one learns to control the states of the brain by learning to control his or her brain waves. Small sensors attached to the scalp pick up the brain waves and send them to two computers. While the therapist monitors the actual brain wave signals on one computer, the patient learns to manipulate these brain waves, which are displayed on another screen in the form of a game. By learning to move the "Pacman" around the screen with mind power, the patient actually alters his or her brain's state of functioning. Neurofeedback works well with attention-deficit disorder, headaches, chronic pain, premenstrual syndrome (PMS), and other conditions.

Polarity Therapy

Polarity therapy asserts that balancing the flow of energy in the body is the underlying foundation of health. Practitioners use gentle touch and guidance in diet, exercise, and self-awareness to help clients balance their energy flow, thus supporting a return to health.

Polarity therapy involves hands-on energy work that is similar to acupressure and based in the ayurvedic tradition of medicine. Practitioners work on the prana, or bioenergetic field of the body, with the goal of clearing away blocks to the free flow of this energy and bringing the bioenergetic field into balance. Practitioners claim that polarity therapy addresses physical, psychological, and spiritual aspects of being. Polarity therapy incorporates diet and exercise (primarily hatha yoga) into its treatment program. The term *polarity* stems from the belief that the human energy system operates within an interplay of positive, negative, and neutral forces of energy.

Reiki

Reiki is an ancient art of laying on of hands. It is thought to have originated in Tibet 5000 years ago and was renewed in the 1800s in Japan. *Reiki* is Japanese for "universal life energy." The knowledge that an unseen energy flows through all living things and is directly connected to the quality of health has been a part of the wisdom of many cultures since ancient times. Reiki is a simple, natural, and safe method of spiritual healing and self-improvement that has been taught to thousands of people of all ages and backgrounds. Simply, the word Reiki describes a spiritually guided universal life force energy that is focused on helping to heal body, emotions, mind, and spirit. Methods of teaching Reiki vary between masters. Reiki is "taught" by having an attunement passed from the master to the student.

TREATMENT

Practitioners of this ancient healing system use light hand placements to channel healing energies to the recipient. Reiki techniques and philosophy vary regarding this simple, hands-on energy healing process: The Usui System of Reiki Healing uses light hand placements to channel healing energies to the whole person—physically, mentally, and spiritually. Reiki Plus incorporates hand placements on the head to tap into the collective unconscious, along with nutrition counseling.

Reiki is commonly used to treat emotional and mental distress as well as chronic and acute physical problems and to assist the recipient in achieving spiritual focus and clarity. Reiki can be beneficial in varying degrees. It is a natural healing technique that often but not always feels like a flow of high-frequency energy into and through a practitioner and out through the hands into another person, whether at a distance or in the same room. Some people experience a warm feeling while others envision a white light searching their body to reach the troubled area. Reiki is intelligent and knows exactly where an affliction is located. Practitioners of Reiki purport to increase the recipient's resistance to illness or pain by acting as a power source for natural healing using divine energy to channel light (energy) from the practitioner to the recipient (vessel). Reiki then moves to the source of disease to improve the body's own defenses.

Reiki practitioners claim that this modality has aided in healing virtually every known illness and injury, including serious problems like cancer and heart disease as well as skin problems, cuts, broken bones, headaches, colds, sunburn, insomnia, lack of confidence, and self-esteem.

Reiki is commonly used to relax muscles, increase blood hemoglobin levels, calm the mind, and ease pain. Clients use Reiki to deal with stress, grief, cancer, fractured limbs, and acquired immunodeficiency syndrome (AIDS). A full treatment takes 90 minutes and treats all major organs and systems of the body.

Robert Jaffe Advanced Healing Energy

Developed by a physician, this healing approach uses "heart-centered awareness," clairvoyant perception, and a variety of energetic healing techniques to identify, understand, and transform energy patterns that are believed to cause disease. The therapy is used to treat physical disease as well as emotional and spiritual disorders.

SHEN Therapy

SHEN (specific human energy nexus, "nexus" referring to the "biofield"—the web or energy body that supports the human body) therapy seeks to release deeply embedded painful emotions through the use of light hand placements.

Inspired by ancient hands-on healing techniques and the theories of modern physics, Californian Richard Pavek developed SHEN 20 years ago as a therapy for a wide range of physical and psychological conditions. Neither a strictly cognitive psychological modality nor bodywork, SHEN is more accurately described as energy work.

Using a nonmanipulative laying-on of hands, the practitioner applies his or her energy flow to the client's clothed body, thus seeking to "unblock" the client's energy flow. This practice is reputed to assist the biofield in its normal flow through the body. Emotional traumas are released and many physical disorders are healed. SHEN therapy is primarily used to treat chronic pain syndromes, physioemotional disorders such as stress-related disorders (e.g., gastric problems and migraine headaches), and general anxiety disorders (often associated with childhood sexual or physical abuse). SHEN is reported to work well with eating disorders, PMS, migraines, chronic pain, anxiety, irritable bowel syndrome (IBS), depression, and stress disorders. It is also known as SHEN physioemotional release therapy.

Spiritual Healing

Practitioners of both spiritual healing and shamanic healing often regard themselves as conductors of healing energy or energy from the spiritual realm. Both may call upon spiritual "helpers" such as power animals (characteristic of the shaman), angels, inner teachers, the client's higher self, or other spiritual forces. Both forms of healing can be used as part of treatments for a range of emotional and physical illnesses.

Therapeutic Touch

Therapeutic touch was developed in the early 1970s by Dolores Krieger, a professor of nursing at New York University, and Dora Kunz, a "natural healer." Krieger and Kunz first taught the technique to Krieger's graduate nursing students, and it remains primarily a nursing intervention today. It has been taught at more than 100 colleges and universities since the 1970s and is currently offered in about 70 health care facilities nationwide. Krieger says she has taught the technique to more than 43,000 health care professionals and several thousand lay persons.

Controversy over therapeutic touch focuses on the "energy field" that its practitioners seek to balance. Krieger claims that the field can be sensed through "hand chakras," centers of consciousness posited in Indian mystical writings. As proof of the field's existence, other proponents cite images of an energy aura taken with Kirilian photography, a technique in which the hands are placed on film and a low current produces the picture.

PRACTITIONERS

Practitioners say that this modern version of "laying on of hands" heals by correcting imbalances in the energy field that emanates from the body. Very controversial, mainstream critics respond that there is no evidence that such a field exists. Proponents contend that therapeutic touch can heal wounds, relieve tension headaches, and reduce stress. According to Nurse Healers Professional Associates (NHPA), the therapy's leading advocacy group, it also reduces pain and anxiety, promotes relaxation, and facilitates the body's natural restorative processes.

Therapeutic touch is usually employed as a supplement to, rather than a replacement for, standard medical therapies. For example, it is sometimes used to relieve discomfort between scheduled doses of pain medication for hospitalized patients. It is also employed by hospice nurses to relieve pain in terminally ill patients and to help the family accept the impending death of their loved one.

HOW THE TREATMENTS ARE DONE

Despite its name, therapeutic touch rarely involves physical contact between practitioner and patient. Instead, the therapist will move his or her hands just above the body (see Figure 13-3). The client sits or lies down before the procedure begins. No disrobing is necessary. The session is conducted in four steps:

1. *Centering.* The practitioner begins by "centering" his or herself. Centering involves attaining a quiet, meditative state in which the practitioner focuses on and attunes to the client's needs. Experienced practitioners can usually complete this process within a few minutes.

2. *Assessment.* The practitioner will then move their hands from head to foot along the body, holding them 2 to 4 inches away. This technique

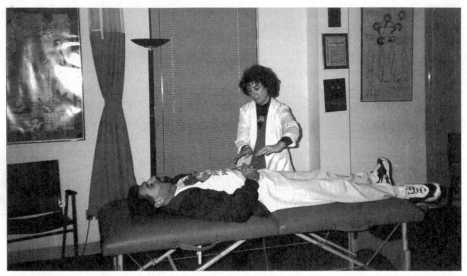

Figure 13-3 A nurse administering therapeutic touch to a patient

assesses the condition of the energy field that is thought to surround the body. Clues to the status of the field include feelings in the palms of the hands and other intuitive or sensory cues that signal areas of congestion or blockage.

3. *Treatment.* Once a blocked area is discovered, the practitioner moves their hands in a flowing motion from the top of the location down and away from the body. This action is repeated until the practitioner no longer feels the blockage.

4. *Evaluation.* After resting, the practitioner gets the client's response to therapy and reassesses their energy field to ascertain that no blockages remain.

Some practitioners add a fourth step to the treatment—energy transfer, which calls for the therapist to place one hand on the back, in the kidney area, and the other hand 2–3 inches from the corresponding location on the client's abdomen while visualizing energy passing between the hands.

Depending on the problem and the medical condition of the patient, the following recommendations should be followed:

Treatment time. Most sessions take 10–20 minutes; few exceed 30 minutes. Treatment stops when the practitioner no longer senses problems in the energy field or feels the client has had enough.

Treatment frequency. A headache in an otherwise healthy person may require only one session; a person with a chronic illness may require multiple sessions.

For frail, sick, and very young or very old patients, proponents recommend keeping the sessions short and conducting them more frequently.

ADVICE TO PATIENTS

When patients approach you about a referral for energetic therapies, you will want to have some understanding about the range and scope of the modalities. For example, the public demand for magnetic devices for painful conditions is booming, with people in North America spending about $200 million in 1999, with international sales at $5 billion. Magnets to relieve pain have been used by some since antiquity, but only recently have scientists begun to test how well they really work. Absolute scientific documentation confirming the existence of energetic fields surrounding and within the body is still not available. However, there are many testimonial and anecdotal reports that substantiate its use.

RESEARCH BOX: Effect of Therapeutic Touch on Osteoarthritis of the Knee

A single-blind, randomized, control trial was conducted to determine if therapeutic touch is effective in the treatment of osteoarthritis of the knee. Patients were between the ages of 40 and 80, had a diagnosis of osteoarthritis of at least one knee, had not had knee replacement, and had no other connective tissue disease. The patients were randomized to therapeutic touch, mock therapeutic touch, or standard care. The main outcome measures were pain and its impact, general well-being, and health status measured by standardized, validated instruments, as well as the qualitative measurement of an in-depth interview. Twenty-five patients completed the study. The treatment group had significantly decreased pain and improved function as compared with the placebo and control groups. The qualitative in-depth interview confirmed this result. Despite the small numbers, significant differences were found in improvement in function and pain for patients receiving therapeutic touch.

Source: Gordon, A., Merenstein, J. H., D'Amico, F., & Hudgens, D. (1998). The effects of therapeutic touch on patients with osteoarthritis of the knee. *Journal of Family Practice, 47*(4), 271–277.

(Continued on next page)

Magnets for the Treatment of Chronic Low Back Pain

Low back pain is one of the most frequent and expensive medical conditions in the United States. It is estimated that 85% of people will complain of low back pain during their lifetime, and currently more than 5 million people are disabled with this condition.

This study compared the effectiveness of one type of therapeutic magnet, a bipolar permanent magnet, with a matching placebo device for patients with chronic low back pain on a population of 20 (19 men and 1 woman) with stable low back pain with a mean of 19 years duration and no past use of magnet therapy for the condition.

For each patient, real and sham bipolar permanent magnets (300 gauss) were applied on alternate weeks for 6 hours per day, three days a week, for one week with a one-week washout period between the two treatment weeks. The magnets were held into place with an abdominal binder connected via Velcro straps.

Pretreatment and posttreatment pain intensity on a visual analog scale (VAS), sensory and affective components of pain on the pain rating index (PRI) of the McGill Pain Questionnaire, and range-of-motion (ROM) measurements of the lumbosacral spine were compared by real versus sham treatment.

Mean VAS scores declined by 0.49 (SD = 0.96) points for the real magnet treatment and by 0.44 (SD = 1.4) points for the sham treatment ($p = 0.90$). No statistically significant differences were noted in the effect between real and sham magnets with any of the other outcome measures (ROM, $p = 0.66$; PRI, $p = 0.55$).

The conclusion of this study is that application of one variety of permanent magnet had no effect on this small group of subjects with chronic low back pain.

Source: Collacott, E. A., Zimmerman, J. T., White, D. W., & Rindone, J. P. (2000). Bipolar permanent magnets for the treatment of chronic low back pain. *Journal of the American Medical Association, 283*(10), 1322–1325.

Magnet Therapy for Diabetic Peripheral Neuropathy

The pathophysiology of diabetic peripheral neuropathy (DPN) is complex and poorly understood. Typically, it begins insidiously, producing symptoms of numbness, tingling, and/or burning and progressing to pain and disability. Given the poor results with conventional pharmacological treatments, alternative therapies directed at slowing or halting the process are becoming attractive.

This randomized, double-placebo crossover study that entailed four phases was done to test the effectiveness of magnet therapy in neuropathic pain and to assess the role of placebo. Secondary objectives were to quantify nerve conduction electrophysiological changes and neurological examination changes over a four-month period. There were 24 initial patients, and 19 completed the four-month trial. Ten patients had advanced refractory DPN and 9 did not have DPN. All patients had failed to improve with various conventional pharmacological treatments [e.g., analgesics nonsteroidal anti-inflammatory drugs (NSAIDs), anticonvulsants, and tricyclites]. Acupuncture was also tried by a few individuals. In the control group, individuals had peripheral neuropathies secondary to multiple myeloma, alcoholism, or ischemia.

Patients randomly received an active magnetic foot insole (475 gauss) for one foot and a similar appearing sham insole on the other foot. Subjects scored their complaints of burning, numbness, and tingling pain independently in both feet twice a day using a standardized VAS scoring system. After 30 days, the sides of the active and sham magnetic insoles were switched for an additional four weeks. At the end of a month, the subjects received two new active magnetic foot insoles (475 gauss) and for eight weeks continued rating their levels of pain twice a day.

Improvement was significantly more pronounced in the diabetic cohort, 90% versus 33%, at the end of the four months ($p < 0.02$). During the first month, the placebo response was noted to be the same in both groups (22%) for symptoms of burning and numbness and tingling, whereas in the second month, the placebo effect was greater in the DPN cohort (38% versus 22%). At the end of four months, improvement was significantly more pronounced in the diabetic cohort for burning ($p < 0.05$) and numbness and tingling reduction ($p < 0.05$). Neuropathological differences identified severe axonal damage principally in the diabetic cohort, whereas mild demyelinating changes were seen principally in the group that did not have DPN.

These findings are predictive of success in the use of magnet therapy for DPN. The constant wearing of magnetic devices was able to dramatically suppress the neuropathic symptoms of burning pain, numbness, and tingling in the diabetic cohort (90%) as compared to the non-diabetic cohort (33%).

Source: Weintraub, M. I. (1999). Magnetic bio-stimulation in painful diabetic peripheral neuropathy: A novel intervention. *American Journal of Pain Management, 9,* 8–17.

SUMMARY

Hundreds of alternative and complementary therapies exist in the contemporary health care system. Many have their roots in antiquity while others are new inventions. Still others are on the frontier of tomorrow. The energetic therapies detailed in this chapter serve to awaken interest and open doors. Since these therapies may be of interest to your patients, you may want to begin exploration of the traditions, practices, training methods, and documented effectiveness of these modalities. Many of the therapies are ripe for research investigation as health care professionals continue to compile data to support the use of alternative and complementary therapies.

ASK YOURSELF

1. What are five or more energy therapies that may be used in an alternative or complementary care practice?
2. Which therapies discussed in this chapter have research to support their effectiveness?
3. What type of person might benefit from a referral for an energetic therapy?
4. Why is there controversy about some of the energy therapies?

REFERENCES

Bradford, N. (Ed.). (1997). *Alternative health care.* Holt, MI: Thunder Bay Press.

Bratman, S. (1999). *The alternative medicine sourcebook: A realistic evaluation of alternative healing methods.* Los Angeles, CA: Lowell House.

Cassileth, B. R. (1999). *The alternative medicine handbook: The complete reference guide to alternative and complementary therapies.* New York, NY: Norton.

Dossey, B., Keegan, L., & Guzzetta, C. (2000). *Holistic nursing: A handbook for practice.* Gaithersburg, MD: Aspen.

Fugh-Berman, A. (1997). *Alternative medicine: What works.* Baltimore, MD: Lippincott Williams & Wilkins Healthcare.

Jacobs, J. (Ed.). (1996). *The encyclopedia of alternative medicine.* Boston, MA: Journey Editions.

Jager, M., & Buchman, D. (1999). *Alternative healing secrets: An A-to-Z guide to alternative therapies.* New York, NY: Grammercy.

Ronald L. (1998). *Magnet therapy: The pain cure alternative.* Roseville, CA: Prima.

Livingston, J. D. (1996). *Driving force: The natural magic of magnets.* Cambridge, MA: Harvard University Press.

Thomas, R., & Shealy, C. N. (Eds.). (1996). *The complete family guide to alternative medicine : An illustrated encyclopedia of natural healing.* Los Angeles, CA: Element Books.

RESOURCES

Energy Work

Bio-Electro-Magnetics Institute
2490 West Moana Lane
Reno, NV 89509–3936
Phone: 702-827-9099

Information on magnet products, services, repairs, and conferences about magnet therapy.

Colorado Center for Healing Touch, Healing Touch Program
12477 W. Cedar Dr.
Lakewood, CO 88828
Phone: 303-989-0581
E-mail: ccheal@aol.com
Web site: www.healingtouch.com

Offers sources of individual practitioners, literature, and ongoing courses.

Healing Touch International
12477 W. Cedar Drive, Suite 202
Lakewood, CO 80228
Phone: 303-989-7982
Fax: 303-980-8683
E-mail: htiheal@aol.com
Web site: www.healing touch.net

Offers ongoing classes in the United States and abroad from beginning to certification in healing touch.

Nurse Healers Professional Associates
1211 Locust St.
Philadelphia, PA 19107
Phone: 215-545-8079
Fax: 215-545-8107
E-mail: nhpa@nursecomine.com
Web site: http://www.therapeutic-touch.org

Primarily focuses on therapeutic touch. Nurse Healers, the procedure's leading advocacy group, offers a list of its roughly 1500 members, but recommends checking the individual practitioner's background. If you are offered therapeutic touch at a health care facility, you might want to ask whether the organization follows Nurse Healers' policies and procedures.

Nurse Healers Professional Associates International
11250 Roger Bacon Dr., Suite 8
Reston, VA 20190
Phone: 703-234-4149
Web site: http://www.therapeutic-touch.org

Provides information on therapeutic touch.

Reiki Alliance
P.O. Box 41
Cataldo, ID 83810
Phone: 208-682-3535

Rubenfeld Synergy Center
115 Waverly Place
New York, NY 10011
Phone: 800-747-6897
Web site: http://www.members.aol.com/rubenfeld/synergy/index.html

Provides information on the Rubenfeld synergy method.

Flower Essence

Flower Essence Society
P.O. Box 1769
Nevada City, CA 95959
Phone: 530-265-9163
Web site: http://www.floweressence.com

CHAPTER 14

Eastern Therapies

Chapter Objectives

- Discover the range of modalities related to Eastern therapies.
- Become familiar with a variety of Eastern therapies used in some alternative and complementary therapy practices.
- Compare and contrast the quality and quantity of various Eastern therapies.

INTRODUCTION

The Eastern therapies are those modalities that arose in the Far East, specifically Asia and the Indian subcontinent. Many of these therapies are thousands of years old but were only introduced to North American culture in the past few decades. The therapies in this chapter include:

Traditional Chinese medicine

Acupuncture

AMMA Therapy

TRADITIONAL CHINESE MEDICINE

The therapies used in traditional Chinese medicine (TCM) have evolved from a philosophical worldview (see Chapter 1). There are a variety of ancient and modern therapeutic methods used in TCM, including acupuncture, herbal medicine, massage, moxibustion (heat therapy), and nutritional and lifestyle counseling, to treat a broad range of both chronic and acute illnesses (see Figure 14-1). All of the therapies in this chapter have their roots in TCM.

According to data of recent archaeological excavations, the history of TCM begins in the Neolithic period (10,000–4000 years ago). Its fundamental principles may be interpreted on the basis of two classical theories of Chinese thought: the yin-yang theory and the five-phases theory. The former states that our reality is the product of the continuous interaction and transformation of the yin and yang principles. The latter recognizes the existence of five emblematic groups in

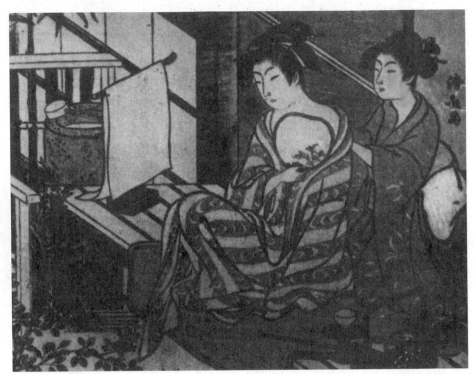

Figure 14-1 The art of massage was practiced by the Japanese centuries ago. This illustration shows a woman being given a shoulder and back massage by her servant. (From the Louvre collection. Courtesy of the New York Public Library picture collection.)

which everything regarding humankind and nature may be classified. The five phases interact in two different ways: the cycle of production (Sheng) and the cycle of control (Ke). The theoretical basis of traditional Chinese medicine are described in the *Huang Di Nei Jing* (*Yellow Emperor's* Classic of Internal Medicine) written during the period 475–225 B.C. as a dialogue between the mythical Emperor Huangdi and his physician Qibo (Cavalieri & Rotoli, 1997). The book is divided into two parts: the Suwen (questions about living matter) and Lingshu (the vital axis). Each part is composed of 81 sections. In this book are set correspondences between phases and organs, viscera, feelings, body fluids, flavors, foods, colors, and so on. We can also find the description of blood (Xue) and energy (Qi) circulation and the pathways of main, collateral, and curious vessels. The origins of disease are also reported in the *Huangdi Neijing*. As regards the psychological point of view, special attention is dedicated to dreams and their possible causes and to the description of various kinds of mental illness.

RESEARCH BOX: Effectiveness of Traditional Chinese Medicine in Alzheimer's Disease

The effects of TCM on dementia, cerebral blood flow, and cerebrospinal fluid (CSF) examination were investigated. Ten patients with Alzheimer's disease (AD) who agreed to take TCM were studied. The TCM was given for three months and the Mini-Mental State Examination (MMSE), P300 examination, cerebral blood flow examination, and CSF examination were performed before and after taking the TCM. The scores of the MMSE, and blood flow in the cerebral cortex in AD improved with treatment with the TCM. The concentration of alpha-aminobutyric acid in the CSF decreased with treatment with the TCM. The improvement is not considered to be a placebo effect.

Source: Oishi, M., Mochizuki, Y., Takasu, T., Chao, E. & Nakamura, S. (1998). Effectiveness of traditional Chinese medicine in Alzheimer disease. *Alzheimer Disease and Associated Disorders, 12*(3), 247–250.

ACUPUNCTURE

Acupuncture is the insertion of very fine needles (sometimes in conjunction with electrical stimulus) into the skin. The purpose of this stimulation is to influence physiological, emotional, and psychological functions in the mind and body. Based on Taoist principles (see Chapter 1), acupuncture aims to restore the patient's overall energy balance.

Overview

Although the ancient medical art of acupuncture may be new to many Westerners, acupuncture and related treatments are over 5000 years old. For many people, the combination of Eastern therapies, such as the use of herbs and acupuncture together, is not merely a treatment but forms a complete and comprehensive medicine.

Yin and yang theory is an important concept in acupuncture treatment, particularly in relation to the Chinese theory of body systems. Originally discovered from viewing natural phenomena, yin and yang are the metaphorical descriptions of opposite forces that, when balanced, work together. In nature, any upset in the balance will result in natural calamities, and in living things, this lack of balance results in disease.

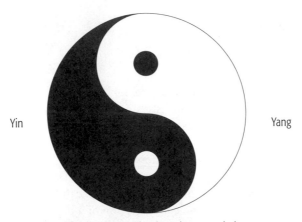

Figure 14-2 The yin and yang symbol

Yin is signified by female attributes described traditionally as passive, dark, cold, moist, that which moves medially, and that which is deficient of yang. Yang is signified by male attributes, such as light, active, warm, dry, that which moves laterally, and that which is deficient of yin. Nothing is completely yin or yang. The most striking example of this is the human person. A man or woman is the combination of his or her mother (yin) and his or her father (yang). He or she contains qualities of both. Figure 14-2 shows the universal symbol describing the constant flow of yin and yang forces.

THEORIES OF HOW ACUPUNCTURE WORKS

The process of exactly how acupuncture works is unknown, however, numerous theories abound. Some of these theories are:

- *Augmentation of immunity theory.* Acupuncture raises levels of triglycerides, specific hormones, prostaglandins, white blood counts, gamma globulins, opsonins, and overall antibody levels.
- *Endorphin theory.* Acupuncture stimulates the secretions of endorphins in the body (specifically enkaphalins).
- *Neurotransmitter theory.* Certain neurotransmitter levels (such as seratonin and noradrenaline) are affected by acupuncture.
- *Circulatory theory.* Acupuncture has the effect of constricting or dilating blood vessels. This may be caused by the body's release of vasodilaters (such as histamine), in response to treatment.
- *Gate control theory.* The perception of pain is controlled by a part of the nervous system that regulates the impulse that will later be interpreted as pain. This part of the nervous system is called the "Gate." If the gate is

hit with too many impulses, it becomes overwhelmed, and it closes. This prevents some of the impulses from getting through. The first gates to close would be the ones that are the smallest. The nerve fibers that carry the impulses of pain are rather small nerve fibers called "C" fibers. These are the gates that close during acupuncture.

HISTORY

The first record of acupuncture is found in the *Huang Di Nei Jing* (*Yellow Emperor's Classic of Internal Medicine*). This is the oldest medical textbook in the world and is thought to have been written about 4700 years ago. It was probably compiled from even earlier theories by Shen Nung, a physician and medical theorist, considered by many to be the father of Chinese medicine. Shen Nung documented theories about circulation, pulse, and the heart over 4000 years before their discovery in European medicine.

Shen Nung theorized that the body had energy running through it (see Figure 14-3). This energy is known as qi (pronounced "chee"). Qi is the motive force of all essential life activities, including the spiritual, emotional, mental, and physical

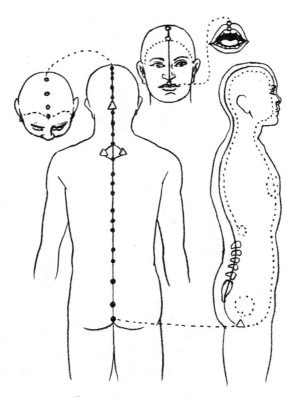

Figure 14-3 The meridian pathways

aspects of one's being. Qi travels throughout the body along "meridians," or special pathways (Fugh-Berman, 1997). The meridians (pathways or channels as they are sometimes referred to) run bilaterally; that is, they are the same on both sides of the body. There are 14 main meridians running vertically up and down. Of these, 12 are organ meridians and 2 are unpaired midline meridians.

Practitioners

According to the National Commission for the Certification of Acupuncturists and Oriental Medicine, there are more than 50 schools of acupuncture in the United States, and several medical schools now include acupuncture courses. There are currently over 10,000 licensed acupuncture practitioners in the United States. Thirty-eight states and the District of Columbia either license, certify, or register acupuncturists and officially recognize the practice of acupuncturists. Twenty-two of these states license, register, or certify acupuncturists to work independently. Doctors of acupuncture are licensed as licensed acupuncturists in most states while some states require practitioners to be medical doctors. The laws in these states vary. For example, some jurisdictions include the practice of Chinese herbology within the practice of acupuncture. In some states acupuncturists are regulated by a state board of acupuncture; in others they are under the department of health, licensing, or education or the board of medical examiners. Practitioners may be called licensed acupuncturist (LAc or LicAc), registered acupuncturist (RAc), certified acupuncturist (CA), acupuncturist, doctor of Oriental medicine (DOM), or doctor of acupuncture (DAc). However, in each case, state licensure means an individual has met eligibility requirements established by the state to practice acupuncture and/or Oriental medicine.

CERTIFICATION

The American Association of Acupuncture and Oriental Medicine (AAAOM) was formed in 1981 for American acupuncturists who are committed to high ethical and educational standards and to regulate the profession and ensure the safety of the public. As the umbrella organization representing the acupuncture profession in the United States, the AAAOM assisted in the formation of both the National Commission for the Certification of Acupuncturists (NCCA, now NCCAOM) and the National Council of Acupuncture Schools and Colleges (NCASC, now CCAOM) in 1982. The NCCAOM was established to develop and administer a national certification process based on nationally recognized standards of competence and education. Since 1985, the NCCAOM has been administering this examination, which represents professional recognition of a diplomate's demonstration of the knowledge and skills necessary for safe and effective acupuncture practice.

The North American Society of Acupuncture and Alternative Medicine is open to all licensed acupuncturists or those having an interest in pursuing a career in acupuncture or alternative medicine. This group offers Certification Examination in Pain Medicine. The American Board of Pain Medicine (ABPM) was founded in 1991 as the American College of Pain Medicine. In 1994, the name was changed to the American Board of Pain Medicine to reflect the nomenclature of other medical specialty boards. Physicians who have successfully completed the ABPM credentialing process and examination are issued certificates as specialists in the field of pain medicine and designated as diplomates of the ABPM.

Treatment

Acupuncture points are specific locations where the meridians come to the surface of the skin and are easily accessible by "needling." Since it is theorized that energy flows up and down these pathways, the connections between them ensure that there is an even circulation of qi. Those that ascribe to the theory and practice of acupuncture believe that a person's health is influenced by the flow of qi in their body. If that flow is insufficient, unbalanced, or interrupted, illness may occur. Acupuncture is said to restore the balance opening the pathways.

During the initial visit to an acupuncturist, the practitioner takes a patient's case history and performs a physical examination that also involves pulse taking (12 pulses, 6 on each wrist) and examination of the tongue. Acupuncture is most widely used for pain relief (e.g., as an "analgesia" in surgery that enables the patient to remain conscious or to relieve arthritis or lower back pain), but it has also been proven effective in treating many other ailments of an acute, chronic, or degenerative nature, such as arthritis, Meniere's disease (ringing in the ears), and headache.

Treatment is rendered by painlessly inserting long, thin needles at specific points along the body's meridians, or energy channels, in order to regulate the flow of chi, or vital energy. The activating force behind chi is the constant movement of energy between the poles of yin and yang. In the body, yin organs, such as the stomach and bladder, are hollow and involve absorption and discharge. Yang organs, such as the heart and lungs, are solid organs that regulate the body. If the yin-yang balance between the organs is disrupted, the flow of chi is blocked and the body becomes ill.

Acupuncturists can use as many as nine types of acupuncture needles, though only six are commonly used today. These needles vary in length, width of the shaft, and shape of the head. Most acupuncture needles are disposable. Practitioners employ precise methods for inserting needles. Points can be needled anywhere in the range of 15–90 degrees relative to the skin surface, depending on the treatment called for. In most cases a felt sensation is desired. This sensation, which is not pain, is called deqi (pronounced "dah-chee").

The following techniques may be used by an acupuncturist immediately following insertion: raising and thrusting, twirling or rotation, a combination of raising/thrusting and rotation, plucking, scraping (vibrations sent through the needle), and trembling (another vibration technique). These techniques are not arbitrary but rather are carefully chosen based on the ailment. This specialized technique is the Chinese medical equivalent of the Western prescription. There are several related procedures that fall into the range of acupuncture treatments:

1. Electro-acupuncture is the use of very small electrical impulses sent through the acupuncture needles. This method is generally used for analgesia (pain relief or prevention). The amount of power used is only a few microamperes, but the frequency of the current can vary from 5 to 2000 Hz. The higher frequencies are generally used for surgery (usually abdominal), and the lower frequencies for general pain relief. The first reported successful use of electro-acupuncture was in 1958 in China for a tonsillectomy. Today, it is a common method of surgical analgesia in China. Other modern methods for stimulating acupuncture points include using lasers and sound waves (sonopuncture).

2. Auriculotherapy, also known as ear acupuncture, is the second most commonly used treatment in the United States (see Figure 14-4). It is based on the theory that since the ear has a rich nerve and blood supply, it also must have connections all over the body. For this reason, the ear has many acupuncture points that correspond to many parts and organs of the body. Auricular acupuncture has been successful in treating problems ranging from obesity to alcoholism and drug addiction.

3. Moxibustion is the treatment of conditions by applying heat produced by burning specific herbs to acupuncture points (see Figure 14-5). Acupuncture and moxibustion are considered complimentary forms of

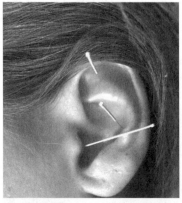

Figure 14-4 Auricular acupuncture. (Photo courtesy of Photodisc.)

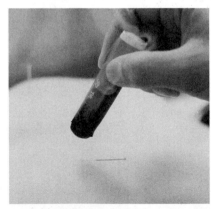

Figure 14-5 An acupuncturist lighting a cigar moxa during a moxibustion treatment. (Photo courtesy of Photodisc.)

treatment and are commonly used together. Moxibustion is used for ailments such as bronchial asthma, bronchitis, certain types of paralysis, and arthritic disorders.

4. Cupping is a technique involving the stimulation of acupuncture points by applying suction through a metal, wood, or glass jar in which a partial vacuum has been created. This approach produces blood congestion at the site and is used to draw out deleterious energy. Cupping is used for low backache, sprains, soft tissue injuries, and helping relieve fluid from the lungs in chronic bronchitis.

CONDITIONS ADDRESSED

The World Health Organization (WHO) recognizes acupuncture and TCM's ability to treat over 43 common disorders, including:

- Gastrointestinal disorders, such as food allergies, peptic ulcer, chronic diarrhea, constipation, indigestion, gastrointestinal weakness, anorexia, and gastritis
- Urogenital disorders, including stress incontinence, urinary tract infections, and sexual dysfunction
- Gynecological disorders, such as irregular, heavy, or painful menstruation, infertility in women and men, and premenstrual syndrome (PMS)
- Respiratory disorders, such as emphysema, sinusitis, asthma, allergies, and bronchitis
- Disorders of the bones, muscles, joints, and nervous system, such as arthritis, migraine headaches, neuralgia, insomnia, dizziness, and low back, neck, and shoulder pain
- Circulatory disorders, such as hypertension, angina pectoris, arteriosclerosis, and anemia
- Emotional and psychological disorders, including depression and anxiety
- Addictions, such as alcohol, nicotine, and drugs
- Eye, ear, nose, and throat disorders
- Supportive therapy for other chronic and painful debilitating disorders

Advice to Patients

Advise your patients to ask prospective acupuncturists where they studied and how they were licensed. Acupuncture schools are federally accredited by the Accreditation Commission for Acupuncture and Oriental Medicine (ACAOM). If your patient lives in a regulated jurisdiction, they should seek a licensed acupuncturist. If they live in an unregulated jurisdiction, they should seek a practitioner that is board

TABLE 14-1	Frequently Asked Questions and Answers about Acupuncture

QUESTION	ANSWER
What can I expect?	Many conditions may be alleviated very rapidly; however, conditions that have arisen over a course of years will be relieved only with slow, steady progress. As in any form of healing, the patient's attitude, diet, determination, and lifestyle will affect the outcome of a course of treatment. Patients are encouraged to actively participate in their healing process. Although acupuncture can treat many conditions, there are circumstances that can be dealt with more effectively by Western medicine. In such cases, the acupuncturist will recommend that a Western medical doctor be contacted. Acupuncture and Oriental medicine should be seen as complementary to Western medicine.
Is acupuncture safe?	In the hands of a comprehensively trained acupuncturist, safety is assured. Acupuncture needles are sterile and are either disposable or autoclaved between treatments. Preference in the type of needles should be discussed directly with the practitioner.
Is acupuncture painful?	Acupuncture is not the same as receiving an injection, since the main source of pain from injections is the larger diameter, hollow needle and the medication being forced into the tissue by pressure. Acupuncture needles are very fine and flexible, about the diameter of a human hair. In most cases, insertion by a skilled practitioner is performed without discomfort. There may be an experience of heaviness or electricity in the area of insertion. Most patients find the treatments very relaxing and many fall asleep during treatment. In some cases, the practitioner may also recommend herbs or dietary, exercise, or lifestyle changes.

certified by the NCCAOM. Some patients will want more information and may ask numerous questions. Table 14-1 offers some suggested answers to the most frequently asked questions by patients.

Research

Acupuncture is a rapidly poliferating field in the U.S. alternative health care field, and as such, there is new research each year.

Three different studies found acupuncture beneficial in the prevention of postoperative nausea and vomiting (al-Sadi, Newman, & Julious, 1997; Andrzejowski & Woodward, 1966; Ferrara-Love, Sekeres, & Bircher, 1996). Another investigation found that acupuncture reduced vomiting in hospitalized pediatric patients (Schwager, Baines, & Meyer, 1996).

RESEARCH BOX: Effect of Acupuncture in Neurogenic Bladder of Spinal Cord Injury Patients

Eighty patients with spinal cord injury (SCI) and neurogenic bladder were studied. Among them, 28 (70%) cases in the control group and 32 (80%) cases in the electroacupuncture group achieved ultimately balanced voiding and were selected for further analysis. The acupuncture group received electroacupuncture at four acupoints—chung chi (conception vessel CV3), kuan yuan (CV4), and bilateral tzu liao (urinary bladder UB32)—in addition to a conventional intermittent catheterization program (ICP), whereas the control group underwent a conventional bladder training program with ICP only. The results revealed that the time of achieving balanced voiding was statistically significantly shorter with electroacupuncture than in the control group: 57.1 ± 22.6 vs. 85.2 ± 27.4 days ($p < 0.005$) for upper motor neuron lesions and 55.4 ± 22.6 vs. 83.4 ± 26.1 days ($p < 0.01$) for lower motor neuron lesions. However, there was almost no difference between upper motor neuron lesions and lower motor neuron lesions. The time at which acupuncture commenced also influenced the results. In those who received acupuncture within three weeks after injury, the total number of days to achieve a balanced bladder was significantly reduced, as compared to those who received acupuncture three weeks after injury (46.6 ± 13.2 vs. 65.8 ± 15.4 days, $p < 0.005$). This study implied that acupuncture might be beneficial in the management of neurogenic bladder of SCI, and the earlier the patient received electroacupuncture therapy, the sooner the bladder balanced. On the other hand, the researchers also found that complete spinal cord injury, either with pronounced detrusor-sphincter dysynergia in upper motor neuron lesion or with persistent areflexic bladder in lower motor neuron lesion, was not affected by acupuncture.

Source: Cheng, P. T., Wong, M. K., & Chang, P. L. (1998). A therapeutic trial of acupuncture in neurogenic bladder of spinal cord injured patients—a preliminary report. *Spinal Cord, 36*(7), 476–480.

Pain is the major complaint of the estimated one million U.S. consumers who use acupuncture each year. Although acupuncture is widely available in chronic pain clinics, the effectiveness of acupuncture for chronic pain remains in question. One study's aim was to assess the effectiveness of acupuncture as a treatment for chronic pain within the context of the methodological quality of the studies (Ezzo, Berman, Hadhazy, Jadad, Lao, & Singh, 2000). MEDLINE (1966–1999), two complementary medicine databases, 69 conference proceedings, and the bibliographies of other articles and reviews were searched. Trials were included if they were randomized, had populations with pain longer than three months, and used needles rather than surface electrodes. The study concluded that there is limited evidence that acupuncture is more effective than no treatment for chronic pain and there is inconclusive evidence that acupuncture is more effective than placebo, sham acupuncture, or standard care.

One rare complication of acupuncture was reported in an 83-year-old woman (Kirchgatterer, Schwarz, Holler, Punzengruber, Hartl, & Eber, 2000). She developed syncope and cardiogenic shock shortly after an acupuncture procedure into the sternum. Echocardiography revealed cardiac tamponade, and pericardiocentesis disclosed hemopericardium. Due to hemodynamic instability, thoracotomy was indicated. A small but actively bleeding perforation of the right ventricle was found and successfully closed. Although acupuncture represents a relatively safe therapeutic intervention, this case report should remind all acupuncturists of possible and sometimes life-threatening adverse effects.

Three different and extensive Conchrane Database Systems Review investigations had findings that acupuncture was not effective. The investigations found:

1. Acupuncture was not superior to sham acupuncture in smoking cessation at any time point (White, Rampes, & Ernst, 2000).

2. There is not enough evidence to make recommendations about the value of acupuncture in asthma treatment (Linde, Jobst, & Panton, 2000).

3. The evidence summarized in this systematic review does not indicate that acupuncture is effective for the treatment of back pain (Tulder, Cherkin, Berman, Lao, & Koes, 2000).

AMMA THERAPY

AMMA Therapy is a specialized form of Oriental bodywork that uses traditional Oriental medical principles to assess and evaluate imbalances in the energetic system. Its origin can be traced back thousands of years to an ancient healing system rooted in the principles of TCM. Therapeutic bodywork along with acupuncture and herbal medicine has been an integral part of the medical system in China for thousands of years.

Overview

AMMA Therapy was developed by Tina Sohn, cofounder of New York College, after she had trained for years in "amma" techniques in her native Korea. What emerged is a complex and highly refined system of bodywork therapy employing a wide variety of massage techniques and manipulations and the application of pressure, friction, and touch to points and channels on which points are found. Rooted in the same fundamental medical principles as acupuncture and herbalism, AMMA Therapy focuses on the balance and movement of energy within the body. The techniques of AMMA Therapy aim to remove blockages and free the flow of energy in the body, thereby restoring, promoting, and maintaining optimum health.

Practitioners

A beginning practitioner of Oriental bodywork relates to a patient from a viewpoint that focuses mainly on the physical body, utilizing and incorporating some basic knowledge of the energy system (Dossey, Keegan & Guzzetta, 2000). Much of the focus is on muscle tissue and blood and lymphatic circulation. An AMMA Therapy treatment involves general manipulation of the primary channels and major points. The practitioner seeks to produce a state of increased qi, blood circulation, lymphatic drainage, and muscular relaxation that is designed to leave the patient feeling revitalized and refreshed.

The National Nurse Certificate Program in AMMA Therapy is endorsed by the American Holistic Nurses Association.

TRAINING REQUIREMENTS

AMMA therapists study Oriental and Western medicine. Becoming an AMMA therapist requires education in the theory, principles, and practical application of Oriental and Western medicine, along with hours of intensive practice, integration, and application of one's growing knowledge to the treatment of patients seeking preventive therapy as well as those with the most serious medical conditions. The principal site of preparation of AMMA therapists in the United States is at the New York College in Syosset, New York.

Many students begin AMMA training after they receive a degree in massage therapy. They may continue their training through the bachelor's degree program in AMMA Therapy. The in-depth advanced-level program offered at New York College focuses on assessment and diagnostic skills for the Oriental medicine practitioner. The program is geared to graduates of massage therapy programs who wish to better understand and treat underlying causes of patients' distress.

Treatment

AMMA Therapy seeks to restore, promote, and maintain optimum health through the treatment of the physical body, the "bioenergy" and the emotions. It is used to address a wide range of medical conditions. There is very little published information about AMMA Therapy effects in patients. However, one article did discuss its positive effects on patients with chronic fatigue syndrome as an alternative management approach for this syndrome (Young, 1993).

An AMMA Therapy assessment uses both Western and Eastern knowledge of techniques, combining traditional Oriental medical principles for assessing energy imbalances with a Western approach to organ dysfunction. A diagnosis is based on the four traditional methods: looking, asking, touching, and smelling. This includes an assessment of every facet of the mind-body complex, including the observation of the tongue, the taking of various pulses, palpation, and evaluation of, for example, the diet and the complexion. Every symptom reflects the internal state of the body and can be used in assessment, providing information about the psychological state of the patient as well as the prognosis of the disease or imbalance. Once a comprehensive assessment is made and energy imbalances and organ dysfunctions diagnosed, the AMMA therapist relies on the sensitivity and strength of the hands and fingers to appropriately treat the body to remove blockages, free the flow of energy, and bring healing energy to problem areas.

Advice to Patients

AMMA therapy is a newly developed modality based on ancient principles. Tell your patient that because of this, they may want to ask the therapist about their length of training and exactly what kind of outcomes to expect.

SUMMARY

Traditional Chinese medicine (TCM), acupuncture, and AMMA Therapy are becoming more widely used each year. The Eastern therapies detailed in this chapter may serve to awaken interest and open doors. If you think one or more of these therapies may be of interest to you or your patients, then begin exploration of its tradition, practice, training methods, and documented effectiveness. Many of the modalities are ripe for research investigation as health care professionals continue to compile data to support or challenge the use of alternative and complementary therapies.

ASK YOURSELF

1. What Eastern therapies may be used in an alternative or complementary care practice?
2. How would you feel if one of your patients asked for a referral for an Eastern therapy?
3. Which therapies have research to support their effectiveness?
4. What are controversies involving the effects of acupuncture? Discuss them.

REFERENCES

al-Sadi, M., Newman, B., & Julious, S. A. (1997). Acupuncture in the prevention of postoperative nausea and vomiting. *Anaesthesia, 52,* 658–661.

Andrzejowski, J., & Woodward, D. (1996). Semi-permanent acupuncture needles in the prevention of post-operative nausea and vomiting. *Acupuncture Medicine, 14,* 68–70.

Cavalieri, S., & Rotoli, M. (1997). *Huangdi Neijing:* A classic book of traditional Chinese medicine. *Recenti Progressi in Medicina, 88*(11), 541–546.

Dossey, B., Keegan, L., & Guzzetta, C. (2000). *Holistic nursing: A handbook for practice.* Gaithersburg, MD: Aspen.

Ezzo, J., Berman, B., Hadhazy, V. A., Jadad, A. R., Lao, L., & Singh, B. B. (2000). Is acupuncture effective for the treatment of chronic pain? A systematic review. *Pain, 86*(3), 217–225.

Ferrara-Love, R., Sekeres, L., & Bircher, N. G. (1996). Nonpharmacologic treatment of postoperative nausea. *Journal of Perianesthesia Nursing, 11,* 378–383.

Fugh-Berman, A. (1997). *Alternative medicine: What works.* Baltimore, MD: Lippincott Williams & Wilkins Healthcare.

Kirchgatterer, A., Schwarz, C. D., Holler, E., Punzengruber, C., Hartl, P., & Eber, B. (2000). Cardiac tamponade following acupuncture. *Chest, 117*(5), 1510–1511.

Linde, K., Jobst, K., & Panton, J. (2000). Acupuncture for chronic asthma. *Cochrane Database of Systematic Reviews, 2,* CD000008.

Schwager, K. L., Baines, D. B., & Meyer, R. J. (1996). Acupuncture and postoperative vomiting in day-stay pediatric patients. *Anaesthesia and Intensive Care, 24,* 674–677.

Tulder, M. W., Cherkin, D. C., Berman, B., Lao, L., & Koes, B. W. (2000). Acupuncture for low back pain. *Cochrane Database of Systematic Reviews, 2,* CD001351.

White, A. R., Rampes, H., & Ernst, E. (2000). Acupuncture for smoking cessation. *Cochrane Database of Systematic Reviews, 2,* CD000009.

Young, A. (1993). Amma therapy: A holistic approach to chronic fatigue syndrome. *Journal of Holistic Nursing, 11*(2), 172–182.

RESOURCES

American Association of Oriental Medicine
433 Front St.
Catasauqua, PA 18032
Phone: 610-266-1433
Toll free: 888-500-7999
Fax: 610-264-2768

National Acupuncture Detoxification Association Literature Clearinghouse
Box 1927
Vancouver, WA 98668–1927
Phone: 360-260-8620

National Certification Commission for Acupuncture and Oriental Medicine
11 Canal Center Plaza, Suite 300
Alexandria, VA 22314
Phone: 703-548-9004
Fax: 703-548-9079

National Commission for the Certification of Acupuncturists
1424 16th St. NW, Suite 601
Washington, DC 20036
Phone: 202-232-1404

New York College, AMMA Therapy Program
6801 Jericho Turnpike, Suite 300
Syosset, NY 11791–4413
Phone: 800-922-7337

North American Society of Acupuncture and Alternative Medicine
816 Frederick Road
Catonsville, MD 21228

Miscellaneous Therapies

Chapter Objectives

- Become familiar with a variety of the miscellaneous therapies used in some alternative and complementary therapy practices.
- Compare and contrast the quality and quantity of various therapies.

INTRODUCTION

Most of the alternative and complementary therapies can fit into categories, such as bodywork or energetics, but some seem to stand alone. The modalities in this chapter are of that variety and thus find their way into a miscellaneous category. The therapies included in this chapter are:

Aquatherapy/hydrotherapy

Aromatherapy

Astrology

Breathwork

Chanting

Chelation therapy

Colon therapy

Feng shui

Holotrophic breathwork

Iridology

Kinesiology

Applied Kinesiology

Educational kinesiology

Health kinesiology

Light therapy

Pet therapy

Rapid eye technology

PRACTITIONERS

The practitioners of these therapies range from the self-trained to professionals with advanced degrees and certification. Often a professional will develop interest in one or more of the miscellaneous alternative therapies and add that skill to his or her professional ones. Some of the therapies have certificate or certification programs, but others do not.

AQUATHERAPY/HYDROTHERAPY

Aquatherapy is using water in all of its various physical forms (liquid, solid, and vapor) and temperatures (hot, cold, and tepid) to heal (Keegan & Keegan, 1998). Here, ways in which water affects the senses and the psyche are considered.

RESEARCH BOX: Use of Hydrotherapy in Rheumatoid Arthritis

This study evaluated the therapeutic effects of hydrotherapy, combining elements of warm-water immersion and exercise. It was predicted that hydrotherapy would result in a greater therapeutic benefit than either of these components separately. One hundred thirty-nine patients with chronic rheumatoid arthritis were randomly assigned to hydrotherapy, seated immersion, land exercise, or progressive relaxation. Patients attended 30-minute sessions twice weekly for four weeks. Physical and psychological measures were completed before and after intervention and at a three-month follow-up. All patients improved physically and emotionally, as assessed by the Arthritis Impact Measurement Scales 2 questionnaire. Belief that pain was controlled by chance happenings decreased, signifying improvement. In addition, hydrotherapy patients showed significantly greater improvement in joint tenderness and in knee range of movement (women only). At follow-up, hydrotherapy patients maintained the improvement in emotional and psychological state. Although all patients experienced some benefit, hydrotherapy produced the greatest improvements. This study, therefore, provides some justification for the continued use of hydrotherapy.

Source: Hall, J., Skevington, S. M., Maddison, P. J., & Chapman, K. (1996). A randomized and controlled trial of hydrotherapy in rheumatoid arthritis. *Arthritis Care Research, 46*(5), 206–215

Hydrotherapy is the traditional use of hot and cold water for physical healing. Hydrotherapy is often prescribed by a naturopath and involves the use of various hot- and cold-water treatments, including baths, saunas, saltwater treatments, whirlpools, and hot and cold compresses and packs. Water can be used as a stimulant or relaxant, and as a way to cure insomnia or a hangover. Hydrotherapy is effective in treating a wide range of digestive, circulatory, and respiratory diseases.

Aquatherapy is broader and more inclusive than hydrotherapy. Use of aquatherapy may involve a trip to the seashore or lakeside to rest and reflect in a peaceful atmosphere that includes the visual, esthetic, and physical use of water.

AROMATHERAPY

Aromatherapy is an ancient healing art with 5000-year-old roots in ancient Egypt. It is the art and science of using pure essential oils for various therapeutic purposes, primarily those related to smell. Practitioners claim that essential oils can heal emotional and physical imbalances when applied so that one can inhale their aroma and/or absorb their essence. Aromatherapy uses essential oils (pure extracts of volatile oils that have been distilled from roots, stems, leaves, flowers, wood, or fruit of plants) to treat emotional disorders such as stress and anxiety as well as a wide range of other ailments. Oils are inhaled, massaged into the skin in diluted form, or placed in baths. Aromatherapy is often used in conjunction with massage therapy, acupuncture, reflexology, herbology, chiropractic, and other holistic treatments. Essential oils are highly concentrated and believed to harness concentrated plant energy that can trigger a healing response from the limbic system of the brain (see Figure 15-1). The concentrated oils are usually diluted or mixed with other oils.

ASTROLOGY

Astrology is the study of the positions of the planets in the solar system and their possible influence on human affairs. Based on this information, an astrological counselor can work with a client to provide individualized insights into emotional, professional, and health matters or into the client's personality. While astrology is not scientifically validated, many people plan their lives in accordance with astrologists' advice. Professionals simply need to be aware of this and be more knowledgeable about the practice so they can help patients incorporate it into their personal health care regime.

ESSENTIAL OIL NAMES

COMMON	LATIN	COMMON	LATIN
ANGELICA	Angelica archangelic	JASMINE	Jasmine officinale
ANISEED	Pimpinella anisum	JUNIPER	Juniperus communis
BASIL	Ocimum basilicum	LAVANDIN	Lavandula fragrans
BAY	Pimenta racemosa	LAVENDER	Lavandula officinalis
BENZOIN	Styrax benzoin	LEMON	Citrus limonum
BERGAMOT	Citrus bergamia	LEMONGRASS	Cymbopogon citratus
BIRCH	Betula lenta	LIME	Citrus aurantifolia
BLACK PEPPER	Piper nigrum	LOVAGE ROOT	Levisticum officinale
BOIS DE ROSE	Anibo rosaeodora	MACE	Myristica fragrans
CAJEPUT	Melaleuca leucadendron	MANDARIN	Citrus nobilis
CAMPHOR	Cinnamomum camphora	MARJORAM	Origanum marjorana
CARAWAY SEEDS	Carum carvi	MELISSA	Melissa officinalis
CARDAMOM	Elettaria cardamomum	MUGWORT	Artemisia vulgaris
CARROT	Daucus carota	MYRRH	Commiphora myrrha
CEDARWOOD	Cedrus atlantica	MYRTLE	Myrtus communis
CHAMOMILE-BLUE	Ormensis multicolis	NEROLI (orange blossom)	Citrus bagaradia
CHAMOMILE-GERMAN	Matricaria chamomilla	NIAOULI	Melaleuca viridiflora
CHAMOMILE-MIXTA	Anthemis mixta	NUTMEG	Myristica fragrans
		ORANGE	Citrus aurantium
CHAMOMILE-ROMAN	Anthemis nobilis	OREGANO	*Origanum vulgare*
CINNAMON BARK	Cinnamonum zeylanicum	PALMAROSA	Cymbopogon martini
		PARSLEY	Petroselinum sativum
CINNAMON	Cinnamomum zeylanicum	PATCHOULI	Pogostemon patchouli
		PENNYROYAL	Mentha pulegium
CISTUS	Cistus landaniferus	PEPPER	Piper nigrum
CITRONELLA	Cymbopogon nardus	PEPPERMINT	Mentha piperanta
CLARY SAGE	Salvia sclarea	PETITGRAIN	Citrus aurantium
CLOVE	Eugenia caryophyllata	PIMIENTO	Pimienta officinalis
CORIANDER	Coriandrum sativum	PINE	Pinus sylvestris
CUMIN	Cuminum cyminum	RAVENSARA	Ravensara aromatica
CYPRESS	Cupressis sempervirens	ROSE BULGAR	Rosa damascena
DILL	Anethum graveolens	ROSE MAROC	Rosa damasacena
ELEMI	Canarium luzonicum	ROSEMARY	Rosmarinum officinalis
EUCALYPTUS	Eucalyptus globulus	SAGE	Salvia officinalis
EUCALYPTUS LEMON	Eucalyptus citriodora	SANDALWOOD	Santalum album
		SAVORY	Satureia montana
EUCALYPTUS PEPPERMINT	Eucalyptus dives	SPEARMINT	Mentha spicata
		SPIKE	Lavandula spica
EUCALYPTUS RADIATA	(same—Eucalyptus dives)	SPRUCE	Picea mariana
		TAGETES	Tagetes patula
EVERLASTING	Gnaphalium polycephalum	TANGERINE	Citrus reticulata
		TARRAGON	Artemisia dracunculus
		TEA TREE	Melaleuca alternifolia
FENNEL	Foeniculum vulgare	THEREBENTINE	Pinus martimus
FIR	Abies balsamea	LEMON THYME	Thymus hiemalis
FRANKINCENSE	Boswellia thurifera	RED THYME	Vulgaris thymus
GALBANUM	Ferula galbaniflua	THYME	Thymus
GERANIUM	Pelargonium graveolens	VALERIAN	Valeriana officinalis
GINGER or GINGER ROOT	Zingiber officinale	LEMON VERBENA	Citroidora lippia
GRAPEFRUIT	Citrus paradisi	VETIVER	Vetiveria zizanoides
HOPS	Humulus lupulus	VIOLET LEAF	Viola odorata
HYSSOP	Hyssopus officinalis	YARROW	Achillea millefolium
IMMORTELLE (Italian Everlasting)	Helichrysum angustifolium	YLANG-YLANG	Cananga odorata

Figure 15-1 Some of the essential oils used in aromatherapy

AURA-SOMA COLOR THERAPY

Color therapy was developed in England by herbalist, podiatrist, and massage therapist Vicki Wall. This modality is based on the premise that life depends on light, the harmonics of which are color. The therapy utilizes brightly colored, two-toned, liquid-filled "balance" bottles that the client systematically chooses. The top of each bottle contains essential oils held in a base oil; the bottom half contains herb extracts in spring water. Both halves are suffused with gem essences. When the bottles are shaken, a temporary emulsion is formed. This emulsion is then applied to the relevant chakra center of the body. Although effective in treating physical symptoms, aura-soma color therapy is intended to help clients regain balance at all levels of being.

BREATHWORK

Breathwork is a general term for a variety of techniques that use patterned breathing to promote physical, mental, and/or spiritual well-being. Some techniques use breath in a calm, peaceful way to induce relaxation or manage pain, while others use stronger breathing to stimulate emotions and emotional release.

CHANTING

Proponents of chanting believe that vocalization can lower blood pressure, reduce stress, and improve health. And one does not even have to be able to carry a tune to reap the benefits. Contemporary medical research has shown that chanting and other forms of vocalization oxygenate the cells, lower the blood pressure and heart rate, increase lymphatic circulation, boost levels of melatonin, reduce stress-related hormones, and release endorphins. One study conducted in Paris found that women with breast cancer were able to significantly reduce or even eliminate tumors through chanting several hours each day for a month. Vocal sound has proven to be effective in treating schizophrenia, eating disorders, hyperactivity, arthritis, heart disease, and Alzheimer's disease.

The pioneering work of French physician and researcher Alfred Tornatis has been especially instrumental in showing the powerful effects of treating the nervous system with sound. His research demonstrates that certain types of high-frequency sounds energize the nervous system and stimulate the middle ear, while other low-frequency sounds deplete it. In sound clinics, practitioners of this healing technique have successfully treated a wide variety of problems, including depression, learning disabilities, sleep disorders, and extreme neurological injuries, by "reeducating" and "feeding" the ear with charged sounds. The treatment protocol for tens of thousands of Tornatis's patients has included listening to chants.

Proponents believe that chanting has the capacity to open our hearts and lift our spirits as well as ease suffering and give voice to our deepest yearnings. They also believe that chanting can help us find peace amidst a whirlwind of emotions and bring us closer to each other and to God.

CHELATION THERAPY

Chelation therapy is the process of administering a series of intravenous drips of ethylenediaminetetraacetic acid (EDTA), a synthetic amino acid with high levels of magnesium and potassium that purportedly helps detoxify the body by removing heavy metals and toxins from the blood. Typically administered in an osteopathic or medical doctor's office, chelation therapy is designed to detoxify the body. Chelation therapy ostensibly removes artery blockage to the heart as well as artery blockage to the brain; hence, it is primarily used in the treatment of cardiovascular disease by offering an alternative to bypass surgery and angioplasty. Advocates of this modality claim that it reduces high blood pressure and helps reverse age-related degenerative diseases; however, it has yet to go through the FDA evaluation process. Therefore, some doctors are hesitant to incorporate its use into their practices. Prior to treatment patients are screened for kidney disease. Kidney patients should not undergo chelation therapy.

COLON THERAPY

Perhaps one of the most controversial of all the alternative therapies is colonic irrigation. This modality is practiced primarily by chiropractors, but other health care providers also use it. Some colon therapists have independent practices devoted exclusively to colonic irrigation.

Colon therapy involves the cleansing of the large intestine with warm purified water. This is a method of detoxifying the colon through a series of colonic irrigations using water and sometimes herbal tinctures. Recipients generally seek out colon therapy for two main reasons: for digestive problems like constipation and to cleanse the body of bacteria and toxins. High levels of toxicity in the body can create symptoms of fatigue, nausea, and lethargy. During therapy, the entire colon tract is cleansed, eliminating the buildup of toxins, wastes, and bacteria that can clog intestinal walls. A single colonic treatment is said to be equivalent to several enemas in removing unwanted debris from the colon. Some people use colon therapy in conjunction with a juicing or herbal medicine program to treat the whole body.

There is a dearth of information in scientific journals, but one report was published in the *New England Journal of Medicine* (Istre et al., 1982). From June

1978 through December 1980, at least 36 cases of amebiasis occurred in persons who had had colonic irrigation therapy at a chiropractic clinic in western Colorado. Of 10 persons who required colectomy, 6 died. Of 176 persons who had been to the clinic in the last four months of 1980, 80 had received other forms of treatment. Twenty-one percent of the colonic irrigation group had bloody diarrhea, as compared with 1% of the nonirrigation group ($p = 0.00013$). Thirty-seven percent of the colonic irrigation group who submitted specimens had evidence of amebic infection on either stool examination or serum titer, as compared with 2.4% in the nonirrigation group ($p = 0.00012$). Persons who were given colonic irrigation immediately after a person with bloody diarrhea received it were at the highest risk for the development of amebiasis. Tests of the colonic irrigation machine after routine cleaning showed heavy contamination with fecal coliform bacteria. The severity of disease in this outbreak may have been related to the route of inoculation.

The National Council Against Health Fraud (NCAHF) (1995) published a position paper on colonic irrigation. It sums up the history, treatment, and controvery about colonics. In colonic irrigation, very large quantities of liquids are infused into the colon via the rectum through a tube, a few pints at a time, in an effort to wash away and remove its contents. Colonic irrigation differs from an ordinary enema, which involves infusing a lesser amount of liquid into the rectum only. A "high colonic" may involve the use of 20 or more gallons pumped by a machine or transmitted with an apparatus that relies upon gravity to achieve its purpose. Liquids used in colonics may include coffee, herbs, enzymes, wheat grass extract, or many other substances. Proponents of the procedure advertise that "all disease and death begin in the colon," that colonics "detoxifies" the body, and that regular "cleansing" is necessary to maintain one's health. None of these claims are true.

The idea that all disease and death begin in the colon is one of the oldest health misconceptions known to humankind. The ancient Egyptians associated feces with decay and decay with death. This caused them to write in ancient papyri that decay began in the anus. The Egyptians were obsessed with preserving corpses. Embalmers observed the putrification by bacteria (a normal process within the intestines after death) and followed the practice of removing the stomach and intestines as part of the embalming process. One of seven medical papyri and 81 of 900 prescriptions referred only to the anus. The connection between food and fecal matter was easily made. Worry about decay governed daily life. Herodotus noted that for three consecutive days in every month they purge themselves, pursuing after health by means of emetics and drenches; for they think that it is from the food they eat that all sicknesses come to men. Although the more than 700 items in the ancient Egyptian pharmacopoeia were worthless by modern standards, it did contain many items that could induce diarrhea (Majno, 1975).

In the nineteenth century, the intestinal toxicity theory became popular. The idea was that poisons from putrifying intestinal bacteria entered the body through the gut wall. Constipation was to be avoided. Numerous remedies were advocated by the health gurus of the day. Yogurt was said to create a friendlier form of bacteria. Bran was advocated for "roughage" to speed up the elimination process. The folk saying "an apple a day keeps the doctor away" is rooted in the idea of increasing roughage. Hydropaths advocated drinking large amounts of water to wash out the alimentary canal from above. One doctor even performed surgery to reshape the colon for more rapid elimination. The laxative industry grew prosperous on the idea of bowel "regularity."

Today, we understand more clearly the importance of dietary fiber, hydration, and so forth. Medical scientists also know that these have nothing to do with intestinal toxicity. Early in this century a medical researcher produced all of the symptoms of constipation (dry mouth, lethargy, etc.) by packing the rectum with sterile cotton. Studies done in the 1920s found that "high colonic irrigations" were useless and did not reach very high, even when fairly long tubes were employed. Studies in the 1930s found that colonic irrigation was contraindicated for treating ulcerative colitis, an intestinal disorder that permits bacterial contamination of the body through the gut wall.

In 1985, the Infectious Disease Branch of the California Department of Health Services stated that "neither physicians nor chiropractors should be performing colonic irrigations. We are not aware of any scientifically proven health benefit of this procedure, yet we are well aware of its hazards" (Kizer, 1985). Hazards include illness and death by contamination of colonics equipment (Istre et al., 1982); death by electrolyte depletion (Ballantine, 1981; Eisele, 1980). In addition to the physiological upsets, the colonic apparatus can perforate the intestinal wall, leading to septicemia (bacterial contamination of the blood), a very serious disorder.

Colonics is currently popular among some groups of people. Although the practice of "cleansing" and "detoxification" has no physiological significance, it does have emotional meaning to some people. Just as the ancient Egyptians did, people who practice colon therapy may temporarily relieve their health anxieties by colonics, laxatives, and purges.

A 1991 survey by the Wisconsin Board of Physician Quality Assurance found that colonic irrigation is poorly regulated. Thirty state boards of medical examiners and six boards of osteopathic medicine responded to a mail survey. Only 11 of the 36 considered colonic irrigation to be "the practice of medicine," meaning that they could regulate its practice as such. The others either had no position or made vague comments. Examining boards may discipline those they license for unprofessional conduct and/or file charges against nonlicensed people who engage in activities defined by law as within their governance. Some boards do not do the latter. They expect justice departments to prosecute imposture as fraud. The lack of attention often provides a gap within which practices such as colonic irrigation can flourish.

The NCAHF agrees with the assessment of the California Department of Health Services. Colonics has no real health benefits but does have a number of serious hazards. Advise your patients to avoid both colonics and practitioners who employ this procedure.

FENG SHUI

Feng shui (pronounced "fung shway") is the ancient Chinese practice of configuring home or work environments to promote health, happiness, and prosperity. Feng shui consultants may advise clients to make adjustments in their surroundings—from color selection to furniture placement—in order to promote a healthy flow of chi, or vital energy.

HOLOTROPHIC BREATHWORK

Holotropic (which means "moving toward wholeness") breathwork combines accelerated breathing and evocative music to induce a nonordinary state of consciousness. Holotropic breathwork loosens psychological defenses and leads to a release of unconscious material, which is facilitated by focused bodywork that involves massage and pressure at areas of accumulated tension in the body. This can free blocked energies, resulting in the healing of old psychological traumas.

IRIDOLOGY

Iridology is a diagnostic system based on the premise that every organ has a corresponding location within the iris of the eye that can serve as an indicator of the organ's health or disease. Iridology is used by naturopaths and other practitioners, particularly when a diagnosis achieved through standard methods is unclear. In 1904, Dr. Henry Lahn introduced iridology to the United States with his book *Iridology: The Diagnosis*. Lahn proposed that the eyes were the "windows to the soul" of one's health, claiming that the eyes, especially the irises, reveal indications of physical and psychological disorders. By examining the iris, Lahn claimed, an iridologist could detect disease tendencies that may not yet have begun to manifest as symptoms. According to Bernard Jensen, author of *The Science and Practice of Iridology*, the purity or brightness of eye coloring is key. The colors are bright and clear when the person is healthy and "defiled and dull" when unhealthy or suffering from toxicity.

KINESIOLOGY

Kinesiology is the study of muscles and their movements.

Applied Kinesiology

Applied kinesiology is a system that uses muscle testing procedures, in conjunction with standard methods of diagnosis, to gain information about a patient's overall state of health. Practitioners analyze muscle function, posture, gait, and other physical aspects of the patient and inquire about lifestyle factors that may be contributing to a health-related problem. Nutritional supplements, muscle and joint manipulation, and lifestyle modification (including diet and exercise) may then be used as part of a treatment plan.

HISTORY

Applied kinesiology (AK) was founded by Michigan chiropractor George J. Goodheart, Jr. In 1964, Goodheart claimed to have corrected a patient's chronic winged scapula by pressing on nodules found near the origin and insertion of the involved serratus anterior muscle. This finding led to the origin and insertion treatment, the first method developed in AK. Successive diagnostic and therapeutic procedures were developed for neurolymphatic reflexes, neurovascular reflexes, and cerebrospinal fluid flow. Later, Goodheart incorporated acupuncture meridian therapy into the AK system. Additionally, the vertebral challenge method and therapy localization technique were added to the AK system. Research on the topic is in its infancy (Gin, Green, & Goodheart, 1997).

PRACTITIONERS

Applied kinesiology was originally devised for use by health care providers who are licensed to diagnose, such as chiropractors, osteopaths, dentists, medical doctors, and nurse practitioners. Approximately 5000 people, mostly chiropractors, practice AK in the United States. However, some nonprofessionals also practice the modality. The International College of Applied Kinesiology teaches doctors how to perform applied kinesiology.

TREATMENT

This therapy is based on the theory that organ or glandular dysfunctions can be caused by muscles that have improper amounts of tension or tone. Applied kinesiology corrects dysfunction by applying acupressure to "reflex points" on a specific muscle. Applied kinesiologists also correct dysfunctions through chiropractic manipulation as well as changes in dietary habits, which are sometimes thought to create the muscular imbalances. Poor posture, injuries, physical and environmental stresses, and allergies are also thought to cause such imbalances.

Proponents say that AK can cure many ailments, from headaches to yeast conditions to asthma. Chronic headaches, for example, could signify problems with the neck muscles. The practitioner applies force to a muscle location on the arm or leg while the patient resists the pressure. If the patient cannot resist the force, the muscle and related organ are deemed too weak. To treat the problem, the practitioner applies pressure to a reference point in order to stimulate or strengthen the weakened muscle and related organ. An applied kinesiologist may also conduct oral nutrient tests. If a test food or nutrient is "good" for the patient, specific muscles will respond with strength; if the food or nutrient is "bad," specific muscles will respond weakly, possibly indicating allergies. Treatment may consist of nutritional supplements or a special diet. Those treated successfully often state that improvement occurs immediately after a muscle-balancing adjustment or after eliminating allergy-causing foods.

Educational Kinesiology

Educational kinesiology (Edu-K) is a synthesis of integrated movements called "Brain Gym" and other holistic processes that integrate the subsystems of the brain. It is based on the principle that all knowledge and wisdom are easily available when the brain and body are integrated. Edu-K uses muscle checking to provide feedback regarding the client's issues. Other techniques include working with meridian systems, meditation, and age regression.

Health Kinesiology

This system of body-mind energy work was developed by physiological psychologist and scientist Jimmy Scott. Utilizing a basic foundation of acupuncture, AK, and Touch for Health, Scott created a technique that he felt had even deeper implications than any of these systems individually. Health kinesiology's broad applications range from treating electromagnetic and psychological issues to enhancing spiritual awareness. Health kinesiology has been found to be particularly helpful with stressors and past traumas.

Advice to Patients

Advise patients to check practitioner's credentials and where they were trained.

Research

Research on kinesiology is in its infancy despite the fact that the International College of Applied Kinesiology states over 2000 papers have been published. There are very few articles in the peer-reviewed professional journals, and most of them are inconclusive.

RESEARCH BOX: Interexaminer Agreement for Applied Kinesiology Manual Muscle Testing

Two trials of the interexaminer reliability of AK manual testing were conducted. On the first trial three clinicians, each with greater than 10 years experience with muscle-testing procedures, tested 32 healthy individuals to estimate their agreement on the strength or weakness of right and left piriformis and right and left hamstring muscles. Significant agreement between examiners was found for piriformis muscles, but little significant agreement was noted when hamstrings were tested. In a second study, the same three examiners tested 53 subjects for strength or weakness of the pectoralis and tensor fascia lata muscles bilaterally. Significant interjudge agreement was found for pectoralis muscles, but no significant concordance could be found when the tensor fascia lata was examined.

Source: Lawson, A., & Calderon, L. (1997). Interexaminer agreement for applied kinesiology manual muscle testing. *Perceptual and Motor Skills, 84*(2), 539–546.

Correlation of Applied Kinesiology Muscle-Testing Findings with Serum Immunoglobulin Levels for Food Allergies

This pilot study attempted to determine whether subjective muscle testing employed by AK practitioners prospectively determines those individuals with specific hyperallergenic responses. Seventeen subjects were found positive on AK muscle-testing screening procedures, indicating food hypersensitivity (allergy) reactions. Each subject showed muscle-weakening (inhibition) reactions to oral provocative testing of one or two foods for a total of 21 positive food reactions. Tests for a hypersensitivity reaction of the serum were performed using both a radio-allergosorbent test (RAST) and immune complex test for immunoglobulin E and immunoglobulin G against all 21 of the foods that tested positive with AK muscle-screening procedures. These serum tests confirmed 19 of the 21 food allergies (90.5%) suspected based on the AK screening procedures. This pilot study offers a basis to examine further a means by which to predict the clinical utility of a given substance for a given patient based on the patterns of neuromuscular response elicited from the patient, representing a conceptual expansion of the standard neurological examination process.

Source: Schmitt, W. H., Jr., & Leisman, G. (1998). Correlation of applied kinesiology muscle testing findings with serum immunoglobulin levels for food allergies. *International Journal of Neuroscience, 96*(3/4), 237–244.

Muscle Test Comparisons of Congruent and Incongruent Self-Referential Statements

This study investigated differences in values of manual muscle tests after exposure to congruent and incongruent semantic stimuli. Muscle testing with a computerized dynamometer was performed on the deltoid muscle group of 89 healthy college students after repetitions of congruent (true) and incongruent (false) self-referential statements. The order in which statements were repeated was controlled by a counterbalanced design. The combined data showed that approximately 17% more total force over a 59% longer period of time could be endured when subjects repeated semantically congruent statements ($p < 0.001$). Order effects were not significant. Overall, significant differences were found in muscle test responses between congruent and incongruent semantic stimuli.

Source: Monti, D. A., Sinnott, J., Marchese, M., Kunkel, E. J., & Greeson, J. M. (1999). Muscle test comparisons of congruent and incongruent self-referential statements. *Perceptual and Motor Skills, 88*(3, Pt. 1), 1019–1028.

LIGHT THERAPY

Light has several well-proven uses in healing. Regular sessions with a light box are an excellent remedy for winter depression, known as seasonal affective disorder (SAD), ultraviolet light is frequently used in the treatment of psoriasis, natural light is a potential remedy for jaundice in newborns, and for everyone sunlight is a leading source of vitamin D.

Light has been used as a medicine for millennia. In the sixth century B.C., Charaka, an Indian physician, treated a number of diseases with sunlight. Hippocrates and other ancient Greek physicians had their patients recuperate in roofless buildings, where they could soak up the rays of the sun. By the 1890s, European sanatoriums were prescribing incandescent electric "light baths" to treat many physical and psychological conditions, and Niels Finsen, a Danish physician, was using ultraviolet light to treat tuberculosis.

Light therapy as we know it today appeared in the 1980s, when doctors realized that people deprived of light sometimes developed symptoms such as depression, lethargy, inability to concentrate, and difficulty sleeping. Researchers speculated that the problems stemmed from a disruption of the patient's circadian rhythm, an internal 24-hour "dark-light cycle" that governs the timing of hormone production, sleep, body temperature, and other functions. Circadian rhythm is regulated by the pineal gland, which in turn is controlled by the presence or absence of external light. During the first hours of darkness, the pineal gland produces the hormone melatonin, a substance that promotes sleep and, according to some researchers, may even strengthen the immune system. When you disturb the circadian rhythm by sleeping during the day, traveling across time zones, or getting insufficient exposure to light, your health begins to suffer. The two most striking examples of the phenomenon are jet lag and SAD.

Seasonal Affective Disorder (SAD)

Seasonal affective disorder strikes 4 to 6 of every 100 people, most of them women over 20 years of age, although children also develop the disorder. The victims, who usually live in northern climates, generally feel fine during the spring, summer, and early fall, when the days are long, but become sleepy, gain weight, crave carbohydrates, and grow unhappy as the days get shorter. Some develop insomnia, lose their sex drive, grow irritable and moody, and find it impossible to complete tasks. Children may become hyperactive or have problems learning and concentrating.

To reset the body's internal clock, researchers tried giving SAD patients regular doses of full-spectrum or bright white light from late autumn to early spring. They speculated that the extra light would suppress overproduction of melatonin (the suspected cause of SAD) and keep the melatonin cycle in sync. This theory has not been substantiated, but the success of the treatments are anecdotally good.

The "white" lights used in SAD light treatments match the radiation obtained from natural sunlight shortly after sunrise or before sunset but do not contain any ultraviolet wavelengths.

Most people take the treatments at home, although some receive therapy in an office or clinic. Those treated by a therapist lie on a couch under a lamp that emits at least 2500 lux of illumination, about half the brightness of full sunlight. To receive any benefit from this therapy, the eyes are open during the entire session

For home treatments, most people buy a light box (see Table 15-1). While most of these lights are 2500 lux, some may be as bright as 10,000 lux. For those not wanting to purchase a light box, any high-intensity fluorescent lamp that does not emit ultraviolet rays can be used.

The treatment time ranges from 15 minutes to 3 hours, depending on the brightness of the light source. With a 2500-lux source, approximately 2 hours per session is needed. A 5000-lux light requires 30–90 minutes, a 10,000-lux source, 25–45 minutes.

Therapy usually begins in the fall and lasts until early spring. It is best to have the sessions in the early morning or at dusk. One session per day is usually sufficient, although some therapists recommend twice-daily sessions for the first few days or until the condition improves.

TABLE 15-1	**Steps to Using Light Therapy at Home**

1. Buy a light box measuring approximately 2 feet by 2 feet and enclosed. Add a full-spectrum or bright white light.
2. Place the light box on a table or other flat surface where it is level with your eyes.
3. Sit about 18 inches from the box, facing the light source, but never looking directly at the bulb. (Some manufacturers recommend that you sit farther away. Be sure to read the directions on the box.)
4. During the treatment session, you can read, eat, work, watch television, or perform other activities as long as you remain facing the light with your eyes open.
5. Never wear sun glasses or goggles during treatment.

Jaundice in Newborns

For jaundice in newborns, intense full-spectrum light (or sunlight) is the recommended treatment (see Figure 15-2). Full-spectrum lights, which are now being installed in many offices, factories, and other workplaces, have also been recommended for ailments ranging from migraines to premenstrual syndrome but have yet to be conclusively proven effective for anything but jaundice.

Advocates of light therapy believe that sunglasses, windows, and pollution are reducing our exposure to the full spectrum of natural sunlight and that indoor

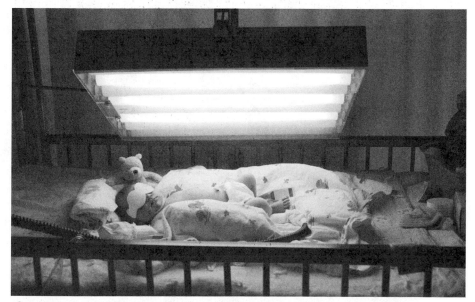

Figure 15-2 Light therapy is used to treat jaundice in newborns.

lighting, usually about 500 lux, is insufficient to compensate for the loss of the 50,000 lux supplied by sunlight. Critics of light therapy point out that none of the theories have been scientifically verified.

PET THERAPY

Pet therapy is the use of animal companions for care, comfort, and health maintenance. Animals are used in a variety of ways in therapy, ranging from Seeing Eye dogs for the blind, monkeys to help quadriplegics, dolphin therapy for brain damage, and the simple benefits of having a pet to care for. Research has shown that having a pet or other positive interaction with an animal can lower blood pressure and reduce anxiety or depression (see Figure 15-3).

RAPID EYE TECHNOLOGY

Rapid eye technology (RET) is an alternative healing program involving the systematic movement of eyes and eyelids, rapid verbal communication, and special imagery work, all of which help to release stressful, negative emotions and belief systems. The purpose of RET is to provide a program of stress relief. It simulates REM (rapid eye movement), thought to be one of the body's natural methods of maintaining health and balance. It is used to treat sufferers of traumatic stress disorder and has been used to treat sexual offenders by integrating their left and right brains. Rapid word input from the counselor helps the client form associations and determine the issues causing stress. Clients are encouraged to release their emotional blocks to wholeness and create new, positive neural pathways that will allow them to function as fully conscious, loving adults.

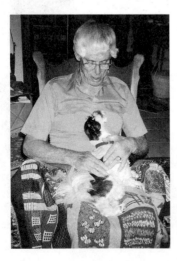

Figure 15-3 Pet therapy provides health benefits to people of all ages. (Photo courtesy of John White, Corpus Christi, TX.)

SUMMARY

Hundreds of alternative and complementary therapies exist in the contemporary health care system. Many have their roots in antiquity while others are new inventions. Still others are on the frontier of tomorrow. The miscellaneous therapies detailed in this chapter serve to awaken interest and open doors. If you think that one or more of these therapies are of interest to your patients, then begin exploration of its tradition, practice, training methods, and documented effectiveness. That way, you will have more knowledge about the practice that your patient may be seeking outside of the conventional health care system. Many of these therapies are ripe for research investigation as health care professionals continue to compile data to support the use of alternative and complementary therapies.

ASK YOURSELF

1. Which five or more miscellaneous therapies may be used in an alternative or complementary care practice?
2. Which therapies are most appealing to you and why?
3. Which therapies have research to support its effectiveness?
4. What are the controversies surrounding the miscellaneous therapies? Discuss them.

REFERENCES

An outbreak of amebiasis spread by colonic irrigation at a chiropractic clinic. *New England Journal of Medicine, 307,* 339–342. (1982).

Ballentine (1981, October). The doctor is in—jail. *FDA Consumer,* pp. 30–31.

Bradford, N. (Ed.). (1997). *Alternative health care.* Holt, MI: Thunder Bay.

Bratman, S. (1999). *The alternative medicine sourcebook: A realistic evaluation of alternative healing methods.* Los Angeles, CA: Lowell House.

Cassileth, B. R. (1999). *The alternative medicine handbook : The complete reference guide to alternative and complementary therapies.* New York, NY: Norton.

Dossey, B., Keegan, L., & Guzzetta, C. (2000). *Holistic nursing: A handbook for practice.* Gaithersburg, MD: Aspen.

Eisele (1980). Deaths Related to Coffee Enemas," *Journal of the American Medical Association, 244,* 1608–1609

Franklin (1981). Questions and answers: Colonic irrigation. *Journal of the American Medical Association, 246,* 2869.

Fugh-Berman, A. (1997). *Alternative medicine: What works.* Baltimore, MD: Lippincott Williams & Wilkins Healthcare.

Gin, R. H., Green, B. N. (1997). George Goodheart, Jr., D. C. and a history of applied kinesiology. *Journal of Manipulative Physiological Therapeutics, 20*(5), 331–337.

Istre, G. R., Kreiss, K., Hopkins, R. S., Healy, G. R., Benziger, M., Canfield, T. M., Dickinson, P., Englert, T. R., Compton, R. C., Mathews, H. M., & Simmons, R. A. (1982). An outbreak of amebiasis spread by colonic irrigation at a chiropractic clinic. *New England Journal of Medicine, 307*(6), 339–342.

Jacobs, J. (Ed.). (1996). *The encyclopedia of alternative medicine.* Boston, MA: Journey Editions.

Jager, M., & Buchman, D. (1999). *Alternative healing secrets : An A-to-Z guide to alternative therapies.* New York, NY: Grammercy.

Kastner, M., & Burroughs, H. (1996). *Alternative healing: The complete A-Z guide to more than 150 alternative therapies.* Owlet.

Keegan, L. & Keegan, G. (1998). *Healing waters.* New York: Berkley.

Kizer, K. W. (1985). The case against colonic irrigation. *California Morbidity, 38.*

Majno. (1975). *The healing hand.* Boston, MA: Harvard University Press.

Martin, R. R., Lisehora, G. R., Braxton, M., & Barcia, P. J. (1987). Fatal poisoning from sodium phosphate enema. *Journal of the American Medical Association, 257,* 2190–2192.

Thomas, R., & Shealy, C. N. (Eds.). (1996). *The complete family guide to alternative medicine: An illustrated encyclopedia of natural healing.* Los Angeles, CA: Element Books.

RESOURCES

The National Association for Holistic Aromatherapy (NAHA)
2000 2nd Avenue, Suite 206
Seattle, WA 98121
Phone: 888-ASK-NAHA or 206-256-0741
Fax: 206-770-5915
Internet address: www.naha.org

The National Association for Holistic Aromatherapy (NAHA) is an educational, nonprofit organization dedicated to enhancing public awareness of the benefits of true aromatherapy. NAHA is actively involved with promoting and elevating academic standards in aromatherapy education and practice for the profession. NAHA is also actively involved in furthering the public's perception and knowledge of true aromatherapy and its safe and effective application in everyday life. The association also has a publication, Aromatherapy Journal.

PART IV

Healers and
the Healed

The Process of Becoming a Healer

Chapter Objectives

- Become aware that healers work from a set of guiding principles.
- Identify some of the processes described by others.
- Learn five traits common to healers.
- Discover these traits by reading others' stories.
- Consider ways that you can develop more healing traits in your life.

INTRODUCTION

The process of becoming a healer involves a number of factors. It is not enough to master the techniques and skills of the modalities without at the same time addressing some of the underlying core traits of what makes a healer. Some say that these traits are personality characteristics that certain individuals are born with. Others believe that once awareness of these traits becomes conscious, it is possible to develop them. Likely it is a combination of both. Very few people are born as healers; most are taught through self-training, observation, and practice. Over time, healers develop both the skills and the traits necessary for healing.

Healers work from guiding principles. Table 16-1 details four categories of principles and belief systems that are a part of many healers' practices.

In many areas of health care there is a movement to change the process of how practitioners become healers. In medicine there is an attempt to restore "humanism" in medical care and medical education. Doctors are beginning to realize that critical and often neglected factors in healing are the personal development and well-being of the healer. Unexamined attitudes and biases and personal stress can interfere with patient care. Therefore, the profession is undertaking the process of setting new goals and objectives for medical education designed to promote self-awareness, personal growth, and well-being (Novack, Epstein, & Paulsen, 1999). Another approach in the process advocates recruiting medical student applicants with a broad education rather than the basic science student of today. Making these changes will engender a more creative, open-minded medical practitioner (Gunn, 1999).

TABLE 16-1 Healer's Guiding Principles

HEALTH	HEALING	SELF	ENERGY/SPIRIT
Health is a process that may include times of having illness or disease.	Healing involves a transformational change that encompasses the whole person; it requires the involvement of the spiritual, emotional, and intellectual domains as well as the physical body.	There is a unity and interdependence within the mind, body, and spirit.	Human beings are energy fields.
Changes in health can occur through experiential learning or as a change in behavior that occurs as a result of living through an activity, event, or situation.	Any modality or health system that supports healing should be valued.	One's attitudes and beliefs toward life (mental-emotional energy fields or consciousness) are a major etiological factor in health and disease.	Each person is an open energy system with the environment.
Each health system should be respected for the resources and the tools that it offers while being challenged to prove its credibility.	Healing, when viewed holistically, is not predictable in terms of time frame, cause, or outcome.	Both one's health and times of having illness or disease are manifested in one's lifestyle, habits, and conscious awareness as well as in the body's physical being and energy.	Energy fields are constantly interacting.
Health is the dynamic evolution toward balanced integration.	The client-practitioner relationship is one of partnership—equal with differing responsibilities.	The self is empowered by the ability to create or maintain health/disease.	Energy fields can become unbalanced as a response to stress in any of the three domains of body, mind, and spirit.
Health involves a sense of unity between the self and the cosmos.		Experiential learning is essential to changing one's lifestyle for high-level wellness.	The human spirit is the core of the person.
Health is influenced by the environment (interpenetrating external energy fields) and genetics (transgenerational energy fields).		The division of the whole person into three domains of body, mind, and spirit is an illusion.	Spiritual health is necessary for physical, mental, and emotional well-being.

HEALTH	HEALING	SELF	ENERGY/SPIRIT
Wellness encompasses increasing openness (acceptance of diversity) and increasing harmony (coherent, high-frequency energy fields).		Body, mind, and spirit share one consciousness.	The Source (known in different terms as God, Allah, Jehovah, or the Holy Spirit) is experienced or known through joy, beauty, love, light, peace, power, and life.

Adapted from Keegan (1994).

Nursing has a slightly different perspective. There may be an actual process to becoming a holistic nurse (Slater, Maloney, Krau, & Eckert, 1999). The transformation begins with separation from mainstream nursing and concludes with reintegration into the profession as a holistic nurse. The growth of the nurse follows a reasonable and perhaps predictable course. Figure 16-1 illustrates the seven-step process. The process of holistic nursing has advanced to the level that it may be time to formally differentiate between certified holistic nurses, practitioners of a

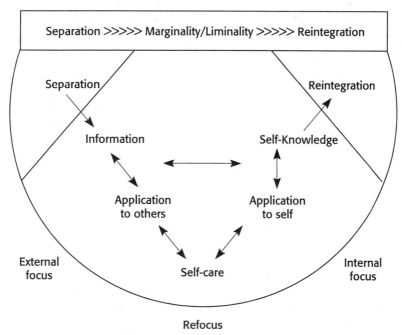

Figure 16-1 Model of the journey to holism. [From Slater, V. E., Maloney, J. P., Krau, S. D., & Eckert, C. A. (1999). Journey to holism. *Journal of Holistic Nursing, 17*(4), pp. 365–383. Used with permission.

healing modality, and healers (Wardell & Engebretson, 1998). Other health care professionals are having similar insights and making comparable changes in curricula, conceptualizations, and practices.

DEVELOPING HEALING TRAITS

There are many paths to becoming a healer. Whatever the process or route taken, healers usually develop some common traits. The following traits are qualities of healing: authenticity, forgiveness, love, altruism, and compassion.

Living from a Place of Authenticity

All of us, at some time or another, wrestle with questions of authenticity. Are we who we say we are? Do our actions represent what we profess to believe or are we being hypocritical? Is our behavior contradictory to professed beliefs? Do we walk the path of authenticity or is there subtle or even frank ambiguity between our attitudes and our behaviors?

To be an effective healer, one must be authentic. In the mystical, metaphoric realm where there is still conjecture about how actual healing occurs, one thing is certain: A healer must be genuine. Within this illusive realm there is no room for self-serving or charlatan activities. Only those with genuine intent become healers.

Those who live from a place of authenticity generally exhibit three universal qualities that are inherent in the healing process: forgiveness, love, and compassion.

Forgiveness

Most people carry grudges, unforgiven issues, mostly silenced and/or repressed, that are operant in our lives. Grudges are derived from emotional hurts that have not been healed but instead have shifted from a conscious initial hurt into mostly subconscious chronic wounds. Perhaps one of the most dramatic and powerful aspects of our humanness is how we continue to carry the burden of our hurts, rejections, criticisms, and disappointments, ostensibly inflicted on us by others. How often do you hear statements such as "my mother was so cruel, and 1 have had to suffer the consequences ever since," or "I can never trust another man again after what he did to me," or "watch out, even your best friend may betray you." These and many similar variations are typical in the contemporary world, and they all smack of the need to forgive.

A memorable book first written by Laura Huxley (1995) during the 1970s, and later reprinted in the 1990s, breaches this subject. *You are not the target* is a series of essays that describe how often we "react" when people snap at us or seem rude and inconsiderate. When we have made a genuine effort to be helpful or kind or have accidentally done something and evoked a hostile reaction, it is important to remember that in most cases we are not at fault but are simply a target for another's pent-up frustrations. This psychological system is analogous to the Oriental physical defense system of akido, in which you deflect onslaught blows instead of combating them as you would in the defense system of karate. Rather than "reacting," the preferable action is to deflect the verbal assault by letting it bypass our stored memory bank. If we "take it on," we accept someone else's unresolved and chaotic issues. Both verbally and physically, we can learn to deflect rather than combat assaults.

To carry this concept a step further, consider an additional step, the act of forgiveness. When we understand the need for forgiveness and actively practice it, we will each do a part in releasing some of the "held" anger and resentment prevalent in the world today. If each of us practiced forgiveness and release in our own daily life, the mass holding of negative energies might shift.

If we agree in theory that forgiveness is a laudable goal, then where and how do we begin? Remember the old adage, "charity begins at home." Forgiveness, similar to charity and other virtues, probably works best when we start with the basics, when we begin with the self.

HEALING STORY: Healing through Forgiveness

Flora was seated with her group in a semicircle at the base of a huge, stone fireplace on the Saturday night of a woman's wellness weekend workshop. Each participant took a turn at telling a story of a primary empowering event in her life. Flora chose to tell a story about her mother, Olivia.

Olivia's mother locked her in dark closets, beat her with a hairbrush, and eventually tried to compete with Olivia for the men in her life. In early adulthood Olivia banned her mother from her life, swearing to never speak to her again. She married and soon thereafter had a baby she named Flora. Shortly following the birth of her child, her husband left her for another woman. Poor, embittered, and alone, Olivia struggled for survival, taking a full-time day job and part-time evening work and placing Flora with a family in a neighboring town. She was only able to visit Flora on her one free Sunday each month. When Flora was old enough to ask about her father and grandmother, she was told that they were "no good" and they were better off without them.

Flora soon learned that men were wicked and old women were meddlesome; to survive, you had to work hard, be wary of men, and be very certain about whom you trusted. Although Olivia's gentle child loved her mother, she also grew to love her grandmother, who eventually was allowed to care for her when Olivia was at work.

(Continued on next page)

As Flora matured to womanhood, she saw the furrows of anger and resentment crease Olivia's tired face. Taught that one's own mother could be meddlesome, Flora was now finding that Olivia was annoying. Through counseling and group therapy, she learned about the concept of forgiveness. Flora was determined to integrate this practice in her daily life. The first person she consciously chose to forgive was her mother. During therapy Flora recognized that she was taking on characteristics similar to her mother's. She began to understand the vicious cycle that had been created and firmly resolved to break the cycle with her generation. Flora committed herself to making operant the phenomenon of forgiveness in her life. She saw where she must begin. Forgiveness, she realized, begins at home.

Thus Flora began a conscious effort to forgive her mother. Flora knew that Olivia could never accept the fact that maybe she had been wrong about men or about her own mother. Consequently, she did not endeavor to change her mother's actions or belief patterns. The person she worked on was herself. She diligently worked to create a mental image of her mother as a young and helpless girl who had no doubt been molded by trauma that swept through her developmental years. Olivia had, after all, done the best possible job she could with the circumstances she faced and the insights she had. Flora completely forgave her mother, although not verbally or in any physically demonstrative fashion that Olivia was ever aware of. Flora forgave Olivia in her heart. Because of this, she softened toward her mother, now elderly, and on whatever occasions were appropriate she found ways to honor her. In time the two women became close, and there even seemed to be a physical change in Olivia. Olivia lived alone in a city apartment, and during Flora's visits, they would stroll through the city streets and visit old haunts. They would link arms, and because of Flora's consistent mental attitude of forgiveness, both of the past and of occasional current irritants, they could also link hearts. Flora became a master of forgiveness in all areas of her life. She did so because she began with the most complex and yet most important place, she began with and achieved mastery at home. From this point Flora projected the ingrained mental behavior of forgiveness into all situations and with people she encountered in her daily life.

Observations and Insights

Consider grudges, hurts, or anger that you may be holding. Would focusing on forgiveness possibly make a difference in your life? How might Flora's life have been different if she had not made a conscious effort to forgive? Consider opportunities that you have to teach and practice concepts of forgiveness in your practice?

Table 16-2 presents a list of ways to forgiveness.

TABLE 16-2 **Twelve Ways to Forgiveness**
Find a quiet place, center yourself, and read through the following list.
1. At first, ask for just the WILLINGNESS to forgive.
2. Later, ask for the POWER to forgive.
3. Ask for the HEALING of another person's deep inner pain that must have caused him or her to hurt you.
4. Visualize the focus person as a "good person." Then also visualize yourself as another good person.
5. Make sure your mind is clean; we tend to despise in others the qualities we despise in ourselves.
6. Make sure that you have made amends to ALL other persons you have harmed, whether you feel they deserve these amends or not.
7. Make a LIST of the other person's GOOD qualities, but do NOT list the bad qualities.
8. Make a habit of SAYING SOMETHING GOOD about this person to another person, even if you have to exaggerate.
9. SEND AWAY thoughts of resentment as soon as they occur, and do not allow them to permeate your thoughts.
10. Make yourself DO A FAVOR for the other person, without letting the source be known.
11. Assume that your forgiveness, whether expressed or not, WILL NOT CHANGE the other person or the attitude toward you; it will ONLY change you.
12. GIVE THANKS for the progress, however small, that you have made in forgiveness and for the spiritual peace it brings.

Love

The Greeks were the first in Western tradition to systematize and describe love. The categories they delineated were eros, agape, and phileo. Eros is a possessive desire. It is the driving force for absolute good and, therefore, the motive underlying education, fine arts, and philosophy. Agape is akin to sacrificial, protective, or brotherly feeling. Philia pertains to the drive for community through friendship. It is possible through each type of love for healing to occur. When people join in eros or romantic love, the components of passion, intimacy, and commitment can and often do serve as a bridge for individual support and transformation.

Relationships demand that each individual be psychologically strong enough to enter such a partnership. The chances of longevity with one strong and one weak partner are remote. Enduring relationships are based on each individual becoming strong, self-reliant, and secure in themselves instead of expecting the significant other to meet all their needs. This means taking care of one's defensive, belligerent, or maladjustive patterns before entering into relationships with significant others. Otherwise, the psychological defense mechanisms of denial, projection, and rationalization might be used to justify an unenlightened perspective. The result is often a lose-lose situation with both partners being hurt and disempowered. If this happens, with sufficient insight, the situation can be turned into a win-win situation by learning to love and honor one's self first.

TOUGH LOVE

Operating from a loving perspective is not always easy. Helen, the nurse specialist in the following story, depicts a quality of "tough love," or love that comes with fortitude and conviction.

HEALING STORY: Healing through Tough Love

"Open up, Mother. I'm going to put your teeth back in now." Juanita's daughter, Maria, had been vigorously scrubbing Juanita's false teeth.

She walked back from the sink and forced Juanita's mouth open to reinsert her dentures. "Now, then, Mother, you look just fine." Maria was clean, brushed, and dressed. "All right, Mother, you rest now while I get your nurse so she can give you your medications."

Maria made her way down the hall to the nurse's station on Unit Two. "Nurse, my mother is ready for her medications now."

"Hello, Maria, how are you today?" the charge nurse asked.

"Okay, I suppose. I'll be okay as long as Mother is all right," Maria answered.

"Say, Maria, one of our nurse specialists here at Havenside has asked me to let her know the next time you were in so she can come and talk to you."

"Why? What about?" Maria said. "I thought everything was just fine."

"Well, yes, everything is fine," said the nurse "it is just that she wants to talk to you."

"Why would I need to talk to a nurse specialist?" Maria asked.

"I'll let her tell you that herself. I'll call her and tell her you're here. Until she arrives, I'll go back to your mother's room with you and give your mother her medications."

Maria waited at the counter as the nurse made her call and then went to the medication room to draw up Juanita's drugs. Maria stared at the rows of elderly people in wheelchairs. Some chatted with one another, but most stared off into the distance.

Maria and the nurse returned to Juanita's bedside. The nurse looked down at Juanita, whose position had not altered since she had turned her two hours previously. She remained contracted, contorted, unresponsive, and mute. The nurse advanced to Juanita's feeding tube, clamped the tube, and inserted the Toomey syringe into the G-button site. Swiftly she pushed the plunger, then switched syringes, and flushed the tube with water before reconnecting the liquid feeding.

Turning to Maria, the nurse said, "Now I'm going to send in the nurse's aide to clean and turn your mother. She has been incontinent again. Why don't you come down to the nurses' station with me. The clinical specialist should be along soon, and you can talk with her in our conference room." Compliantly, Maria moved to follow the nurse.

"See you later, Mother."

Helen, the clinical nurse specialist was standing at the nurses' station when Maria and the staff nurse arrived. "Hello, Maria, my name is Helen. I have been looking forward to meeting you. Let's go into the conference room and sit down." Once seated, Helen said. "You must be wondering why I want to talk to you?"

"Yes, I am," answered Maria.

"As the staff nurse told you, I am a consultant here at Havenside. Officially I am a nurse thanatologist. That means I work with clients and their families to assist them in the dying process."

"I don't see what that has to do with me," said Maria.

"Well, Maria, that is actually part of the reason we are meeting now. The team that cares for your mother has observed that you don't seem to be acknowledging that she's terminally ill. There seems to be some discrepancy between her deteriorating condition and your acceptance of it. Do you understand what I am saying?"

Maria's lower lip quivered. "Mom could go on for a long time, you know."

"Do you really think so?"

"Well, doctors and scientists are always coming up with cures."

"That's true, but let's examine the facts in your mother's case. Juanita is 87 years old. She's been crippled with arthritis for over 20 years and had a debilitating stroke four years ago. She has not recognized anyone or spoken since that time."

"Why are you telling me this? Don't you think I know. After all, I'm the one who has cared for Mother all these years."

"Of course, you have, and that's laudable," Helen said. "I bring this up now because I think it may be time for you to reexamine the quality of your mother's life, not solely the quantity of years she survives. It also may be time for you to reflect on what her passing means to you. You know some people cling to life to the extent that they begin to deny or at least block the fact that death is inevitable. When blocking becomes a pattern, it's difficult to recognize.

Maria, you may not know this, but all of us are actually dying and being reborn all the time. We are composed of billions of cells. Thousands of cells slough off and new ones are reformed on a daily basis, which means we are dying and being reborn on a continual basis. In our circulatory

(Continued on next page)

system red blood cells are replaced every 120 days, all our skin cells are replaced every four weeks, and bone cells are replaced every four days. In fact, every five years we have an entirely new body.

What this means, Maria, is that physical life is a continual renewal process. Your mother's spiritual life may be more difficult to ascertain, but consider this. If the body dissipates and rebuilds, then perhaps so too does the spirit. Is it possible that much of your mother's spirit has already left her and she is simply awaiting your release of her physical form? I raise these questions to you, Maria, because your mother's care team has recognized the holding-on process that is consuming so much of your life's energy. What I am trying to do, Maria, is help you refocus on what death means to you. Once you do that, I think it will be easier for you to talk with us about allowing your mother her final release.

Do you recall your mother's wishes on her living will prior to her stroke? She asked for no heroics, yet for the past two years she has been sustained on internal tube feedings. I don't mean to be harsh, Maria, but I think it's time for you to consider your mother's requests and why we have been prolonging the inevitable."

"Helen, this is so difficult for me. I've tried so hard to be a good daughter."

"You have been an excellent daughter, and, of course, talking about death and dying is difficult. Maria, I bring this topic up because the staff here cares about you and your mother. It may take a little time for you to think about the things I have brought up today, but I think it's important. I want you to think about redirecting our approach to your mother's care. Can we meet again in two days to talk some more?"

"Sure, I guess it's time I faced the facts. Thanks for spending time with me."

Observations and Insights

Helen and the other nurses cared enough about Maria and her mother, Juanita, to force an unpleasant issue to consciousness and to gently but effectively demand that it be acknowledged and dealt with. Consider how you deal with unpleasant issues in your life and ways you can work with clients and patients to help them confront their issues. Sometimes it takes tough love to force an issue to resolution.

Altruism

Altruism, a recognized virtue of doing acts to benefit others, is a concept that has come under scrutiny in recent years. What is in question is the motivation behind the act. Pure altruism without any ulterior motive by the doer is laudable, but it is the sorting out of hidden motives that is difficult. People can deceive themselves when doing good works. While on the surface it appears both to the unexamined self and to others that acts are performed solely for the benefit of the recipient, on analysis, unconscious or hidden motivation by the doer may exist. For example, someone who consistently volunteers for unpopular assignments may be doing so for secondary gains by thinking that he or she may be able to call in favors later on. Rather than doing a noxious job out of sheer altruism, it is instead done in order to gain favor in the eyes of others.

The doer may be seeking some sort of social or psychological remuneration because of the act or acts performed. This is usually at the subconscious level of the doer. The problem with this is that these acts can and often do provoke untoward effects or outcomes rather than the anticipated benefit.

Thus the examined life is the better path. In particular, healers must scrutinize their motivations and actions, and if they become altruistic should do so from the level of basic goodness, not from the place of consciously or subconsciously expecting or anticipating reward.

Compassion

Compassion is more than simple kindness or caring. We can care without having compassion. Compassion leads us to go where it hurts, to enter places of pain, to share in brokenness, fear, confusion, and anguish. Compassion challenges us to cry out with those in misery, mourn with those who are lonely, or weep with those who cry. Compassion means full immersion in the condition of being human.

HEALING STORY: Healing through Compassion

Tomica was in her mid-forties while working at a large hospital in the south. She divorced many years ago after the birth of her son, Tyrone, and was his sole support for 10 years. For the next 7 years Tomica was a cheerful and dedicated employee and a committed mother. While they lived in the south, her son attended the local public high school and Tomica did her best to be a good mother. Following Tyrone's high school graduation, Tomica and Tyrone decided to return home to the northeast.

During this first year back in New England, both mother and son saved all their money after meeting basic living expenses. They located an excellent

(Continued on next page)

school that would meet Tyrone's needs. The only problem was that the tuition, fees, books, and room and board totaled $29,000 a year. The college financial advisor examined the family income but stated that Tyrone was not eligible for financial aid because his father earned a high income. The problem was, however, that the father was estranged from the pair and would not agree to pay anything for college.

Tomica once again in her life took a financial plunge and enrolled Tyrone for the following fall. She had a choice on how to respond to the financial situation, and she did what was needed to empower them both. Now, she not only had to support herself but also had to net an additional $20,000 annually for Tyrone's schooling. Tyrone could earn the other $9000. True to her nature, Tomica sought a new job that would earn the necessary income and at the same time launch an independent business, something she had wanted to do her whole life. So, in Tomica's fifty-fifth year and Philip's twentieth, she went back to work and he started college.

Tomica's specialty was gerontology. She had been a caring person and a good mother all her life, but her true compassionate nature came out with the activity that began with Tyrone's education.

During Tyrone's first year at college she opened her new business, CEI, Creative Education Integration. With her advanced degrees and 30 years of nursing experience she was able to offer educational programs to nursing homes to train their off-the-street personnel in how to give humanistic care to the elderly. To support both her weekday business during its formative years and her son's expenses, Tomica was forced to take a second job. She obtained a job as a staff nurse in a nursing home. This was not a regular position, but to get the pay she required, she agreed to work 12-hour shifts, 7 A.M. to 7 P.M. every Saturday and Sunday for one year. She would only have two weekends off during the year.

Tomica did have clinical experience and certainly knew the theory, but what she encountered and the feelings evoked in her in this setting were not what she had expected. On her first weekend she came to the job feeling energetic and enthusiastic. However, because she was a registered nurse, the director assigned her the more difficult patients. Almost without exception these patients were withered, frail, helpless, cranky, incontinent, deaf, blind, and terminally ill. It was Tomica's assignment to bathe, feed, medicate, and turn and position them, treat their bedsores, and last, but not least, give them nurturing. Her first weekend was exhausting. Even though she had taught and even directed a school of nursing, she was not prepared for the reality of elder care in contemporary American nursing homes. What she encountered jolted her to the core. Here, within the confines of physically isolated, long-term care facilities, were the rejected beings of our technological health care revolution. Mere physical shells of forgotten grandmothers and grandfathers lay curled in embryonic positions. They were thin-skinned skeletons of organisms, only remnants of what once had been. They were beings whose spirits were crushed as calloused personnel carelessly tossed and bumped them about or painted their withered faces with bright lipstick and rouge and then laughed at their helplessness while they sat imprisoned, strapped in, one after another in a row of wheelchairs facing a meaningless series of incomprehensible color flashes on a television screen.

Occasionally a plea of, "Oh God, please help me," emanated from a toothless mouth, interrupting the incomprehensible stream of words flowing from the television. Other times a yellow puddle of fluid would appear on the floor from a diaper or Chux pad overflow from one of the few who had not yet had a permanent, indwelling, urinary catheter insertion.

Tomica did the best she could during her 12-hour weekend shifts. She fed, tended, and observed an isolated, abandoned segment of the population, outcast because of a society who does not know how to deal with them.

Faithfully, each weekend for 50 consecutive weeks Tomica and others like her left the outside world and came to be with the elders. They did so with compassion. Tomica felt a tremendous empathy for these discarded elders, often comparing them to how her own parents might be soon, and she hoped they would receive similar compassionate care as she gave here.

The other thing that happened with Tomica because of her tenure at this nursing home was her developing an awareness of and arriving at a conclusion in favor of the controversial issue of euthanasia, or "mercy killing." During her care she witnessed that many of these beings had moved beyond the state of ordinary, redemptive suffering and, being mere shadows of their former self, were actually almost punished because they had the unfortunate fate of living beyond their normal life span. This is true in most cases because of technological interventions for which they had not asked. Old grandmothers and grandfathers lingered with feeding tubes taped to their noses and catheters between their legs.

Tomica participated mechanically as she was instructed to insert needles into the backs of old hands with tissue-thin skin for the purpose of allowing the drip of antibiotic liquids into sclerotic veins to further prolong their helpless life.

Day after day, week after week, Tomica went there with compassion. She always did her best, but she increasingly asked why. Why are we prolonging the life of these souls who are so frail, so sick, and terminal?

At the end of a year's time Tyrone had successfully completed his first year of college, and Tomica had witnessed suffering she had not known

(Continued on next page)

before. Because of her compassion for their plight, she learned about euthanasic practices in the Netherlands and the Hemlock Society in California. She discovered a group of compassionate consumers sincerely concerned about the issues and practice of humanistic death and dying and learned about living wills and her legal rights to prevent the prolongation of her own life.

Observations and Insights

Initially, it was because of her son that Tomica went to work with the elderly. Once with them, her compassion caused her to lift their spirits and care for their frail bodies as best she could. Is compassion a part of your daily practice? To whom do you show compassion and why do you do so? Are you aware that compassion helps your spirit?

SUMMARY

The process of becoming a healer is multifaceted. Possessing the knowledge and having the skills of modalities and techniques is not enough. In order to most effectively practice those skills, it is important to have the overlay of healing traits. These traits are innate in some but also can be learned and developed. The traits inherent in effective healers include living from a place of authenticity, forgiveness, love, altruism, and compassion.

ASK YOURSELF

1. What are the four categories of guiding principles of a healer?
2. What are the five traits of a healer?
3. In which situations would it be appropriate to use tough love in your personal or professional life?
4. Which healing traits do you most identify with, and which do you have more difficulty identifying with?

REFERENCES

Gunn, A. E. (1999). The healing profession needs healers: The crisis in medical education. *Issues in Law and Medicine, 15*(2), 125–139.

Huxley, L. (1995). *You are not the target.* Metamorphous Press.

Keegan, L. (1994). *The nurse as healer.* Albany, NY: Delmar.

Novack, D. H., Epstein, R. M., & Paulsen, R. H. (1999). Toward creating physician-healers: Fostering medical students' self-awareness, personal growth, and well-being. *Academic Medicine, 74*(5), 516–520.

Slater, V. E., Maloney, J. P., Krau, S. D., & Eckert, C. A. (1999). Journey to holism. *Journal of Holistic Nursing, 17*(4).

Wardell, D. W., & Engebretson, J. (1998). Differentiating holistic practice and speculations for future directions. *Journal of Holistic Nursing, 16*(1), 57–67.

Attitudes and Behaviors
of Healers

Chapter Objectives

- Understand how the attitude of the caregiver affects the individuals they treat.
- Identify traits of caregivers whose attitudes positively impact their patients.
- Discuss how a sense of purpose impacts the healing environment.
- List the behaviors used in healing.

HEALING ATTITUDES

People assume caregiving roles due to a variety of reasons. Some people are abruptly thrust into the role due to an illness of a loved one while others deliberately choose a caring profession: social work, pharmacy, nurse, physician, or allied health worker. Still others assume roles in nursing homes, as a companion, or as a worker in some health care agency. Those who choose the professional route may be surprised to discover that they enter the workplace as a skilled technician. Often schools prepare students for technical or scholarly roles, leaving the more valuable lessons of caregiving to the experiential process. The potential for becoming a healer generally comes after study, experience, and a time of conscious attention to developing healing attitudes and behaviors.

Perhaps the single most important aspect of the attributes of a healer is attitude, for it is from attitudes that behaviors flow. Healing behaviors are manifested by the person who has developed the attitudes delineated here (Keegan, 1994):

- Joy and empowerment through service
- Caring for others as an extension of the self
- A sense of purpose

Joy and Empowerment through Service

When we consider the topic of joy and empowerment through service, the questions that come to mind are whose joy and whose empowerment? The answer gratifyingly is that both the server and the served are empowered. Any time service is performed from an awakened, conscious sense, there is an opportunity for positive attitudes and behaviors to ensue.

Although we still do not have scientific instrumentation to measure it, there are probably positive energies generated from positive thoughts and actions. Hence when we function with joy, we are a conduit for forces of empowerment.

HEALING STORY: Healing through Service to Others

The X-ray technician said, "Take it easy. As you lay down, the table may feel hard."

Beth lowered her heavy upper torso onto the narrow, sheet-covered X-ray table. Automatically, she pulled up her knees to protect her abdomen and lessen the knife-sharp pain that seemed to cut through her back and down to the groin. "You're doing great. You know I had five kidney stones myself," said the X-ray technician. "The first one was a lulu, mostly because I was scared and didn't know what was happening to me. Then they became kind of like anniversary presents, I got one every year for the next five years."

The technician laughed as he moved around the room positioning the equipment and stacking the film in preparation for picture taking. Beth was about to undergo an intravenous pyelogram, and had it not been for this jovial, garrulous man bouncing around his own, well-known territory, she might have panicked. However, despite her pain, she was amused and distracted. Also, he had survived five diagnosed stones, and they were not even sure if she had one yet. "Yeah," he continued "these stones can be a pain, but what the heck, everyone's gotta have some pain in life. Maybe ours is just gonna be kidney stones."

Comforted by his homespun philosophy, Beth relaxed on the metal table. The procedure was rapidly completed, and in time, as is the usual case, she was as good as new.

Observations and Insights

This story is an example of how a healer has the opportunity to perform joyful service through every procedure. Each time this occurs, both the client and the practitioners are empowered.

How did the X-ray technician make Beth feel better? Do you think that his comfortable laughing and talking improved the situation?

Have you ever had a medical experience improved because of a good health care provider? How did their behavior impact you?

Do you think that the X-ray technician was happier because of how he handled the situation?

A JOYFUL DISPOSITION

Mother Teresa, an Albanian Catholic nun, was renown for initiating an order of caregivers who minister to the terminally ill in hospices in India and Nepal. The criteria for selection to serve in her order are not the same as those in health care agencies in developed countries. The primary quality she looked for in her workers is a joyful disposition. The belief is that joyful service empowers. This is true no matter if the service is to assist one in healing and growth or to assist them in the transition process from living to dying. Mother Teresa was one of many

HEALING STORY: Healing with Humor and Skill

Jane smartly slapped the syringe, pushing the plunger in an exacting fashion to flip out the single, remaining air bubble as she held the small, calibrated tube high between her eyes and the ceiling light. She softly whistled a simple tune as she did this procedure, which was automatic to her now. She swiftly turned toward Sam and said, "Pull your britches down and roll over. This will just take a moment. Great, now take a deep breath. This will feel like a bee sting." With a quick, decisive movement she thrust the syringe deep into the gluteal muscle and with firm thumb pressure plunged the liquid medication into his body. The needle was out and discarded in the Sharps container before Sam could say "Ouch." He turned toward her and she was mock dancing with empty, upturned hands waving in the air, her whistle replaced by a jazzy song.

What could have been a serious, melodramatic incident was being transformed. Jane was a healer. It was not that she intended mockery or to make light of Sam's situation; it was just that it was natural for her to be cheerful. She was one of those people who without conscious awareness or practice just seemed to have a knack for balancing a situation. In Sam's case she naturally eased a possibly tense situation by music and movement, all done spontaneously and without premeditation. It was just her style.

Observations and Insights

In what ways did Jane's behavior make what could have been an embarrassing, hard situation better? Do you try to put patients at ease? What are the benefits you see when you do?

Sam probably felt much more comfortable with Jane than with another nurse after the injection. Why do you think Sam would feel better?

who have recognized that a joyful disposition is one of the basic ingredients to becoming an effective healer.

CULTIVATING A JOYFUL DISPOSITION

What if a happy disposition does not come naturally; can it be cultivated? In many instances the answer is yes. Most of us are inclined to repeat behavior that has been rewarded. This is as true in joyful service as in any other endeavor. The value in cultivating this attitude is not only that the recipient of the service feels better when in contact with the server, but also that the server reaps rewards. Contrast the personal joy of Jane, in the preceding story, as she momentarily loses herself in singing and dancing to the attitude of another caregiver who might react to the same situation by begrudging her time and the fact she had to be at work at all. Individuals like this would more than likely project their personal dissatisfaction not only to the other individual but also in the entire work environment.

Caring for Others as an Extension of the Self

Watson (1988, 1999) and Benner and Wrubel (1989) are among those who popularized the term *caring*. Mayeroff (1972) may have begun the movement when he listed and defined eight major ingredients for caring as follows:

1. *Knowledge.* In caring we need to know who the other is, what the needs are, and what will help. We need to know about ourselves, our strengths, and our limitations. Some things we will know cognitively, others intuitively.
2. *Alternating rhythms.* We move between past experiences and the present situation, between narrow and wide frameworks, between attention to detail and attention to the whole. Both are necessary and both are part of caring.
3. *Patience.* It is not that we wait passively for something to happen; it is that we give it our attention while allowing the person to go at their own pace.
4. *Honesty.* This is a positive, often active confrontation between ourselves and the other. We need to see the other as they are, not as we would like them to be.
5. *Trust.* This involves the appreciation of the other. Sometimes we care too much and overprotect and do not trust that the other can coparticipate. By trusting, we have confidence in our ability to help.
6. *Humility.* Humility is seeing others as existing for themselves, not simply to satisfy our needs. We treat each person and each situation as unique and relate with humility to each event.

7. *Hope.* Hope is not wishful thinking, but an expression of the fullness of the present. The process of caring is possible because hope is always present.

8. *Courage.* When caring we go into the unknown. Courage makes risk taking possible, but courage is not blind. It is informed by knowledge of the past and the present and by trust in our own and the other's ability to grow.

Canadian nurse-philosopher Roach (1987) established the "Five C's of Caring," which grew out of her general statement that caring is the human mode of being. She believes that caring is the basic element of being a person, that when we do not care, we lose our "being," and that caring is the way back into "being." Her five C's are as follows:

1. *Compassion.* A way of living born out of an awareness of one's relationship to all living creatures.

2. *Competence.* A state of having the knowledge, judgment, skills, energy, experience, and motivation required to respond adequately to the demands of one's professional responsibilities.

3. *Confidence.* The quality that fosters trusting relationships.

4. *Conscience.* A state of moral awareness; a compass directing one's behavior according to the moral fitness of things.

5. *Commitment.* A complex, affective response characterized by a convergence of one's desires and ones obligations and by a deliberate choice to act in accordance with them.

All of these concepts of caring are interwoven with the theory and anecdotes threaded throughout this text. Caring is an integral part of being a healer. The evolving focus on caring and healing may well be an exemplar to the growing field of alternative medicine. We are exploring ever deeper aspects of human science that include many ways of knowing as well as many ways of healing. This shift in focus toward caring and healing is a vision of the future (Watson, 1995). In more recent work, Watson (1999) proposes a reconstruction for the twenty-first century by calling for nursing to reclaim its caring-healing identity in the postmodern/transpersonal world. Dossey (2000) tells nurses to consider Florence Nightingale's heritage and rediscover caring/healing roots from the nineteenth century. She depicts Nightingale as a mystic, visionary, and healer and describes how contemporary healers can learn from her legacy.

A Sense of Purpose

Purpose involves the conscious direction and flow of a person's inner visions toward achieving a stated potential. Health care practitioners are accustomed to

HEALING STORY: Healing through Caring

"There, Maria, calm yourself. Look at me and take a deep breath. You can control yourself. Look at me as I speak," Lisa said.

"But I miss my mother so much," Maria sobbed. "It's hard being away from her."

Little, 11-year-old Maria quivered as her weepy brown eyes met Lisa's. They sat together in the middle of a boisterous, bustling summer camp dining room, a first-time camp staffer and a young girl from Mexico City. Maria felt totally displaced, alienated from her reality of city life and her native tongue and abandoned by the mother she adored. When the sounds of the dining room became too loud, Lisa led Maria outside.

They crouched down beside a huge, granite rock, the roar from the dining room blending into background noise. Lisa put her arm around Maria and picked up the conversation where they had left off.

As Maria's eyes filled with tears, she placed her right hand over her abdomen, "My stomach hurts so much," she wailed.

"I know it hurts," Lisa replied. Maria had a stomach ulcer and was on a specific regimen for treatment and control of symptoms. "Maria, do you notice how it hurts more when you cry?"

"Yes," Maria sobbed, burying her face in her knees, simulating a fetal position.

"Maria, I believe your heart and your stomach are connected. When your heart is sad and unhappy, your stomach hurts. What do you think about that?"

"Yes, you are right, my heart is sad."

"Maria, if you understand the connection, then we must find a way to help you have a happy heart. I think we both agree that is what is important and that is what will make your stomach better."

"But, I miss my mother; I love her so much."

"What a lucky mother you have to have such a sweet little girl to love her as much as you do." Lisa's heart went out to this small, miserable child. She was literally sobbing her heart out, a very unhealthy state, particularly for someone with stomach ulcers. Lisa looked at her and saw a part of herself reflected back. Her inner child, her own little-girl self related to this child who had come without any warning into her life.

"Maria, your mother is wiser than you suspect. When she tells you she has your best interests at heart, you must believe her. There are many important lessons to learn in this life, and your mother is aware of things you don't know yet." Maria watched Lisa intently, wondering if this new person would quiet her deep, unrelenting misery?

(Continued on next page)

"Maria, in this life people you love come and go. Sometimes you love someone so much, and that someone, for one reason or another, finds they must go away. If that person is the only one you love, then your heart can be broken by their absence. It can be a very sorrowful thing, and you can suffer greatly. That, Maria, is what is happening to you now. I understand your pain for I have experienced it myself."

Lisa told her the story about when she was a camper her age and about her own homesickness. As she spoke, she became a little girl again, and it was through these moments and this medium of dialogue and storytelling that the two connected. Lisa became an actual extension of Maria, and Lisa saw Maria as an extension of herself

Lisa continued, "Maria, what is important for you to do is to begin to love other people. You cannot go home now and your mother is not here, but other people are here. Do you think you can learn to love other people? Can you love me?"

"Oh yes," she fervently declared, "I do love you, but I miss my mother."

"Of course you miss her, but what is important now is to put your thoughts of her into a special safe place, maybe a small, magical locket that you can wear around your neck. Save and treasure your thoughts and memories, but store them in safekeeping for the next few weeks. Now is the time, and here is the place to learn new skills. To have a happy heart, you must learn to love other people. Know that I love you."

"And I love you," she said as the hoard of girls just dismissed from the dining hall came stampeding out. Lisa gave her a wink as Maria smiled and ran off with her friends for evening games.

Observations and Insights

There are many parts to an individual psyche. The mature grown-up incorporates the child within, the adult, and the parent. These parts correlate with the id, ego, and superego theory of mid-twentieth-century psychology. A person may not actually be a parent but integrates aspects of the critical and/or supportive parent into the judgmental aspect of the mature psyche. Likewise, even though the physical child has developed to adulthood, the psychological aspects of the playful and/or hurt child remain in the grown-up. Consequently, an adult working with a child has their own psychological child within and can put forth those aspects of themselves to more quickly and easily relate to the child.

In this case, Lisa extended her own inner child to help Maria make sense of her plight. Because of Lisa's concern, Maria felt the connection, the bridge building between them.

To become a healer in the fullest sense, one must experience the trials of many of life's challenges. To feel another's suffering, it is beneficial for

the healer to have some sense of the sorrow of the other. To compre-hend the suffering of loss, of sickness, and of sorrow, the healer must have developed empathy and a sense of connectedness with others. Through Lisa's extension to this child, she established their interconnect-edness and took on her sorrow. Lisa helped her and, by so doing, once again experienced the interconnectedness of all matter, mind, and spirit.

meeting goals and objectives. Purpose, while applicable to these finite ends, implies direction at a broader or higher level. Practitioners who work with pur-pose superimpose the guiding principle of health and healing onto all other clini-cal goals and objectives.

One of the major plights of many people in the modern world is their sense of purposelessness, boredom, and apathy. However, most healers have embarked on their own self-healing and crossed the river of ennui and apathy. In so doing, they have emerged with a clear and definite purpose. Healers are people who make a difference. What kind of people become all they can be, what kind of people become healers? Can everyone, regardless of station in life, have a sense of pur-pose? People with exceptional ability exist at every level, even the lowest levels of an organization, and in every walk of life. People in the process of becoming can be found in every type of job.

BEHAVIORS OF HEALERS

The behaviors of healers are born out of their skills, knowledge, and experience. Perhaps the most important quality that guides the development of healing behaviors is the healer's attitude. Some significant behaviors of healers include:

- Being fully present
- Listening
- Empathy
- Attention to detail

Being Fully Present

Healers use all their senses to be completely present during successful healing encounters. Being fully present includes developing listening skills, attending to detail, and learning the art of empathy (see Figure 17-1).

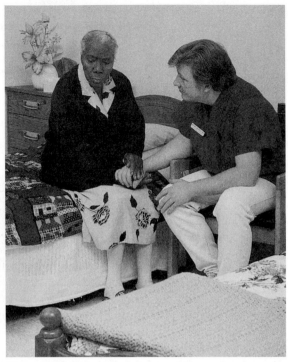

Figure 17-1 Being fully present is an important key to a successful healing encounter.

The following is a list of ways to increase "being fully present":

- Situate your body so you directly face the person with whom you are working.
- Focus eye contact on the person receiving attention.
- Focus mental thoughts on the immediate event.
- Block distracting motion, words, and sounds from entering your conscious attention.

HEALING STORY: Healing through Presence

"Help, somebody help us, Saul's bleeding." Not unaccustomed to trauma, Luis, a therapist at the local hospital, tossed down his popcorn and quickly entered the roller-skating rink. Three swift skate strokes later he arrived at Saul's side, and sure enough, there was blood gushing from his face. Following a quick physical assessment, Luis ascertained that he had no other major injuries except the overt bleeding from his nasopharnyx region.

"Okay Saul, get up. I'm going to take you over to the bench." Luis looked directly into his eyes. He met Luis's gaze and followed his authoritative direction. Together, skate to skate, they wobbled their way to the side. Within seconds Luis had Saul lying on a bench. Oblivious to anything else, he kept his attention fixed on Saul and commanded one of the gaping onlookers to get some ice and paper towels from the concession stand. "The rest of you move back so we will have some more room."

"Now breathe deeply and think of something pleasant," Luis said. "I'm going to move my hand for a moment and look into your mouth." As he moved his hand to release the pressure over Saul's mouth, blood gushed from the area of his upper lip. He replaced his hand and said, "Saul, now I want you to slow your breathing. I have my hand over your mouth, so breathe deeply through your nose. Here we go now, in through your nose, pause, and now out." After a few more breaths he felt his panic begin to subside. He stopped trembling. "Saul, you're going to be okay." Just then, someone dropped a paper towel filled with ice onto Luis's lap. Without looking up, Luis thanked them, and placed the ice pack over Saul's lip. "Now, let's continue, breathe in deeply and release it, good, that's the idea. Now again." After a few more times he said, "Saul, the ice has been on a while now, so I'm going to release my hand, remove the ice, and take another look." This time the bleeding had clearly stopped. There was a small laceration on the lip where the tooth had punctured the skin when he fell to the wooden floor. Obviously, there would be no need for emergency care. Realizing that the bleeding had stopped, Saul sat up.

"I feel much better now. Can I have a drink?"

"Good idea." Luis sent another child to get Saul a soda. The hovering crowd began to disburse. Saul and Luis sat chatting as the soda arrived.

They sat a few more minutes as he gulped the drink and then Saul said, "Can I skate again now?"

"It's all right with me," Luis replied, "but don't you want to call home and tell them about your fall."

"Naw, I feel fine now. I'll tell them when I get home." So with a puffy, red lip and tear-stained cheeks little Saul, whom Luis had never seen before and would likely never see again, shyly thanked him. Before Luis could answer, Saul skated off into rink and became indistinguishable in the crowd from which only minutes ago he had emerged.

Observations and Insights

During the healing process healers are rarely distractible. The act of healing requires full presence. Being fully present is a skill that can be acquired but rarely has to be. That is because during the healing act

(Continued on next page)

itself the healer's attention naturally focuses on the act and on the person, which is the nature of healing. During the time Luis was with Saul he had no cognition of the people surrounding him, how long the healing act took, or the fact that the care took place in a setting with an extraordinarily high noise level. This healer's attention was completely focused on the child and the desire to stop the bleeding.

Listening

An essential aspect of communication is active listening. Active listening includes eye contact, attentive nonverbal behavior, and a genuine effort to be empathetic (see Figure 17-2). Listening of this type prepares the healer to clearly reflect the client's thoughts and feelings so that a genuine understanding between the client and the healer will occur.

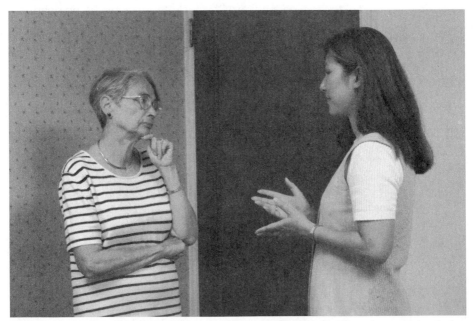

Figure 17-2 Active listening and concentrating on the interaction with the client enhance communication.

HEALING STORY: Healing through Listening

"Diane, this is Betty Barnes, could I talk to you for a few minutes?" Diane was busy, but knew if Betty were calling, it must be important.

"What's up?" Diane said. "It's been a year since I've heard from you. Are you okay?" Betty was one of those numerous people in life whom you get to know and like, but the relationship stays on an acquaintance level only because there is not enough time to devote to fostering a meaningful friendship. Diane wanted to keep up with Betty, but did not get to see or talk to her often.

"I've had some hard times lately," Betty replied. "I'm having so much trouble and facing some difficult decisions, and I just wondered if you would see me professionally, to counsel me?"

Diane was quick to reply, "Betty, I closed my client-based counseling practice last year and I am no longer doing that, but I will talk to you as a friend. Can you come over?"

"I couldn't bother you like that. I'll only come if I can pay you."

"Nonsense, I wouldn't charge you even if I still had my practice." The last time Diane had talked to her, Betty was adjusting to the financial strains of a divorce and was between jobs. "How about at three o'clock this afternoon?"

"Are you sure? I don't want to impose on you."

"Don't worry, come over then and we will have tea and talk. See you then." Diane hung up the phone knowing Betty must be in some sort of pain; she was not someone who easily asked for help. Diane readjusted her afternoon schedule and went back to work.

Promptly at three o'clock Betty arrived, leaning on a cane and carrying a rubber, air-filled ring encased in a pillowcase. Diane gave her a hug and said. "Let's go back to my office and sit down." She was already brewing a pot of herbal tea for her guest.

"If you don't mind, I'd like to stand for a while. I had to sit in the car on the way over here and I can't sit for very long at a time anymore. Mostly I have to lie flat, but I brought my special cushion along for when I do sit." Diane's mental wheels churned; Betty only lived a 15-minute drive away; she must be in intense pain.

"Okay, come walk down the hall with me while I get the tea tray." Betty hobbled along behind her. "Betty, you are obviously having more physical problems than when I saw you last," Diane said as she contemplated the possible reason Betty had come. Diane had known Betty for about five years, mostly professionally, and had always liked her spunky nature and willingness to try new, innovative approaches. She worked well with

(Continued on next page)

people and had many of the attributes of a healer herself. Now, at what should be the peak of her life at age 35, Betty was in trouble. Back in Diane's cozy office, Betty circled the chair, adjusted her cushion, and carefully lowered her tiny frame over the circle of air.

"My back is worse. I'm in pain all the time. I didn't renew my teaching contract last year. None of my colleagues know the severity of my pain. I'm so embarrassed, they think I took the year off to travel. I thought I'd be better by now. It's been six months, but I'm no better, and the money is running out. My parents have offered to help, but I want to be independent." She raced on, with all the pain and misery of six months of confinement flowing out, as Diane sat across from her transfixed by the outpouring of suffering. Betty continued, "I've been to the pain clinic, and they have me on some potent analgesics, but full relief is seldom. What I want is your opinion and advice about the options I've delineated." She looked at her watch, "but I don't want to take up too much of your time."

"Betty, relax. I have the time to spend with you now." Settling back she took her first sip of the now cold tea. Betty didn't seem to notice.

"I guess the divorce hit me harder than I expected it to. I feel so alone. He took everything, but I didn't care. At least I don't have to see him now. I just never expected it. And now all this pain to boot. How could life have been so rosy, and now it's so bleak? But I don't want to get mired down in self-pity, so here are what I see as options. First, what do you think about this Pain and Rehabilitation Center in California. I've heard the doctors there can turn around chronic pain. Is this true?" She thrust a brochure about the clinic into Diane's hand. "Second, since I can't hold a job now, what do you think about taking charity from my family? They have offered to let me move back in with them, but it would make me feel so dependent. What would you do in this case? The other thing I would like to do is study and read, but that seems so lazy, what do you think? Honestly, I feel so weak for not being able to come to terms with these issues by myself, but if you don't mind, I really would value your opinion."

Over the next few minutes Diane responded to her questions and gave her the feedback she requested. Betty affirmed that Diane's opinions matched her own, yet Diane was unsure at the time if she only said that to please her. Diane sensed that the other thing Betty needed and was reticent to ask for was someone to really listen to her. Any sincere listener would have been moved to compassion and been willing to direct her to get the care she so obviously needed. They talked for an hour. Then as promptly and politely as she arrived, Betty left.

Diane did not hear from her again for another year, when, once again, as unexpectedly as the previous year, Betty called. "Hi," she said, "I called to tell you I followed all of your suggestions and I am much better. I went to the pain clinic and was able to get long-term relief. I moved in with my parents and have spent the year in seclusion reading and studying. At this point I am about to reenter the outside world, and I wanted you to be the first to know. I simply wanted to thank you for the answers and information you gave me last year. In a way, you saved my life. I shall be eternally grateful." After a few pleasantries they hung up. A few months later Diane saw Betty in the grocery store, still with a cane, but with a smile and an obvious sense of independence, a trait she prized over many others.

Observations and Insights

The desire and ability to listen is one of the behaviors of healers. One never knows when important moments, windows of healing opportunities, will emerge. Through the vehicle of genuine listening healing can be evoked.

- *If Betty came to see you, how would you have responded? What options would you have suggested to her?*
- *How did Diane's behavior help Betty? Many times people simply want someone to bounce their feelings off of. Do you listen when your patients or friends have problems?*

LISTENING TRAPS

Sometimes even healers become so involved and rushed in trying to accomplish their work that they forget some of the essentials of effective listening and lapse into poor listening skills. Answer the list of questions in Figure 17-3 and rate yourself to check your listening skills. Answer yes, no, or sometimes. If you have a predominance of "yes" or "sometimes" responses, you might consider working on your listening skills.

Empathy

Empathy is the art of communicating to others that we have understood how they are feeling and what makes them feel that way. It is closely related to listening but goes a step beyond. Some of the benefits of empathy include:

- Increases the feeling of being connected to another
- Fosters self-esteem in those to whom you extend yourself

	YES	NO
■ Does your mind tend to wander and think about something else when your client is talking to you?	____	____
■ Are you so involved in your own feelings that it is impossible to let go of your own thoughts and really listen to another?	____	____
■ Do you mentally tune the other person out to prepare your own response to the issue under discussion?	____	____
■ Do you tend to jump ahead of the speaker and reach conclusions before you have heard the speaker out?	____	____
■ Do you often think you know what the other person is going to say before he or she has finished saying it?	____	____
■ Are you in a hurry to impart your ideas to the conversation or relate your experiences when the other is talking?	____	____
■ Do you have a tendency to finish sentences or supply words for the other person?	____	____
■ Do you get caught up with insignificant facts and details and miss the emotional tone of the conversation?	____	____
■ Do you listen with half your attention tuned toward giving advice, solving the problem, or figuring out what to say to make the other person feel better rather than allowing the person to finish speaking before trying to solve their problem?	____	____
■ Do you realize that good listening skills take consistent effort?	____	____

Figure 17-3 Listening skills check list

■ Demonstrates to another that you genuinely accept them as they are

■ Assists the other to increase self-awareness

■ Allows the client to be less critical and increasingly caring toward themselves

HEALING STORY: Healing through Empathy

Four health care students approached a bed in a semidarkened room. A fragile, elderly woman was lying semiconscious, her withered face turned upward and unseeing eyes gazing into a dimension beyond the huddled group. The fluorescent lights flickered on as one of the students began to prepare the patient for a demonstration of how to do a neurological status check. The conversation flowed over the body of the bedridden Mrs. Smith, who remained silent. As the lights grew brighter, the instructor noticed a quiet, withdrawn woman sunken in a corner of the couch adjacent to the bed. The instructor left the group and walked over to her.

"Hello, my name is Ms. Ostralski and I am here with the students to care for Mrs. Smith. Are you a relative?"

"Yes, I'm her daughter, Mrs. Lanshen." She pulled herself up, became animated, and continued. "Do you know what is going to happen to my mother? She has been here three days, and I don't know anything."

"Do you live here in town?" the instructor inquired. At this point the students were getting squirmy, wondering when their instructor would finish this conversation and get back to the task for which they entered the room.

"Yes, we've lived here for years. However, Mother lived in a distant town until three weeks ago. We have just finished closing up her house and moving her here to live with us. Everything has been going well, until this. Now I just don't know what to do." She reached in her purse for a tissue and wiped the corners of her eyes as her voice became tremulous. "We finally thought we had things stabilized, and now this." Tears began to flow and the wide-eyed students observed their instructor to see what she would do next.

"Mrs. Lanshen, have you just come from work?" It was about 6:00 P.M. and she was well dressed.

"Yes, I have" she said, gaining composure. "I work full time and I have Mom, and now I do not know what to do? Can I expect that she will get better? Will she have to go to a nursing home? Only a few days ago we were talking about moving into a larger home so there would be more room for mother. Now this."

Mrs. Smith was 89 years old, and like so many others in her age group, she had suffered a stroke. She was paralyzed on the left side of her body, incontinent of urine, and unable to feed herself without assistance. Her speech was intermittently incoherent and her activity curtailed. Within a brief period her daughter witnessed her vigorous, independent mother become feeble, dependent, and possibly on the verge of death. "Will she get better?" her daughter implored.

(Continued on next page)

"Mrs. Lanshen, it is difficult to assess how your mother will progress. Generally, there is some improvement in the condition with time. She will require special care in the future. Have you thought about placing her in a nursing home?"

"Yes, I know one in our area, and my husband and I have discussed it."

"Good. I'm sure that once you have more facts from the medical team, you will be able to proceed by working with the Social Service office here in this hospital. They will be able to assist you in making the necessary transport, admission, and financial arrangements. When that time draws closer, there will be someone to work with you specifically."

The instructor noticed how tired she appeared. "Mrs. Lanshen, I'll bet you haven't been home from work yet. Let's inquire about when the doctor will be here so you can talk to him."

"That would be great. For two days I've been here after work until 8:00 P.M., and I haven't seen him yet. I could rest so much easier if I knew what to expect."

The instructor sent one of the students out only to discover that Mrs. Smith's doctor had gone home for the day. He had been in to see her before her daughter had arrived. They relayed the information to Mrs. Lanshen and told her they would inform the charge nurse as well as place a note on Mrs. Smith's chart for the doctor to call her daughter tomorrow. They procured her telephone number at home and at work and wrote a note to follow through with verbal and written communication.

Mrs. Lanshen stood up. "I feel so much better now. You're the first person to talk to me about Mom in two evenings. I feel she is in good hands so I can go now."

"Do go and get some rest now; we will take good care of your Mom." The instructor gave her a pat on the back as she discarded her tissue and gave us all a big smile.

"Thank you all" she said as she swiftly left the room, closing the door behind her.

"Now," the instructor said to the students, "let's proceed with the neurological status exam."

Observations and Insights

Empathy, the capacity for participating in another's feelings or ideas, is an integral behavior of healers. Empathy should not be confused with sympathy, which means a relationship between people wherein whatever affects one similarly affects the other. During sympathy there is mutual or parallel susceptibility to the prevailing condition. Sympathy is not conducive to the healing process; empathy is.

Too often in the technological health care delivery system empathy is abandoned or neglected in the cause of expediency. In the above situation the daughter and the mother are part and parcel of the same package. The mother may be in the bed, but the daughter requires as much, if not more, empathic attention to be healed.

Attention to Detail

When we attend to the details of care, we make sure that all aspects are considered. As we become increasingly meticulous in caring for others, we also note that organization and order improves in our own lives. The benefits of attention to details include:

- Organizes our practice
- Assures an orderly completion of work
- Improves the odds of successful outcomes
- Provides a system for inclusion of all aspects of the endeavor

HEALING STORY: Healing through Attention to Detail

"Take a deep breath and think of something pleasant. One, two, three, now," and with that Janice, with one quick, well-planned motion injected an 18-mm intravenous needle into the subclavian space just above her client's right collarbone. As Marsha lay silent on the bed, Janice deftly threaded approximately 6 inches of sterile transparent filament into the vein she had skillfully entered. Within seconds she connected the thread of tubing protruding from the chest to the prepared line coming from the liquid-filled plastic pouch on a stand above Marsha's bed. Just as quickly she procured a readied dressing complete with prophylactic antibiotic ointment and secured the entire apparatus snugly onto her client's chest. Next Janice wrote the date, time, and her initials on a label. This way, she assured Marsha, anyone can tell at a glance when this procedure was started, the relative degree of freshness of the site, and when the topical dressing should be changed. This sounded good to Marsha, and it also felt as if Janice knew what she was doing.

(Continued on next page)

Janice is an intravenous (IV) therapy nurse. For the past 11 years she has been one of eight nurses responsible for starting, maintaining, and properly terminating all the IVs at Community Hospital. To get her job, Janice first became a registered nurse with a firm knowledge of anatomy and physiology. She worked in a variety of staff nurse positions and became comfortable in dealing with several different personality types, fear levels, and pain thresholds. She became a confident, disciplined, and attentive caregiver. One day Janice read about IV therapy nurses at another hospital and decided to approach the administration about the possibility of starting a program at Community Hospital. Much to her delight, and the patient's benefit, her proposal was accepted and Janice was given the position of organizing the IV Therapy Department. To do the best possible job, Janice joined the Association of IV Therapy Nurses, and after attending her first meeting, she voraciously read everything she could on the topic and immediately began manipulative skill building on plastic surrogate dummies. Within a few short weeks of her new appointment Janice was proficient with IVs and ready to begin using her new skills. Within two months she mastered several techniques and began an in-service program to teach four other nurses who had expressed interest in this new field. She wrote a curriculum, teaching objectives, and outcome criteria. She taught the classes, supervised the clinical practice, and determined who passed and who required more training. Janice was a stickler for detail. She knew skills were important, and so did the other nurses. One by one she built up the department until she had all three shifts covered all the time. It became known in the community that if you want expert IV nursing care, Community Hospital offers it. The hospital infection rate decreased and patient satisfaction increased.

Janice was low keyed, not well known by name, but a very important person who will be long remembered as a disciplined professional because of the skillful care rendered through attention to detail.

Observations and Insights

Attention to detail is a behavior common to healers. Without this attention, procedures, techniques, and care rendered are inclined to be sloppy and fraught with flaws. Without attention to detail an important step in a procedure may be glossed over or inadvertently omitted altogether, thereby rendering a technique or procedure that still might work but with increased hazards to the recipient. For example, if Janice were not attentive to and expert at each step in the IV procedure, several things could happen. If her needle insertion technique was not mastered, then she could cause damage as she probes for veins, contaminate the sterile field setting up a site for infection, or cause suffering to the unwary recipient of her services. Because Janice believes that she is a nurse healer, she values the importance of her technical skill as a significant component of a healer's repertoire. She, and others like her, conscientiously practice and perfect skill building until it is tight and masterful. These healers recognize that attention to detail is an important part of their healing regimen.

SUMMARY

Our attitudes can affect everything in our lives and as health care providers can affect the lives of others. Throughout this chapter we have seen examples of how the behavior and attitude of the health care provider can affect their patients with comfort, compassion, and peace of mind in highly stressful situations. Learning to be kind, compassionate, and understanding is not hard, it is already within us all, but we must learn to utilize and recognize those parts of ourselves and use that to help others.

ASK YOURSELF

1. What are three significant attitudes of healers?
2. What are four significant behaviors of healers?
3. How do attitudes influence the development of behaviors?
4. How do the attitudes and behaviors of healers that you know compare with those of the healers in the stories in this chapter.

REFERENCES

Benner, P., & Wrubel, J. (1989). *The primacy of caring.* Menlo Park, CA: Addison-Wesley.

Dossey, B. (2000). *Florence Nightingale: Mystic, visionary, healer.* Springhouse, PA: Springhouse.

Keegan, L. (1994). *The nurse as healer.* Albany, NY: Delmar.

Mayeroff, M. (1972). *On caring.* New York: Harper & Row.

Roach, M. S. (1987). *The human act of caring.* Ottawa: Canadian Hospital Association.

Watson, J. (1988). *Nursing: Human science and human care.* New York: National League for Nursing.

Watson, J. (1995). Nursing's caring–healing paradigm as exemplar for alternative medicine. *Alternative Therapies in Health and Medicine, 1*(3), 64–69.

Watson, J. (1999). *Postmodern nursing and beyond.* London: Churchill Livingstone.

Healing Ourselves
and Our Environment

Chapter Objectives

- Become aware of why healing ourselves is important.
- Relate to another's story and find similarities in your own life.
- Build self-care knowledge skills.
- Discover why healing our environment is part of a healer's journey.

INTRODUCTION

The process of healing is multifaceted. One reason is because more than one person is involved in the healing process. First there is the healer, second there is the recipient or group of recipients, and third there is the environment in which both the healer and the recipient(s) dwell. In many instances, all three may be impaired and thus all three have to be healed. The healer may be overtaxed and unable to fully focus due to stress, the recipient may seek help for a physical or mental impairment, and the environment may be impaired due to musty air, contaminated carpets, sick building syndrome, or noxious noise and fumes in the air. Healing then involves healing the healer, healing the client/patient, and healing the environment. The most important place to begin, and the entity that we have most control over, is to heal ourselves.

HEALING YOURSELF

Very little attention was given to the needs of caregivers a generation ago. The fact that health care practitioners had serious self-care needs was first acknowledged in the 1970s and 1980s. At that time, it was primarily nurses who aroused interest in the topic, a profession that itself had only begun to examine and take care of itself during the 1960s and 1970s. Prior to that time, many caregivers worked tirelessly and either burned out and left the profession or worked in a state of chronic fatigue. In the 1980s and 1990s a host of seminars, retreats, and conferences were given on "Healing the Healer" or "Care for the Caregiver."

Books and magazine and journal articles on self-care became popular, and for the first time, caregivers and health professionals began to pay attention to meeting their own health needs. Many proceeded to move beyond basic self-care and focused on their own self-actualization.

Self-Care Begins with Assessment

The first step in the self-care process is self-assessment. Before you decide on a course of action, it is important to determine the baseline. Self-assessment tools now exist as part of many treatment regimens and can be found in a number of reference books. Assessments cover facets of the body, mind, and spirit and have to do with actualizing our human potentials. Assessing your strengths and weaknesses in the area of your potentials takes some time and attention and spending a few minutes apart from current demands.

CIRCLE OF HUMAN POTENTIAL

The dance of life involves many possibilities. The circle of human potential is composed of six areas: physical, mental, emotional, spiritual, relationships, and choice (see Figure 18-1). The circle is an ancient symbol of wholeness. The circle in this model has six separate but equally important parts. When any part is incomplete, the entire circle loses its completeness since all parts create the whole.

People are complex feedback loops. As we become aware of these feedback loops, we are able to understand our body-mind connections. Think of all the life experiences that run through your body, mind, and spirit and consider ways that you can enhance your lifestyle behaviors to help develop and support all your potentials.

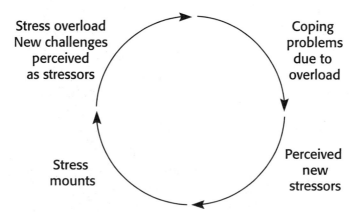

Figure 18-1 Circle of human potential

HEALING STORY: Healing with Alternative Therapies

Maya is a 54-year-old health care professional. Two years ago she had an episode of atrial fibrillation interspersed with periods of tachycardia and shortness of breath. She went to a cardiologist who examined her, took an electrocardiogram, and put her on a Holter monitor for 24-hour cardiac readings. On the return visit she was told that she had developed an ectopic focus on the electrical stimulation area of the heart. Her options were (1) begin taking a beta blocker to counteract the arrhythmia, (2) have cardiac surgery consisting of an ablation (cauterizing the extra foci node on the exterior wall of the heart), or (3) wait and do nothing and see what happens next.

Maya took this information and considered the alternatives. She looked back over the previous few years and reflected on her general heath status, what she had done wrong and where and how she could alter certain lifestyle behaviors. She realized that this was not a sudden occurrence, but rather a gradual building of symptoms that finally erupted in the crescendo of a marked arrhythmia. For the past two years, her workload had increased, she had accepted more professional external committee and organizational activities, and had growing children that continually required psychological and physical needs. During this period she had paid little attention to the fact that she was going through menopause and had not added any vitamin, mineral, herbal, or hormonal supplements. She concluded that she was depleted in several areas of her human potential. She sought the guidance of a close friend and medical colleague who was knowledgeable of alternative and complementary therapies. Together, they worked out a noninvasive, nonpharmaceutical approach to Maya's immediate medical problem. Maya reported back to the cardiologist that she was going to try an alternative approach and bypass the medication and/or surgical route. The cardiologist wished her luck but added that he did not think highly of her choice and would await her return to his office when her chosen alternative route failed.

Maya and her health care provider strategized the following approach:

■ Include the following supplements in her diet:

   (a) Vitamins and minerals
   (b) Calcium: necessary for cardiac contractions
   (c) Magnesium: necessary for cardiac contractions
   (d) Potassium: necessary for cardiac contractions
   (e) Full-potency multivitamins: necessary for augmentation of food vitamins

    (f) Complement of trace minerals: add to the arsenal of helpful supplements

    (g) Antioxidants: necessary as the body ages

■ Begin taking the herbal supplement co-enzyme Q10: a strong antioxidant that feeds cells so the body can operate at an optimum level. This substance is known to revitalize heart function and relieve heart disease symptoms.

■ Reduce stress.

■ Resign from the extra committees and organizations: Be candid and explain the reason why she was resigning to the people involved.

■ Get more sleep: Turn off the television in the evenings and spend 10 hours in bed.

■ Reduce the amount of care and concern given to the children; ask them to accept more responsibilities.

■ Add relaxation modalities to her monthly regimen.

■ Schedule a monthly massage, more often if needed or desired.

■ Take time after work or between jobs to purposely lounge and do nothing.

■ Change the family's diet to reduce sugar, fats, and artificial substitutes and increase quantities of fresh, whole foods.

These changes were discussed with Maya's family, close friends, and employer. She decided that it was no secret that she was in this condition so candidly explained her plight to those it affected. Frankly she felt so bad that she thought if she did not do something dramatic and soon she might actually die from heart failure. She purposely did not begin an exercise regimen. At the time she instituted these measures, she still had constant tachycardia and needed to get that under control prior to doing anything physical. Fortunately, the acute episode occurred at the end of an academic school year, and she gave notice that she would not teach summer school but would take the summer off and rest.

For those three summer months, Maya lounged in a hammock, read books, and ate fresh, whole foods. Even then, at the beginning of the summer, any extra physical exertion would initiate the arrhythmia. However, as the summer progressed, she shed a few pounds, became increasingly relaxed, and began to feel stronger. The intervals between the episodes of tachycardia decreased and she felt herself growing stronger and increasingly conscious of her purpose for living. She began, for example, to literally "smell the roses" and see flocks of birds that had been all around her for years but she had been too busy to enjoy.

At summer's end, the arrhythmia had subsided and Maya returned to her teaching job. She purposely reduced her load and continued to find ways to disengage from activities that initiated the stress response. At the

(Continued on next page)

same time she added relaxation modalities and kept up her supplements, massages, and meditation program. By late fall, she decided she was well enough to begin an exercise program and did so gradually.

Two years later, Maya felt stronger than she had in years. Her energy level was high, the arrhythmia had ceased, and her exercise tolerance was good. Her children had become increasingly self-sufficient and had even acquired scholarships to help finance their college education.

In looking back over the experience, Maya began to see what seemed at the time to be a terrifying and life-threatening event as an opportunity for growth and self-care she would not have otherwise had. Looking back, she believed the "event" was a "wake-up call" that forced her to pay conscious attention to her life. Because of the conscious attention she was able to initiate enlightened self-care and heal herself.

Observations and Insights

Maya's story is characteristic of many people. In our fast-paced, technological world it is easy to become so preoccupied with the demands of everyday living that attention to self-care does not become a priority until an individual is confronted with an illness. Unfortunately for many, not all people respond as well as Maya did to her lifestyle reversal. Are you one of those millions who are on the treadmill of life and have not paused long enough to take a good, close, introspective look at your self-care assets and deficits?

Personal Options to Stay Fit

Try some of the following ideas to prevent setbacks and stay fit:

- *Determine your motive, goals, and expectations.* Burnout researchers often support the fact that what brings you to work is also what burns you out. Often it is the most idealistic, altruistic, and committed providers who burn out first.

- *Take advantage of ongoing education.* Take time to attend classes for the acquisition of new knowledge. Take the opportunity to improve communication and conflict resolution skills that will enhance empathy and relationships with others.

- *Develop self-awareness and a personal philosophy of life.* Before getting into difficult situations, it is important to know your own basic belief system.

- *Promote interdisciplinary collaboration and develop a support network.* The challenge for an interdisciplinary team is not just to work more closely with each other but to work together toward a common goal. When one member in the group needs help and support, other members can give it. Opportunities to give and receive support are enhanced since they contribute to morale and camaraderie under stressful working conditions.

■ *Listen to your body.* Learn to consciously tune into the subtle signals your body sends to tell you in advance of an illness. Eat and drink in moderation and rest when your internal feedback loop sends signals that you have done enough.

CHRONIC DISEASE AND SELF-CARE

Approximately 80% of all illnesses in the United States fall under the category of chronic disease, meaning that such conditions tend to last for long periods of time and to regularly recur. Unlike acute conditions, which usually respond well to conventional medical care, chronic health ailments usually will not resolve until their underlying systemic causes are addressed, not just their presenting symptoms. Such an approach to health is one of the hallmarks of holistic medicine and includes paying attention to diet, nutrition, lifestyle, home and work environments, prevention, exercise, and social and spiritual factors, along with a variety of treatment approaches that can be used separately or in tandem with each other. Using a holistic approach in conjunction with some of the alternative and complementary therapies works very well in the self-care arena.

Many treatment approaches lend themselves well to self-care enhancement, especially with regard to ailments that are self-limiting and not life threatening. Examples of such approaches include but are not limited to dietary measures, nutritional supplementation, herbal remedies, aromatherapy, massage, traditional Chinese medicine (TCM), flower essences, aquatherapy, and a regular exercise program (see Chapters 6–15 for a description of most available modalities).

As you begin to use some self-care options, you may experience a period of acceptance and rejection of various modalities and approaches as you discover what works best for you. Such a period of adaptation is normal to all new endeavors. Over time, you will increase your understanding of the therapies and be able to utilize them with confidence. As you try new approaches and modalities, be patient and open to a new sense of adventure.

BASIC SELF-CARE APPROACHES FOR MAINTAINING AND IMPROVING YOUR HEALTH

Too many people mistake health and wellness to mean simply the absence of disease. Health is far more than this. Derived from an ancient Anglo-Saxon word that means "to make whole," *health* means "wholeness." And to be whole means to have an abundant supply of energy and overall sense of satisfaction and contentment physically, emotionally, mentally, and spiritually. A person operating on this level arises each day refreshed from a good night's sleep and eager to face the new day. Such people not only have greater levels of energy, they also tend to be happier and to have fuller, more deeper relationships with their spouses or partners, families, friends, and co-workers. As high a standard as that may seem, it is attainable. To achieve it, though, you have to be willing to take the necessary steps that will lead you to health's door.

To be really healthy means:

- Effectively and easily being able to manage stress by accessing your innate levels of creativity to both solve the problems in your life and create further successes and prosperity
- Fully enjoying daily interactions with others
- Having a fuller, more intimate love life
- Feeling connected to your family, friends, and community

Practitioners of the healing arts recognize that our bodies, emotions, and thoughts are all interconnected. Therefore, achieving improvement in one level of our being will create improvement in all the others. This makes it possible, by focusing on the physical, for instance, to resolve emotional problems as well. As an example, consider how easily a feeling of depression or anxiety can be lifted simply by participating in a sports activity that you enjoy, such as golf, tennis, kayaking, or taking a hike in a natural setting.

Some basic components to achieving optimal health include diet, exercise, stress reduction, relaxation and introspection, having a sense of purpose, and a close connection with at least one other person.

Obesity in America

Americans are getting fatter, and that fat kills. As elementary as this statement sounds, research shows that it is overwhelmingly true. Consider the fact that the United States has the highest rate of obesity of any industrialized nation in the world, despite the fact that we also pay the most amount of money for health care of any nation and have the finest medical system on earth (Must, Spadano, Coakley, Field, Colditz, & Dietz, 1999). (Obesity is defined as being 20 pounds or more above one's ideal body weight.) A full 60% of all adult Americans fall into this category, and studies indicate that an even higher percentage of our children are following suit (Ludwig, Pereira, Kroenke, Hilner, Van Horn, Slattery, & Jacobs, 1999). Obesity is a major cause of mortality in the United States and an epidemic that has surged in the past decade and now affects nearly one in five adults, killing some 300,000 a year (Allison, Fontaine, Manson, Stevens, & Van

RESEARCH BOX: Obesity Epidemic in the United States

The increasing prevalence of obesity is a major public health concern, since obesity is associated with several chronic diseases. To monitor trends in state-specific data and to examine changes in the prevalence of obesity among adults, a cross-sectional random-digit telephone survey (Behavioral Risk Factor Surveillance System) of noninstitutionalized adults aged 18 years or older was conducted by the Centers for Disease Control and Prevention and state health departments from 1991 to 1998. The results were that the prevalence of obesity (defined as a body mass index of 30 kg/m^2) increased from 12.0% in 1991 to 17.9% in 1998. A steady increase was observed in all states; in both sexes; across age groups, races, educational levels; and regardless of smoking status. The greatest magnitude of increase was found in the following groups: 18–29-year-olds (7.1%–12.1%), those with some college education (10.6%–17.8%), and those of Hispanic ethnicity (11.6%–20.8%). The magnitude of the increased prevalence varied by region (ranging from 31.9% for the mid-Atlantic to 67.2% for the South Atlantic, the area with the greatest increases) and by state (ranging from 11.3% for Delaware to 101.8% for Georgia, the state with the greatest increases). The conclusion of this study is that obesity continues to increase rapidly in the United States. To alter this trend, strategies and programs for weight maintenance as well as weight reduction must become a higher public health priority.

Source: Mokdad, A. H., Serdula, M. K., Dietz, W. H., Bowman, B. A., & Koplan, J. P. (1999). The spread of the obesity epidemic in the United States, 1991–1998. *Journal of the American Medical Association, 282*(16), 1519–1522.

Itallie, 1999). One study by the U.S. Centers for Disease Control and Prevention showed that the number of Americans considered obese, defined as being more than 30% over their ideal body weight, soared from about one in eight in 1991 to nearly one in three in 1998 (data were calculated using the Behavioral Risk Factor Surveillance System) (Mokdad, Serdula, Dietz, Bowman, & Koplan, 1999).

Other recent research has found that more than 50% of Americans are overweight and 22% are obese, even though weight loss products and services are a $33-billion-a-year industry (Allison et al., 1999). Being overweight has been strongly associated with greater risk of certain illnesses, including heart disease, high cholesterol and blood pressure, diabetes, stroke, and some cancers. Recent studies in the *New England Journal of Medicine* of more than 1 million Americans concluded that obese people run a significant risk of dying early, even if they do not smoke and are otherwise healthy (Manson, Willett, & Stampfer, 1995; Stevens et al., 1998).

UNDERLYING CAUSES OF OBESITY

Why as a nation are we so fat? Could it be that we consume the most fast foods, eat the most sugar, drink the most soda, and eat more hamburgers, hot dogs, and pizza than any other country on earth? Unfortunately, this occurs despite record expansion in memberships in health clubs and use of home exercise equipment.

Growth in the marketing of fast food and snack food and a lack of exercise, are among the reasons Americans are taking in more calories than they burn. Children and adults alike watch more television daily than ever before and are besieged with fatty food advertisements. Physical education has been markedly reduced in our schools, while many neighborhoods lack sidewalks for safe walking. The workplace has become increasingly automated, household chores are assisted by labor-saving devices, and walking or bicycling has been replaced by automobile travel.

CHILDHOOD OBESITY

The old adage "like father, like son" holds true when it comes to obesity. More than a third of the adult population in the United States is overweight, and there is an alarming increase in obesity among children and adolescents (Troiano & Flegal, 1998). About one in four U.S. children are either overweight or borderline overweight, and that figure has doubled over the past three decades. Unfortunately, at present most available treatments for obese children have yielded only modest, unstained results (Epstein, Myers, Raynor, & Saelens, 1998). A study in the *Annals of Human Biology* found that 41% of children who were overweight when they were 1 year old also were obese at age 21 (Hills & Peters, 1998). The earlier we can prevent obesity, the better. It seems, then, that prevention holds the greatest promise to affecting this national malady.

Start Good Eating Habits Early with Children

The U.S. Department of Agriculture (USDA) has issued a new food guide pyramid for children ages 2–6. The pyramid is a more child friendly version of the chart for grownups. It simplifies the headings of each of the six food groups and outlines the number of servings as well as serving sizes. The changes are minor, but the hope is to make proper dietary habits appeal more to children, who too often opt for high-calorie foods with little nutritional value. The early years are the best time to make an impact on the lifelong eating and exercise habits that contribute to health maintenance and disease prevention. Children start forming good eating habits as early as 2 years old, and bad nutrition habits are hard to fix.

So how much should kids eat? Children 1–3 years old should take in nearly 50 calories per pound of body weight. That works out to about 1300 calories a day for a 29-pound child. Children 4–6 years old should have closer to 40 calories per pound of body weight, or about 1800 calories for a 44-pound child. It is a very high calorie intake for children because they are growing, and it takes energy to grow.

The USDA recommends six servings from the grains group, five servings of fruits and vegetables, and two portions each from the dairy and meat groups. Sweets should be eaten sparingly. One slice of bread or a half-cup of rice equals a serving of grain. A half-cup of vegetables or canned fruit equals a serving in that group. A serving in the meat group consists of 2–3 ounces of beef, fish, or poultry.

ENCOURAGE CHILDREN TO EAT WELL

Getting children to eat right when there is so much to tempt them involves some creative thinking on the part of practitioners and parents. Try these guidelines yourself and then try teaching your patients by posting a list of them in your waiting room. Supplement with printed alternative therapies materials.

- *Eat right yourself.* Children are more likely to become obese if both parents are overweight. The parent is still the role model. Children imitate parents, and parents have the responsibility to practice nutritional habits themselves.

- *Start small and sweet.* Some foods simply do not look enticing to children. However, you can accustom your child to certain foods by starting with small portions and arranging them in interesting ways. For example, use celery sticks with a layer of peanut butter in the center for afternoon snacks and call them "peanut butter logs."

- *Familiarity breeds acceptability.* Many vegetables are bitter, so start with sweeter tasting kinds, such as corn, peas, and carrots.

- *Introduce these foods in the right environment.* Eventually, they will become comfort foods that children will come back to later. However, it is not a good idea to hide small bits of one food inside other kinds; this creates mistrust.

- *Monitor children's meals.* On average, children from 2 to 6 years old should eat three meals and three snacks a day at set times. If, however, children are not hungry at the usual hour, simply offer them more food at the next meal.

RESEARCH BOX: Reducing Children's Television
Viewing to Prevent Obesity

Observational studies have found an association between television
viewing and child and adolescent obesity. A randomized, controlled
school-based trial was done to assess the effects of reducing television,
videotape, and video game use on changes in adiposity, physical activity,
and dietary intake. There were 198 elementary-age school children who
received an intervention of an 18-lesson, 6-month-classroom curriculum
to reduce television and video game use. Compared to control groups,
children in the intervention group had statistically significant relative
decreases in body mass index and decreases in television viewing and
meals eaten in front of the television. This simple intervention and
lifestyle modification route may be a promising, population-based
approach to prevent childhood obesity.

Source: Robinson, T. (1999). Reducing children's television viewing to prevent obesity.
Journal of the American Medical Association, 282(16), 1561–1567.

Healthy Digestion

We are what we digest. Proper digestion means that the food we eat is broken
down into its respective parts, ideally, vitamins, minerals, essential fats, amino
acids, enzymes, and fiber, all of which are sorely lacking in the standard American
diet. Then those nutrients must be properly delivered to the bloodstream to be
carried to the rest of the body while waste products get easily eliminated. For true
health to occur from the foods we eat, three important factors, digestion, assimi-
lation, and elimination, must be present on a daily basis. A meal of hamburgers,
French fries, and soda falls far short of achieving these goals. So does any other
fast food meal you might care to name. In order to be healthy, we should get at
least five full servings of fruits and vegetables each day.

Components of a Healthy Diet

Since each person is unique, including individual biochemistry, there is no such
thing as an ideal diet, despite the numbers of books on the bestsellers' list each
year telling us otherwise. No matter how healthy a diet may be, invariably at least
10% of the people who try it will not notice any improvement, and another 10%
will actually feel worse because of trying it. Therefore, before beginning any specific dietary regimen, there are two things you can do to ensure that it will work
for you. When it works for you, it is far easier to model and teach the regimen to

your clients. First, determine your biochemical nutritional needs. Some people, for instance, would benefit most from a vegetarian diet, while on the opposite end of the spectrum, some people become weak or anemic if they abstain from red meat. Second, determine how you will plan your diet. When working with patients and clients, ask them what they do now and then discuss some alternative dietary changes.

The key to healthy eating can be greatly improved by eating whole foods. Whole foods have the least amount of processed, adulterated, fried, or sweetened additives or preservatives and are free of hydrogenated oils. They include all fruits and vegetables, complex carbohydrates (such as whole grains, pasta, or baked potato), seeds and nuts, beans and other legumes, fish and poultry, and dairy products like eggs, cottage cheese, and yogurt. By ensuring that at least 80% of your total food intake each week is made of whole foods, you will be able to tolerate the occasional pizza or cheeseburger here and there.

Eat at least five servings of fruits and vegetables each day to provide your body with the vitamins, minerals, and enzymes they contain. You can easily accomplish this by making a salad or steaming or sautéing a variety of vegetables and snacking on fruits when you get hungry. Also drink six to eight glasses of pure water every day and refrain from coffee, nonherbal teas, sodas, and commercial fruit juices. These are usually prepared with artificial sweeteners and, ironically, contribute to dehydration.

The best oil for most people is olive oil, for its proven health benefits (Willett, Sacks, Trichopoulou, Drescher, Ferro-Luzzi, Helsing, & Trichopoulos, 1995). Olive oil is monounsaturated and therefore cooking will not cause rancidity. However, polyunsaturates are essential (they cannot be made in the body) and are readily available from canola, safflower, sesame, or other seed oils and fresh fish, particularly cold-water, ocean-going fish such as salmon. Use spices according to your personal tastes; garlic, onions, ginger, and cayenne pepper are all recommended (Balentine, Albano, & Nair, 1999; Billing, 1998).

Some people subscribe to the theory of avoiding certain food combinations. Entire books have been written on this subject, yet the basic rules are as follows: Fruits are best eaten alone, not during meals, and water is best when consumed between meals, especially with regard to protein meals, to avoid diluting the digestive juices necessary for proper breakdown of food. In addition, each mouthful of food should be thoroughly chewed before it is swallowed, making it far easier to digest.

It is the quality of the foods you eat that determines the quality of fuel available to your body to perform its countless functions. Eating healthy can dramatically increase your energy levels over time and make a significant difference in how well you respond to disease. Be aware, however, that if you are not used to a whole-foods diet, you can sometimes experience initial feelings of abdominal cramping aches and increased trips to the bathroom because of increased intestinal peristalsis, or even headaches and fatigue. Usually, these symptoms will pass within a day or two as your improved eating habits start to take hold. If they persist or become too discomforting, you may be trying to do too much too soon. In that case, move more slowly into your new diet. Increased consumption of fluids can often also help.

Exercise

Regular exercise is another important component of overall health. Exercising at least three times a week can improve energy levels, aid in digestion, increase circulation, make for deep and restful sleep, stimulate the lymphatic system (the body's filtration and purification system), and promote enhanced levels of overall wellness and balanced mood. Regular exercise of an aerobic nature has been shown to increase serotonin levels in the brain (Imeri, Mancia, Bianchi, & Opp, 2000). Serotonin levels are associated with feelings of calm and well-being, improved brain function, and enhanced sleep (Seifritz, Moore, Trashsel, Bhatti, Stahl, & Gilli, 1996). There are a number of exercise routines from which to choose. A key to successfully following an exercise routine is to teach patients and clients to choose activities that they already enjoy.

Relaxation Techniques

In today's increasingly fast-paced world, one of the biggest obstacles to staying healthy is stress. Of even more concern is that we as a nation are becoming so used to operating under stressful conditions that we no longer are even aware of how habitual our stress has become. Is it any wonder, then, that in the United States more people die of heart attacks on Monday mornings prior to returning to work than at any other time of the week? This statistic validates that our lifestyle can literally kill us.

There are numerous relaxation techniques. Some are presented below. Master these techniques and then teach them to your clients.

DEEP BREATHING

Breathing is one of the easiest stress release methods and is available no matter where you are. The next time you notice that you are stressed or feeling tension in your body, close your eyes for a few moments and allow yourself to take five or six deep breaths. Do not force your breaths. Breathe in deeply, feeling the force in you abdomen. Inhale as fully as you comfortably can, then exhale naturally. Learning to do this on a regular basis throughout the day can pay big dividends and will help to keep stress under control. An additional benefit of deep breathing is that when you pause to do this exercise, you become conscious of the factors that are affecting you and influencing the stress response.

STRETCH BREAKS

Many people work at desks or computers most of the day. At least every hour step away from your desk and take a stretch break. Twist and bend and make your body really stretch comfortably. If you can, go outside into the fresh air as well. Exaggerate a yawn to force more air into your lungs. Instead of interfering with your deadlines, you will find that this simple break will actually help to produce more energy and make you more productive.

EYE BREAKS

Particularly if you are a computer user or read a lot in your work, frequently shift your eyes away from the screen or written page. Look out the window or across the room. A couple of times a day try to recline in a lounge chair. Elevate your feet and put a cool washcloth across your eyes. This aquatherapy technique will cause vasoconstriction of the delicate eye capillaries and restore the vitality to tired, red eyes.

Another useful technique for computer users, which can also help eyestrain, is to sit at your desk and cup both eyes with the palms of your hands. Take a few deep breaths and focus on the soothing energy of your hands moving across your eyes and down your body. This is a wonderful pick-me-up to try three or four times during the day.

MUSIC

Numerous studies have shown that listening to music you enjoy can banish stressful feelings within minutes (Chlan & Tracy, 1999; Watkins, 1997; White, 1999). Ideally, choose music of a relaxed tempo and listen to it while lying down with your eyes closed. The effect physiologically can be very similar to meditation.

NAPS

Many creative and productive individuals take catnaps throughout the day. For those who can fall asleep easily, naps result in more energy. While napping may not be possible at work, laying down for 20 minutes or so after you arrive home can prove extremely refreshing.

USE WATER TO REFRESH AND RESTORE

Water has an amazing capacity to heal. Take a shower upon arriving home and compare this with how you feel when you do not take a shower. Soothing hot baths before retiring are used for relaxation by many different cultures.

Massage

Receiving a massage one or more times each month has been shown to not only relieve stress but also significantly enhance immune function (Ironson et al., 1996). Self-massage is also quite valuable and can be easily learned. Forms of massage such as acupressure, shiatsu, or reflexology are particularly valuable (see Chapter 11). Many instruction books on these techniques are readily available at book stores.

Therapeutic massage involves the manipulation of the soft tissue structures of the body to prevent and alleviate pain, discomfort, muscle spasm, and stress and to promote health and wellness. The American Massage Therapy Association (AMTA) defines massage therapy as a profession in which the practitioner applies manual techniques and may apply adjunctive therapies with the intention of positively affecting the health and well-being of the client.

Massage therapy improves functioning of the circulatory, lymphatic, muscular, skeletal, and nervous systems and may improve the rate at which the body recovers from injury and illness. Massage involves holding, causing movement of soft tissue, and/or applying pressure to the body. It comes in many forms, including:

Swedish—a gentle, relaxing massage

Pressure point therapy—for certain conditions or injuries

Sports massage—focuses on muscle groups relevant to the particular sport

People find that therapeutic massage can help with a wide range of medical conditions (see Table 18-1).

TABLE 18-1	**Medical Conditions Helped by Massage**
Allergies	Insomnia
Anxiety	Depression
Arthritis (both osteoarthritis and rheumatoid arthritis)	Sinusitis
Asthma and bronchitis	Myofascial pain (a condition of the tissue connecting the muscles)
Carpal tunnel syndrome	Stress
Chronic and temporary pain	Sports injuries, including pulled or strained muscles and sprained ligaments
Circulatory problems	
Headache, especially when due to muscle tension	Reduced range of motion
	Emotional distress
Digestive disorders, including spastic colon, constipation and diarrhea	Temporomandibular joint dysfunction (TMJ)

Although massage therapy does not increase muscle strength, it can stimulate weak, inactive muscles and, thus, partially compensate for the lack of exercise and inactivity resulting from illness or injury. It also can hasten and lead to a more complete recovery from exercise or injury. Therapeutic massage can be inappropriate in some cases, such as in people with:

- Inflammation of the veins (phlebitis)
- Infectious diseases
- Certain forms of cancer
- Some skin conditions
- Some cardiac problems

In the case of phlebitis, it is possible that rubbing the extremity may dislodge debris from a vein and precipitate an embolism, massage of persons with certain infectious diseases and cancers may stimulate the lymphatic system to disburse more of the diseased or malignant cells to proximal areas, and some skin conditions will be aggravated with dermal stimulation. The primary care practitioner can help patients decide if they need to avoid use of massage. If your clients have one of these, or some other diagnosed medical condition, have them check with their primary provider before receiving a massage.

Research on the effects of massage therapy has been ongoing for more than 120 years. A surge in research over the past 20 years has resulted in more than 100 published studies. The National Institutes of Health (NIH), the government agency that oversees and conducts medical research in the United States, has funded several studies on the benefits of massage. Among research findings so far:

- Office workers massaged regularly were more alert, performed better, and were less stressed than those who were not massaged. (Field, Quintino, Henteleff, Wells-Klife, & Delnecchio-Feinburg, 1997)
- Massage therapy decreased the effects of anxiety, tension, depression, pain, and itching in burn patients. (Field, Peck, Krugman, Tuchel, Schanberg, Kuhn, & Burman, 1998)
- Premature infants who were massaged gained more weight and fared better than those who were not massaged. (Field, 1995)
- Increased relaxation for hospitalized patients. (Smith, Stallings, Mariner, & Burrall, 1999)

Advise patients that all of the above self-care practices, whether engaged in separately or together, can result in dramatic improvements in health and well-being over time. The key thing to remember is that usually healing is not instantaneous. It often takes years for conditions to develop into chronic disease, so a few weeks or months are sometimes needed to reverse that decline. Suggest that they be patient and gentle with themselves and do not try to do too much too soon.

Encourage them to remember that self-care and the resultant healing is an ongoing process, not something that is achieved once and then forgotten about. Regular practice of the chosen therapies, combined with a proper diet, can yield amazing results over time. Have them experiment with different therapies and see what works best.

HEALING OUR ENVIRONMENT

There is a clear connection between environment and health (Scally & Perkins, 1998). As we move into the next millennium, the importance of environmental health issues escalates. While humans have always had an impact on their environment, their destructive impact began to mount with the advent of the Industrial Revolution and continued throughout the nineteenth century. As the twentieth century closed, soaring world population, overconsumption, and waste production led to an enormous number of anthropogenic toxicants causing widespread environmental pollution of land, water, and air. The issue of environmental degradation and its effects on human health was slow to reach the world's conscience. A major step in addressing this issue occurred in 1972 when the United Nations General Assembly organized the United Nations Conference on the Human Environment in Stockholm. This led to the creation of the United Nations Environment Program (UNEP), which attempts to solve many problems, including cleaning up the Mediterranean; protecting water resources; combating deforestation, desertification, and drought; and phasing out the production of ozone-depleting chemicals (Goehl, 2000).

Numerous people helped bring about this general awareness of environmental issues, for example, Rachel Carson, who is perhaps the best known of the early environmental prophets. The growing awareness of the problem culminated in the convening of the Earth Summit in Rio de Janeiro, Brazil, in 1992. This meeting was attended by nearly 30,000 people from around the world, including more than a hundred world leaders and representatives from 167 countries. The goal of that summit was to address troubling symptoms of environmental decline. One important accomplishment of the summit was the signing of the Framework Convention on Climate Change. Five years later in Kyoto, Japan, an agreement (Kyoto Protocol) was reached that limits greenhouse gas emissions by developed countries (Goehl, 2000).

Data from other countries are also cause for concern. For example, Holland estimates that the long-term effects of particulate air pollution account for almost 60% of the total environment-related health loss. Environmental noise accounts for 24%, indoor air pollution (environmental tobacco smoke, radon, and dampness, as well as lead in drinking water) for around 6%, and food poisoning (or infection) for more than 3%. The contribution of this set of environmental exposures to the total annual burden of disease in the Netherlands is less than 5% (de Hollander, Melse, Lebret, & Kramers, 1999).

Although there is disappointment with the progress to protect the environment, there is a growing awareness of the impact that a polluted environment can have on our health and well-being. Green education continues to be an important need.

Overview of Some Environmental Problems

In large part we live in a polluted environment. In most communities air quality is from poor to bad, ever-present noise has become so prevalent that most people are unaware of it, and it is a constant battle to keep our water clean. There is not one, but a plethora, of environmental concerns. They range from polluted air, use of pesticides and insecticides, noise pollution, and contaminated water.

NOISE

Although its danger is still for the most part unrecognized, noise pollution may be the most common modern health hazard. Studies have repeatedly demonstrated that a high noise level is a significant factor in diminishing office productivity (Heerwagen, Heubach, Montgomery, & Weimer, 1995; Tafalla & Evans, 1997). More than 20 million workers in the United States are exposed to hazardous levels of noise every year, and the majority of them are in the white-collar work environment. Other studies here and in Europe have shown that high noise levels reduce pulse and respiration rates and release extra fats into the bloodstream (Maschke & Harder, 1998).

The danger posed by noise pollution is a function of the volume of sound heard over a period of time. Sound and its intensity are measured in decibels, abbreviated dB. Because the scale is logarithmic, rather than linear, each 10-dB increase is equivalent to multiplying the intensity by 10. The arbitrary zero is the weakest sound that a young, sensitive human ear can hear. Humans begin to perceive irritation around 50–90 dB and actually feel pain around 120 dB. At levels above 70 dB, the autonomic nervous system can become aroused, often without the person's awareness. When exposed for 8 hours to noise at 70 dB, which is the sound level of many typing pools or cafeterias, people may become irritable, distracted, or tense (Schuster & Keegan, 2000). There appears to be sufficient evidence that noise exposure can induce hearing impairment, hypertension and ischemic heart disease, annoyance, and sleep disturbance and decrease school performance. Evidence for other effects such as changes on the immune system and birth defects is limited (Goehl, 2000).

In particular, hospital noise has long been associated with patient fatigue due to sleeplessness, sensory overload, and in some cases even intensive care psychosis.

The more consciously aware health care providers become of this, the better able they are to combat it.

PESTICIDES

Pesticides are high-volume, widely used environmental chemicals and there is continuous debate concerning their possible role in many chronic human health effects. Because of their known structures, known rates of application, and the presence of a large occupationally exposed population, they are not only important in their own right but also are ideal models for the effects of environmental chemicals on the population in general. For reasons that are not always clear, this potential has not been realized. These exposed populations represent an underused asset in the study of the human health effects of environmental contaminants. Chronic effects thought to involve pesticides include carcinogenesis, neurotoxicity, and reproductive and developmental effects (Hodgson & Levi, 1996).

The U.S. Environmental Protection Agency (EPA) has made protecting children's environmental health its highest priority. Data on how and when children may be at risk are vital for accomplishing this goal. Recent examples of the link between research and policy include EPA actions to carry out the recommendations of the National Academy of Sciences on pesticides in children's food, reduce and prevent childhood lead poisoning, and revise national ambient air quality standards for ozone and particulate matter. Today, the Food Quality Protection Act (FQPA), which has made protecting children from pesticide residues in food a national priority, is contributing to the growing need for data for decision making. Further impetus comes from provisions in the FQPA and 1996 Safe Drinking Water Act Amendments for establishing a screening and testing program for potential risks from endocrine disruptors. Success of the U.S. international commitment to protect children is directly tied to the strength and availability of environmental data. To meet such challenges, the EPA is revising key science policies, expanding research opportunities, and adding to the public's right-to-know tools (Goldman, 1998).

For those interested in tapping into the database and pursuing environmental toxicology further, there is the National Library of Medicine's Toxicology and Environmental Health Information Program. This program is responsible for the creation and deployment of both bibliographic and factual files concerned with toxicology, carcinogenesis, developmental and reproductive effects of chemical substances, toxic chemical releases, and the medical and environmental behavior of chemical substances. The two main computer systems that provide bibliographic and factual data banks are Toxicology Data Network (TOXNET) and ELHILL. A number of the files found in the TOXNET system are built and maintained by other federal agencies, such as the National Cancer Institute, the EPA, and the National Institute for Occupational Safety and Health (Fonger, 1996).

Personal Space

All of us live and work in personal spaces. It is these areas that we can most effectively control, and we can actively participate in making them healthy. A healthy space is one that is aesthetically attractive, clean, with low noise, good lighting, and good ventilation. It is sad to realize that many people accept their personal space without conscious attention to the fact that it is dim, dirty, stagnant, and unattractive. Everyone can make their lives better by cleaning up their space. Table 18-2 gives an example of typical problems and solutions. Consider your personal space and your office environment, and whenever appropriate, share this information with patients.

TABLE 18-2 Creating a Healthy Personal Space	
TYPICAL PROBLEM	**SOLUTION**
Stuffy, stagnant room air	• Install openable windows. • Add potted plants for O_2/CO_2 exchange.
Dim lighting	• Use a wide array of new full-spectrum fluorescent and/or incandescent light bulbs.
Cluttered piles of paper	• Sort and toss out unused material. • Organize important documents into file drawers. • Install wall mount book shelves.
Dull room colors	• Paint bright accent colors on selected wall space. • Redecorate.
Musty smells	• Dry clean or wash all wall hangings and curtains. • Shampoo carpet annually. • Whenever possible, open windows and air out room. • Toss litter. • Clean inside drawers and closets.
Too much noise	• Search for noise pollution source. • Let others in your personal space know the value of a noise-free environment. • Sometimes the addition of soft music can muffle harsh, uncontrollable sounds.

Joint Space Work Environments

Pause for a moment and think about your shared work space and the space where you work with patients. How does it hinder and how does it heal? Do you return home at the end of the work day with tension headaches, aching shoulders, or tired feet? Do your patients have to sit in hard, uncomfortable straight-back chairs. Consider the ergonomics of the space. Do you bend over when

TABLE 18-3	Equipment for In-house Staff Healing Room

EQUIPMENT	FUNCTION
Reclining chair	Allows a worker to elevate their feet during break periods.
Foot massager	Electronic vibrations on the soles of the feet provide simultaneous stimulation and relaxation that affects the whole body.
Audio cassette player with earphones	Gives an opportunity to relax and meditate with a choice of music or guided imagery audiocassette tapes.
Rheostat light control	Allows the room guest the ability to turn down the brightness of light while they rest.

sitting on a high stool or do you chart in a poorly lit area? Most people spend their days in inferior work environments that tax their long-term vision, posture, and body alignment.

Work environments can be easily modified to enhance worker health. Consider the case of one hospital that installed healing rooms on each inpatient care unit. These units were not for the patients but for the employees. It does not take much of a budget to create these spaces. Table 18-3 details some of the characteristics of an in-house staff healing room.

One hospital converted an unused storage room to a "staff recovery" room. It was painted a soft lavender, soundproof insulation was added, and a convertible sign was placed on the door stating occupied or unoccupied. Staff on this unit delighted in taking their breaks while engaging in readily available self-care options. As a byproduct to feeling better, staff retention rate greatly improved on this unit.

SUMMARY

The quest for better care begins at home. Healers must give attention to healing themselves. Self-care involves initial and periodic self-assessments, plans of action, and follow-through with specific daily and weekly regimens. A proactive healer then looks at their environment, again does an assessment, and looks for ways to make their personal space better. Once conscious of the difference that improving one's personal space makes, healers can move ahead to help others in work settings and help communities find ways to heal their environment. Opportunities for action at the regional and national level abound for those who can move forward at those levels.

ASK YOURSELF

1. Why is self-care important in my personal and professional life?
2. How can I teach self-care skills to my patients?
3. What are three negative facts about the typical American diet and what can be done to change eating behaviors?
4. For which environmental concern can you institute environmental changes in your personal and professional space? Discuss this concern.

REFERENCES

Allison, D., Fontaine, K., Manson, J., Stevens, J., & VanItallie, T. (1999). Annual deaths attributable to obesity in the United States. *Journal of the American Medical Association, 282*(16), 1530–1538.

Balentine, D. A., Albano, M. C., & Nair, M. G. (1999). Role of medicinal plants, herbs, and spices in protecting human health. *Nutrition Reviews, 57*(9, Pt. 2), S41–S45.

Billing, J., & Sherman, P. W. (1998). Antimicrobial functions of spices: Why some like it hot. *Quarterly Review of Biology, 73*(1), 3–49.

Chlan, L., & Tracy, M. F. (1999). Music therapy in critical care: Indications and guidelines for intervention. *Critical Care Nurse, 19*(3), 35–41.

de Hollander, A. E., Melse, J. M., Lebret, E., & Kramers, P. G. (1999). An aggregate public health indicator to represent the impact of multiple environmental exposures. *Epidemiology, 10*(5), 606–617.

Epstein, L. H., Myers, M. D., Raynor, H. A., & Saelens, E. B. (1998). Treatment of pediatric obesity. *Pediatrics, 101,* 554–570.

Fonger, G. C. (1996). Toxicological and environmental health information from the National Library of Medicine. *Toxicology and Industrial Health, 12*(5):639–49.

Field, T. (1995). Massage therapy for infants and children. *Journal of Developmental and Behavioral Pediatrics, 16*(2); 105–111.

Field, T., Peck, M., Krugman, S., Tuchel, T., Schanberg, S. Kuhn, C., & Burman, I. (1998). Burn injuries benefit from massage therapy. *Journal of Burn Care Rehabilitation, 19*(3); 241–244.

Field, T., Quintino, O., Henteleff, T., Wells-Keife, L., & Delnecchio-Feinberg, G. (1997). Job stress reduction therapies. *Alternative Therapies in Health and Medicine, 3*(4); 54–56.

Goehl, T. J. (2000). Reviews in environmental health, 2000. *Environmental Health Perspectives, 108* (Suppl. 1), 3–4.

Goldman, L. R. (1998). Linking research and policy to ensure children's environmental health. *Environmental Health Perspectives, 106* (Suppl. 3), 857–862.

Heerwagen, J. H., Heubach, J. G., Montgomery, J., & Weimer, W. C. (1995). Environmental design, work, and well being: Managing occupational stress through changes in the workplace environment. *AAOHN Journal, 43*(9), 458–468.

Hills, J. O., & Peters, J. C. (1998). Environmental contributions to the obesity epidemic. *Science, 180,* 1371–1374.

Hodgson, E., & Levi, P. E. (1996). Pesticides: An important but underused model for the environmental health sciences. *Environmental Health Perspectives, 104* (Suppl. 1), 97–106.

Imeri, L., Mancia, M., Bianchi, S., & Opp, M. R. (2000). 5-Hydroxytryptophan, but not L-tryptophan, alters sleep and brain temperature in rats. *Neuroscience, 95*(2), 445–452.

Ironson, G., Field, T., Scafidi, F., Hashimoto, M., Kumar, M., Kumar, A., Price, A., Goncalves, A., Burman, I., Tetenman, C., Patarca, R., & Fletcher, M. A. (1996). Massage therapy is associated with enhancement of the immune system's cytotoxic capacity. *International Journal of Neuroscience, 84*(1–4), 205–217.

Kuczmarski, R. J., Carroll, M. D., Flegal, K. M., & Troiano, R. P. (1997). Varying body mass index cutoff points to describe overweight prevalence among U.S. adults. *Obesity Research, 5*(6); 542–548.

Ludwig, D., Pereira, M., Kroenke, C., Hilner, J., Van Horn, L., Slattery, M., & Jacobs, D. (1999). *Journal of the American Medical Association, 282*(16), 1539–1546.

Manson, J. E, Willett, W. C., & Stampfer, M. J. (1995). Body weight and mortality among women. *New England Journal of Medicine, 338,* 1–7.

Maschke, C., & Harder, J. (1998). Environmental medical action required on exposure to noise. *Gesundheitswesen, 60*(11), 661–668.

Mokdad, A., Serdula, M., Dietz, W., Bowman, B., & Koplan, J. (1999). The spread of the obesity epidemic in the United States, 1991–1998. *Journal of the American Medical Association, 282*(16), 1519–1522.

Must, A., Spadano, J., Coakley, E., Field, A., Colditz, G., & Dietz, W. (1999). The disease burden associated with overweight and obesity. *Journal of the American Medical Association, 282*(16), 1523–1529.

Scally, G. (1998). Perkins C environment and health. *Hospital Medicine, 59*(11), 872–876.

Schuster, E., & Keegan, L. (2000). Environment. In *Holistic nursing: A handbook for practice.* Gaithersburg, MD: Aspen.

Smith, M. C., Stallings, M. A., Mariner, S., & Burrall, M. (1999). *Alternative Therapies in Health and Medicine, 5*(4); 64–71.

Stevens, J., Cai, J., Pamuk, E. R., Williamson, D. F., Thun, M. J., & Wood, J. L. (1998). The effect of age on the association between body mass index and mortality. *New England Journal of Medicine, 333,* 1–7.

Seifritz, E., Moore, P., Trachsel, L., Bhatti, T., Stahl, S. M., & Gillin, J. C. (1996). The 5-HT1A agonist ipsapirone enhances EEG slow wave activity in human sleep and produces a power spectrum similar to 5-HT2 blockade. *Neuroscience Letters, 209*(1), 41–44.

Tafalla, R. J., & Evans, G. W. (1997). Noise, physiology, and human performance: The potential role of effort. *Journal of Occupational Health Psychology, 2*(2), 148–155.

Watkins, G. (1997). Music therapy: Proposed physiological mechanisms and clinical implications. *Clinical Nurse Specialist, 11*(2), 43–50.

White, J. M. (1999). Effects of relaxing music on cardiac autonomic balance and anxiety after acute myocardial infarction. *American Journal of Critical Care, 8*(4), 220–230.

Willett, W. C, Sacks, F., Trichopoulou, A., Drescher, G., Ferro-Luzzi, A., Helsing, E., & Trichopoulos, D. Mediterranean diet pyramid: A cultural model for healthy eating. *American Journal of Clinical Nutrition, 61*(6, Suppl.), 1402S–1406S.

PART V

Body-Mind-Spirit Connection to Health and Illness

CHAPTER
19

Consciousness and Healing

Chapter Objectives

- Discover how shifts in the scientific revolution have affected shifts in consciousness.
- Recognize that increasing consciousness develops in steps over time.
- Learn some theories of awareness from the disciplines of psychology, education, and counseling.
- Become aware of some of the barriers to awareness.
- Discover the roots, process, and rituals germane to healing meditation.
- Learn about the relationship between spirituality and healing.

HISTORY, SCIENCE, AND A SHIFTING PARADIGM

Willis Harman, Roger Sperry, and other contemporary scientific philosophers have speculated that Western society is on the verge of a second Copernican revolution, in which the dominant attitudes will evolve into a belief in consciousness as the primary stuff of the universe. In this context, consciousness, or mind, is defined as the primary force from which all matter and energy derive. This is contrary to positivism, or empiricism, which holds that the only way to know the universe is through the reduction of matter. For empiricists, the brain is the basis for consciousness. Under the new model, no such limit exists.

Five or six such dramatic shifts, including the scientific revolution and the rise of capitalism, have already occurred. Whether or not this global shift takes place, modern medicine has already begun to incorporate aspects of this new framework. Many health professionals are recognizing the significance of perceptions, thoughts, feelings, and the need for love as vital components of well-being. Rather than viewing health as the absence of disease, the goal of the new integrated model is the attainment of optimal well-being (Leighton, 1998). And it is becoming increasingly clear that this state of being is most rapidly achieved through an awakened consciousness.

AWAKENING CONSCIOUSNESS

Life is a series of responses to actions and the reactions they bring. Yet, it is impossible to describe what happens to us in such simple ways. Often events in our lives occur as a propellant to jolt us into making conscious choices. For example, the Dalai Lama left Tibet, not because he or his constituents had done something wrong, but to escape political and religious persecution. As it turned out his fleeing that tiny mountain nation, sandwiched between China and India, led to the consciousness-raising of millions of people worldwide. So far he has spent more than 20 years in exile, and during these years he has taught by word and example the principles of conscious deliberation and conscious acts of healing.

The events in our lives sometimes seem to allegorically twist us like a pretzel. As humans with logical minds, we are always attempting to understand the lesson, to find the reason, or to lay blame for the event that has happened. When we stop at the level of placing blame, we are not propelled forward in our consciousness, but rather stay in the loop of acting and reacting. In a long-term view of things it is, for the most part, unimportant who is right and who is wrong. What does matter is our reaction to events and how effectively we have learned the skills of living.

Attempting to understand why things happen is reasonable; most people want to learn the lesson from an occurrence. However, an answer does not always come. Rather than continue to grapple with the issue, at times the best course is to release the question and/or quandary to our unconscious or superconscious mind. When we release these unanswerable questions, we acknowledge that we cannot and do not need to understand everything. The benefit of this technique is that the conscious mind is cleared of fret and worry and can proceed with temporal tasks while the bigger issue is relegated to another realm. Oftentimes it is weeks, months, or even years later that the troubling, unresolved issue or painful event comes into clear focus. The unconscious or superconscious mind requires time to sort out and return to the conscious mind an understandable image of meaning and perspective.

In almost all situations the art of living consciously is learning to react to events in a way that is reflective of an inner belief that we cannot know the reasons for everything. We can better let go of questioning why things happen in our life when we accept that sometimes the answer cannot be comprehended by our conscious mind. Only when we release and let go can the issue move to a different level for processing.

Mindful Living

Becoming increasingly conscious develops in steps. It is a skill, and like many other skills, it takes practice and repetition to attune the mind to a different way of being (Umlauf, 1997). Consciousness is the essence of mindful living, a Zen Buddhist term. Vietnamese monk Thich Nhat Hanh has a Zen meditation center, Plum Village, in the south of France. Here mindfulness bells ring throughout the day to remind everyone to slow down and be aware of the present moment. Whenever the gong sounds, everyone stops what he or she is doing, takes three breaths and practices a moment of mindfulness. We do not need a gong, however, to experience life more deeply. You can take ordinary moments in your day and, through simple rituals, turn them into moments of mindful awareness (Sury Das, 1999). When you have opportunities, share this perspective with your patients.

Daily Ritual

In many formal centers, indeed in many private homes, the people who live there participate in daily rituals. The ritual described in Figure 19-1 is currently used by many and one that you might want to try in your life. The ritual consists of six parts that are meant to increase mindfulness in daily living. Try this ritual for yourself and/or use it in sessions with patients.

- **Waking up**
  Each day presents a new opportunity to awaken in a sacred manner. You can intentionally begin your day in a more mindful fashion. Each day as you awaken, remind yourself of what it means to truly become and stay awake. The inner light of awareness has the capacity to shine brightly all day. As you arise take three mindful breaths.

  Inhale . . . exhale . . . one.
  Inhale . . . exhale . . . two.
  Inhale . . . exhale . . . three.

  Clear yourself of stale air. Breathe out the residue of last night's dreams and finally expel any negativity you might be feeling.

- **Mindful grooming**
  Before you begin to dress for the day, stand in front of the mirror. Take three breaths in and out, relax for a moment, and look into the mirror with fresh eyes. See who is there. Pay attention to your posture; smile at yourself. As you approach your morning shower, reflect upon the sacred rituals of the bath. Let the water blast at high volume for a minute. Listen to the water. Recognize that water is used to both bless and anoint. You can partake of its blessings through a transformative moment of calm, mindful reflection as you wash. Reflect for a moment with the water running over your head and face. Become aware of your feelings. Drop your hands. Just stand there. Breathe in and out a few times. Relax and feel the hot water running over your head, neck, shoulders, and back. Be aware that you use water not only to physically cleanse yourself, but also to wash away all ills, transgressions, and preoccupations. Close out the bathing ritual and dry yourself with conscious attention to the glory of your body.

  Go to your closet and choose your clothing to complement your desire to go into the day looking and feeling your best. Brush or comb your hair, and put on accessories to complete your self-image of worthiness.

  (Continued on next page)

Figure 19-1 An example of a daily ritual

- **Leaving the house**

   As you get ready to leave your home, consciously approach the door. Stop and stand up straight in front of it. Take three slow breaths. Use your breathing to help you be more conscious. Do you have everything that you need? Walk out and enter the world with your eyes wide open and a smile on your face.

- **Beginning your work day**

   When you arrive at your destination, pause and smile both inwardly and outwardly. Be aware that this is the place that offers you the opportunity to provide for your needs. Give thanks for its being and resolve to do your best work today.

- **Mindful eating**

   Mindfulness while eating is an ancient spiritual practice. In Asia, some Buddhists practice chewing each mouthful of brown rice a hundred times before taking the next bite. Being mindful while eating can help you experience the taste, texture, and temperature of what you put in your mouth; it helps you become aware of how, when, and why you nourish yourself. As you eat your lunch be aware of the source of your food and how it nourishes your body to enable you to be in this place and time. When you sit down to eat, take three breaths to remind yourself to enjoy a moment of mindfulness. Smile and appreciate this little nondenominational moment of grace. Put your hands in front of you and inhabit the moment. Then for the first bite or two, try chewing your food 15 or 20 times. How does it feel? How does this food taste? Are you getting nourished? Be grateful for this moment. By opening up to it, you can fully experience it.

- **Mindful homecoming**

   When you return home, rejoice. Stand in front of your door and appreciate the moment of your arrival. Breathe in and out three times. Mark the passage and completeness of the circle. Feel the satisfaction. Just be there for a moment. Now open the door and step inside. Home is a temple; enter your sacred domain. Come home to yourself.

Figure 19-1 *(Continued)*

AWARENESS IN HEALING

The concept of awareness is well known to health care professionals, but the term often has a different meaning to individuals based on their experiences and beliefs. The word *awareness* is derived from the Old English *gewaer,* which means "watchful." In modern English, awareness generally means to be informed, cognizant, and alert about some subject or event.

Health care professionals know well that they must be knowledgeable and alert to their clients and the constantly changing environment in which they practice. There are several forms of awareness that we all practice in different ways at different times. This awareness is from not only one's knowledge base but also other areas of the mind. Table 19-1 describes three types of awareness.

TABLE 19-1	Three Types of Awareness
TYPE OF AWARENESS	**DESCRIPTION**
Intuitive	Intuitive awareness includes some other ways of knowing and may be felt directly rather than through the linear, logical, and rational methods. For example, the "ah ha" feeling when you "just get it."
Transcendent	Similar to the intuitive, transcendent awareness is not bound by time or matter. It is the exchange of energy that occurs without rational thinking and analyzing. It is sudden and therefore similar to intuitive awareness, yet it permits the closest and most intimate communication among beings. For example, you suddenly know that a loved one is in trouble or needs you.
Cognitive	Cognition is both the process and the product of knowing. For example, you get the answer to a problem through a logical, deductive process.

Each type of awareness is important in the healing process. Each is crucial to the healer as well as the healed. Maximum healing is possible when all types of awareness take place in both the healer and the healed.

Theories of Awareness

Several theories of awareness are found in the disciplines of psychology, education, and counseling. The conceptualizations that follow represent a variety of approaches to this phenomenon and are meant to provide only a brief overview of this concept (Rew, 1996).

PSYCHODYNAMIC THEORY

The classical psychodynamic theory of Freud contains a topographical conceptualization of three levels of awareness or consciousness (Strachey, 1962). These levels of awareness, or consciousness, influence one's behavior and are identified as the preconscious, the conscious, and the unconscious:

- The preconscious level of awareness contains information or memory that is not readily available but that can be recalled with some effort.

- The conscious level of awareness includes that information and knowledge over which the individual has conscious control.

- The unconscious level of awareness includes mental functions that are very difficult in some cases and impossible to recall.

Memories of infant states, including the motivations and behaviors associated with being dependent and self-centered, remain in the individual's psyche. They are, however, incompatible with learned values about adult functioning and in Freud's view create anxiety that must be controlled through defense mechanisms such as repression. These motivations seek expression and often manifest themselves through the individual's dream, impulsive behaviors, and slips of the tongue.

GESTALT PSYCHOLOGY

This discipline is based on the assumption that the "whole determines the parts," rather than the "whole is equal to the sum of the parts." Based on work with brain-injured soldiers, Frederick S. Perls began to develop the theory of focusing on awareness as a way of taking responsibility for one's problems and their solutions. According to Gestalt theorists, personality evolves in three phases. These three phases are the social, psychophysical, and spiritual and are all present at birth (Perls, Hefferline, & Goodman, 1951). Gestalt therapy was designed to help healthy people grow and develop their unique potentials. Most therapy is conducted in groups and focuses on the individual's development of awareness.

CLIENT-CENTERED THERAPY

This discipline was created and advanced most notably by Carl Rogers (1961). A basic assumption of this approach is that the individual has the potential or capacity to be competent. In other words, human beings are motivated toward self-actualization. Three essential components of this approach to helping and healing are genuine caring or empathy of the helper, congruence between the helper's inner experience and the outer expression of this experience in the relationship with the person being helped, and unconditional positive regard for this person. Rogers asserted that when an individual is unaware of the fullness of personal experience, he or she does not act in the most constructive way possible.

PSYCHOSYNTHESIS

This includes the concept of awareness know as the grounding technique (Assagioli, 1971). This means that simply becoming more aware of our motivations and connections between thoughts, feelings, and behaviors is not sufficient for lasting psychological change or growth. Rather, the individual must learn to ground new awareness so that pain or depression does not result from feeling overloaded or overwhelmed by new information and knowledge about oneself.

THERAPEUTIC HYPNOSIS

Hypnosis is conceptualized as transforming an idea into an act. Through hypnosis an individual can become more aware of how misinterpretation of words and events can lead to illness and how obtaining new and unexpected awareness can promote the healing process. Some alternative practitioners use hypnosis as a therapy to help patients bring forth and surface unconscious memories in order to discover the root cause of current behavior that may be motivated by past repressed events. Another form of hypnosis involves a practitioner teaching a client how to use autosuggestion phrases to help overcome habits such as overeating and smoking.

Barriers to Awareness and Healing

A barrier is anything that interferes with movement towards a desired end. Any situation that limits the development of personal awareness acts as a barrier in the healing process. Many factors can hinder the healing process by interfering with a person's awareness. These factors can include cultural beliefs and values, emotions, and social conditions. When your patients do not heal or seem to have failure to thrive, you may consider some of these awareness factors when trying to establish a different approach.

When people are fully aware of their beliefs and values, they have an understanding of how they interpret the world around them. This awareness also enables them to understand that their perceptions of the world may be different from those of other people. Consequently, they will also understand how their minds and bodies and the minds and bodies of others respond to provocation and competition from the environment. The external environment poses a variety of threats and challenges to people, particularly when they encounter new situations, and we know that many health care settings seem foreign and formidable to patients.

HEALING STORY: Healing through Awareness

Harriet was a widow for seven years before meeting Jonathan. Jonathan and Harriet met through mutual friends, and she was swept off her feet by the variety of activities they enjoyed together. After a short three-week courtship, Jonathan and Harriet married, but the whirlwind romance came to a screeching halt. Soon after the honeymoon, Harriet began to experience nausea and occasional diarrhea. Harriet was 74 years old when she was hospitalized for a vague syndrome of stomach distress. Within two months, these symptoms increased in both frequency and severity. She lost her appetite and began to feel despondent. Jonathan settled into a routine of quiet passivity.

Harriet finally made an appointment with her physician, who began by treating the obvious symptoms. However, she soon decided to hospitalize Harriet for observation and tests. The physician, a long-time friend of

(Continued on next page)

Harriet's, suspected that the vague syndrome of stomach distress might possibly be masking the real cause of Harriet's disorder. She requested that nurse counselors visit Harriet and provide consultation. Within 48 hours of her admission to the hospital, and with the encouragement of Ann, the nurse counselor, and her physician, Harriet focused her awareness on what she was really feeling and her beliefs about the expectations of her family. She realized that the symptoms of her stomach distress were really reflections of her feelings about her new marriage and whether her family would support her quick marriage. The symptoms and hospitalization did give her time away from Jonathan and she was able to engage in self-reflection. As her anxiety decreased, she became aware of her true feelings and her behavioral response behind the physical illness. She left the hospital free from her abdominal distress and with the resolve to address her husband and family directly.

Observations and Insights

The story about Harriet illustrates the power of emotion to produce barriers to both awareness and healing. Fear and anxiety are natural and protective emotions. They are associated with strong physiological changes within the body that are difficult to ignore. Because awareness is essential to the process of healing, barriers to self-awareness also become barriers to healing. The outcomes of strong feelings that are not acknowledged and expressed openly and directly by people prevent those people from healing the discomfort and disharmony in their lives. With Harriet and Jonathan, her fear and anxiety over her new marriage led to damage and discomfort in her gastrointestinal system. The more she ignored those feelings, the farther she got from healing the physical symptoms and the disruptions in her interpersonal relationships.

Creativity and Healing Awareness

There are many things to do in order to increase healing awareness; one of those things is to increase your creativity. Often there is a correlation between increasing creativity and improving one's powers of observation. In addition, innovative ways of looking at old situations come from adding insightful ways of viewing the world. One way to stimulate creativity in your patients is to make your practice environment friendly, relaxed, and conductive to putting them at ease. Soft colors and lighting, gentle music, and interesting reading material can help promote an environment that is conducive to alternative discussions.

HEALING STORY: Healing through New Insights

Teresa, a young mother, stood quietly next to a hospital bed where her young son lay. Thoughts and feelings raced through her mind as she considered the outcome of the examination of Jared's spinal fluid. "Could it be meningitis? Will he die? I'm so scared. What about the other children at home? Have they been exposed to this germ?"

Jared's nurse, Mary, came by his bedside to assess his temperature and check his IV. She observed Teresa's worried demeanor and said to her, "You must be feeling exhausted by now. Would it help if I brought you a cup of tea, and we could sit together with Jared for a while?" Teresa smiled and nodded her head.

Mary brought the tea and sat with Teresa. They discussed Teresa's concerns and worries and laughed and talked about small children. Teresa began to feel more relaxed and secure and realized that Jared was in very good hands. By the second day Jared was up, watching television, and feeling much better. Mary came in to take his temperature and Teresa went over and said, "Mary, thank you so much for your time and the tea on Sunday night. I guess I didn't realize how frightened I was and how much I might be hindering Jared's recovery and even making myself sick with my own worries and fears. You really helped me put it all in perspective—and now look how great we are both feeling!"

Observations and Insights

The story of Jared and his mother sounds amazingly simple and straightforward. However, a form of healing took place in this story. Mary recognized that Teresa's anxiety formed a barrier to Jared's healing and could make Teresa sick herself. This awareness on Mary's part might have reflected basic knowledge of human psychology and behavior or it might have reflected personal knowledge based on years of experience with similar patterns of behavior that she had observed between parents and children. Mary intervened first by focusing on Teresa's need for rest, comfort, and diversion. Mary creatively transformed the sick room into a tea party where Teresa's physical and emotional needs could be met. Mary not only brought a hot cup of comforting tea to Teresa, but she took the time to listen and make jokes and put a worried mother at ease.

Healing is not merely restoration or return to a previous health state. Rather, it is a new awareness that is created out of the breakdown in the natural wholeness and harmony between that person and the world.

(Continued on next page)

Patients can be stimulated to engage in creative problem solving as part of the healing process. Divergent thinking involves taking a different path toward a goal; it involves tolerance for ambiguity and entertaining the possibility that there are multiple solutions rather than just one right answer.

HEALING MEDITATION

A great deal of what we learn as health care providers and as ordinary humans we learn through experience. Some of the strongest supporters of meditation are ordinary people who, after struggling uphill against difficult problems in life, discovered meditation.

In strictly behavioral terms, meditation can be described as a process developed to achieve or maintain physical and mental balance that combines the techniques of controlled breathing and focused concentration.

Meditation Process

The technique of meditation couples slow breathing with the simple directive to mentally consider only one thought over a prescribed period of silence. The proper execution of meditation requires voluntary control to slow the rate of breathing while increasing the depth of each respiration.

Our thoughts are usually in constant motion. We are forever judging and entertaining any number of ideas or mental pictures in our mind's eye during every waking moment. This persistent tumbling of ideas is not necessarily a benign event to our bodies. If these ideas and mental pictures are stress producing, they trigger the stress responses of the body. As long as this barrage of ideas is incessant, the stress response is triggered constantly. Initially, the stress level may be low and the stress response relatively minor, but this activation of the alarm system may become constant. The constancy of this process becomes a habitation cycle of increasing wear and tear on the body. Therapeutically, the aim of meditation is to limit this random stream of negative stimulation and interrupt this protective mechanism gone awry.

Modern Medicine and Ancient Therapeutics

Meditation is an ancient technique that can be effectively used by modern health care providers. Although the state-of-the-art medical care is known for its dependence on technology, many health problems are now being attributed to our overstressed emotional or psychic states. No amount of technology can buffer the stresses of our lives or the lives of our patients. When taught to patients as a self-care skill, meditation becomes a useful and effective medical therapy. Even when the patient is only expected to get partial relief from routine care, adding meditation to standard practices can improve patient care outcomes.

Elements of Meditation

- *Practice.* In meditation, a deliberate effort is made to focus consciousness on a single idea, object, or sensation while being perfectly relaxed. The concept of sitting quietly to ponder a single idea is truly alien to many individuals' nature. This is one of the primary reasons that repeated practice is required to be accustomed to meditating.

- *Concentration.* As most of us have observed our own behavior, the ability to concentrate or focus our attention depends upon several factors. Children have more difficult concentrating because they have developmental limits for their attention span. Almost without exception, the ability to totally concentrate depends upon having an environment suited both to the individual and the task. The concentrative effort of meditation is no different in that regard. Meditation is best practiced in places that fit with the concentrative needs of the individual.

- *Environment.* Privacy and a quiet atmosphere are important aspects in selecting a place to meditate regularly. In fact, using the same place and time on a daily basis is very helpful when trying to establish a mediation habit.

- *Willingness.* Like any other healthy habit, meditation demands a commitment to willingness. As with any change in lifestyle, such as beginning an exercise program, practicing that new activity must be persistent and consistent.

Behavioral Aspects of Meditation

Active concentration combined with the control of breathing patterns produces the unique physical responses attributed to meditation. The phenomenon that occurs is in fact a behavioral treatment similar to operant conditioning or desensitization. By repeated use, individuals can decondition themselves to the negative physical experience of repeated stress. It is the repeated experience of stressors that causes the body to lose its ability to extinguish the stress response. Even the most modest attempts at regular meditation deflate the body's responses to that stress. Meditation differs from operant conditioning in that individuals must necessarily deliver the treatment to themselves. The mechanism of desensitization is, however, the same as is used for the treatment of anxiety disorders. The difference in this circumstance is that the anxiety is more diffuse and the causative factors may be less well defined.

Meditation and Behavior Modification

The best technique to reduce or eliminate a bad habit is to break the cycle and put new information into the system. As we all know, the depth and rate of breathing can be controlled to some degree on a voluntary basis. This type of control is relatively easy to practice but does require concentration. Achieving control of breathing is both a skill and a talent that can be enhanced by repeated practice, as prescribed in meditation.

Science has shown that when the breathing rate decreases, the heart rate also decreases (Travis & Wallace, 1999). The heart not only beats more slowly, it also beats more effectively, delivering more oxygen and nutrients to the body with less effort. The technique of voluntarily controlling respiration to reduce heart rate is a scientific fact (Peng, Mietas, Liu, Khalsa, Douglas, Benson, & Goldberger, 1999; Travis & Wallace, 1999). What we also know is that this physical response, slowing of the breathing and slowing of the heart, can be evoked even in the presence of acute stressors such as real physical danger and emergencies. When this technique is used, the body does not transmit messages of stress to any other organs of the body. The deliberate execution of controlled breathing effectively blocks the release of stress hormones as long as the controlled breathing is maintained. Almost anyone can learn the technique of breath control and can employ it in any number of circumstances. Table 19-2 presents a program for effective meditation.

HEALING STORY: Healing through Controlled Breathing

This was the first of her son's baseball games that Latisha had been able to attend for several years. This was the team's first game against one of the best high school baseball teams in the state. Latisha, who was a health care provider, had told the coach she was willing to help with the team. This meant she got to bring the first aid kit and attend to any kids that skinned their knees.

The game went very well; the score was very close, but her son's team lost. However, they were not as disappointed, as one would expect, because it had been against the state champions, and they had come close. As Latisha talked to her son, she noticed one of the boys on the other team wheezing and coughing. Two other students explained that he was asthmatic, and his inhaler was empty.

Latisha looked at him and said, "Hi there. I work at the hospital and I've have asthma too. We're going to sit down here and work to slow down your breathing." She then whispered in his ear, "I know you have had these kinds of attacks before and I'm sure you know what to expect. What I want you to do is to slow down your breathing. I want you to close your eyes. Listen to my voice and nothing else. Now, I want you to breathe along with me. Listen to me breathe in and out." Latisha placed a warm, wet towel around his neck. Within minutes, the boy was pink and breathing easily. She reminded the boy to always bring an extra inhaler in the future and to remember that he has the power to control his breathing in dangerous situations if he needs to.

Observations and Insights

Latisha's baseball-playing patient experienced an asthma attack after a high school baseball game. It is fortunate that Latisha was confident and capable in conveying the breathing techniques used in meditation to quell the boy's symptoms. The fundamental elements of meditation, controlled breathing, and focused concentration create specific physical reactions in the human body. Regular practice of these methods in tandem reinforces this positive and predictable response in the body.

As a therapeutic skill, meditative techniques are an important adjunct to regular medical care. When other treatments are not available, meditation can be an important element in the health care personnel's repertoire. As described in this story, asthma attacks can occur at any time. When there is no medication available, health care providers must innovate by using the resources at hand.

TABLE 19-2 Eight-Step Program for Effective Meditation

1. Find a time that is the same every day, preferably before or after work, or a time when you won't feel a lot of stress.
2. Find an amount of time that is the same every day. If you choose to meditate 15 minutes at lunchtime, then try to keep it consistent and develop a routine. You may want to set a small alarm or a clock radio with soft music that begins to play when your 15 minutes are up.
3. Find a quiet place where others will not bother you.
4. Sit in a comfortable position.
5. Place your hands comfortably on your thighs.
6. You may keep your eyes closed or open.
7. Focus your thoughts on a single picture or object. Do not let distractions or other thoughts interrupt you.
8. Breathe slowly in and out and concentrate on the inhalation and the exhaling process. Work to focus effectively for the entire 15 minutes.

SPIRITUALITY AND HEALING

Toward the end of the twentieth century part of the populace became more suspicious of authority and more open to new ways of doing things. Another segment of the population became increasingly religious, evangelical, and even judgmental. Sometimes these groups clashed, but for the most part, this increasing diversification opened new avenues for exploring and expanding our spirituality.

Forming a Spiritual Group

Over the past few years many people have embarked on individual spiritual paths only to discover that it is difficult to go it alone. Many find that the taped voice of a teacher or an author's printed words, however inspiring, lack a personal dimension. This sense of dissatisfaction and longing for connection often move us to seek out the company of others. Humans are socially oriented, and we enjoy sharing and reflecting our beliefs with others. Many individuals, especially those that may be ill or unable to find a church that they enjoy, need a group that supports the spiritual aspects of their life. These groups can be formed in long-term care facilities, residential living centers, neighborhoods, or communities. When working to form a patient spiritual care group, there are several steps involved:

- *Find a group focus.* A spiritual group focus could be meditation, reading and discussing certain types of spiritual literature, and listening to tapes on different spiritual topics together while having a group tea. This focus will provide a common identity and reason to gather.

- *Tell others about the group.* In order to get members with this like-minded focus, you must find people who share this drive. By telling other patients and encouraging them to join, a small group is created, and more members will join as others hear about the spiritual group.

- *Have the group meetings at the same time each week.* If the group is formed in an area such as an elderly residential living area or neighborhood, you can all decide when would be best. In many cases, it is impossible to meet the needs of everyone, so it should be a time that the majority is comfortable coming. Good times are Wednesday or Sunday evenings, when everyone may feel more relaxed, and an established pattern should be developed.

- *Don't let the group get too large.* Normally groups larger than 12 become hard to manage, and not everyone gets the opportunity to express themselves. If your group continues to grow, you could break into two groups that meet at the same time and then meet once or twice a month for large group gatherings.

- *Group ideas.* Make an agenda for each spiritual meeting. If you are planning on discussing meditation—and practicing it—let the group decide this and make proper plans at least a week ahead of time. Let every member have an opportunity to express their beliefs and to present or plan an evening spiritual meeting.

SUMMARY

To become a fully integrated individual, we must become aware of ourselves, our feelings, and our effect on others. We must integrate the body, the mind, and the spirit to reach our fullest and highest potential as health care providers. We also have the responsibility of showing others how to do the same. Awareness is an important part of our lives—awareness of our motives and drives and awareness of others. As we learn to understand more about ourselves, we will understand more about others and therefore be able to provide care in multifaceted ways.

ASK YOURSELF

1. What does the term *consciousness* mean?
2. What are some ways to awaken consciousness?
3. Do you have an opportunity to tell patients about how they might develop a daily ritual in their life? How would you feel about discussing that with them?
4. What are the three types of awareness? Describe them.
5. What are the four psychodynamic theorists?
6. In what aspect of your practice could you include a meditative experience?
7. Would you ever have an opportunity to form a spiritual group? Would you like to do that?

REFERENCES

Assagioli, R. (1971). *Psychosynthesis.* New York: Viking.
Leighton, C. (1998). A change of heart. *American Journal of Nursing, 98*(10), 33–37.
Peng, C. K., Mietus, J. E., Liu, Y., Khalsa, G., Douglas, P. S., Benson, H., & Goldberger, A. L. (1999). Exaggerated heart rate oscillations during two meditation techniques. *International Journal of Cardiology, 70*(2), 101–107.
Perls, F., Hefferline, R. F., & Goodman, P. (1951). *Gestalt therapy.* New York: Dell.
Rew, L. (1996). *Awareness in healing.* Albany, NY: Delmar.
Rogers, C. R. (1961). *On becoming a person.* Boston: Houghton Mifflin.

Sury Das, L. (1999). *Awakening to the sacred: Creating a spiritual life from scratch.* Derry, NH: Broadway Books.

Strachey, J. (1962). *Sigmund Freud: The ego and the id.* New York: Norton.

Travis, F., & Wallace, R. K. (1999). Autonomic and EEG patterns during eyes-closed rest and transcendental meditation (TM) practice: The basis for a neural model of TM practice. *Consciousness and Cognition, 8*(3), 302–318.

Umlauf, M. (1997). *Healing meditation.* Albany, NY: Delmar.

Stress and Its Consequences

Chapter Objectives

- Learn about the all-pervasive nature of stress in contemporary society.
- Discover some of the main theories of the origin of stress.
- Recognize that there are effective coping mechanisms available to deal with stress.
- Build a personal set of skills to protect yourself against too much stress.
- Understand how important stress management is to being an effective healer.

INTRODUCTION

Stress is epidemic in our society. Over two-thirds of office visits to physicians are for stress-related illnesses (Preville, Potvin, & Boyer, 1998). It is accepted that there is a relationship between stress and heart disease, high blood pressure, coronary artery disease, some respiratory disorders, accidental injuries, and alcoholism leading to cirrhosis of the liver and suicide, all of which are leading causes of death in the United States.

There is substantial evidence from both healthy populations as well as individuals with cancer linking psychological stress with immune suppression. Psychological stress can result in physiological action that effects the natural killer (NK) cells and the role that they may play in malignant disease. In addition, distress or depression is also associated with two important processes for carcinogenesis: poorer repair of damaged DNA and alterations in apoptosis (Kiecolt-Glaser & Glaser, 1999). Conversely, however, there is the possibility that psychological interventions may enhance immune function and survival among cancer patients, and this clearly merits further exploration, as does the evidence suggesting that social support may be a key psychological mediator. Thus psychological or behavioral factors may influence the incidence or progression of cancer through psychosocial influences on immune function and other physiological pathways. In a study of 8059 healthy women (mean age 58 years) with the aim of establishing the presence or absence of a variety of physical and psychological risk factors for mammary cancer, psychological factors seemed to potentiate the effect of physical factors, particularly in the middle range (Grossarth-Maticek, Eisenck, Boyle, Heeb, Costa, & Diel, 2000). In addition to contributing to illness, stress has the ability to aggravate other conditions such as multiple sclerosis, diabetes, herpes, mental illness, drug abuse, family discord and violence (Harenstam, Theorell, & Kaijser, 2000; Calderon, Schneider, Alexander, Myers, Nidich, & Haney, 1999).

Stress not only affects a person's well-being, it also costs the United States massive amounts of money in medical costs, insurance, and lost days of work (Shain, 1999). The medical costs alone have been estimated at well over $1 billion per year. Stress costs industry approximately $150 billion per year in increased health insurance outlays, burnout, absenteeism, reduced productivity, costly mistakes in the office and on the shop floor, poor morale, high employee turnover, as well as family and alcohol- and drug-related problems (Greenberg et al., 1999). Anxiety disorders alone cost approximately $42.3 billion in 1990 in the United States, or $1542 per sufferer. This comprises $23.0 billion (or 54% of the total cost) in nonpsychiatric medical treatment costs, $13.3 billion (31%) in psychiatric treatment costs, $4.1 billion (10%) in indirect workplace costs, $1.2 billion (3%) in mortality costs, and $0.8 billion (2%) in prescription pharmaceutical costs. Of the $256 in workplace costs per anxious worker, 88% is attributable to lost productivity while at work as opposed to absenteeism. Posttraumatic stress disorder and panic disorder are the anxiety disorders found to have the highest rates of service use (Greenberg et al., 1999). From an economic standpoint alone, stress is a major concern in the United States.

However, stress is not always negative; managed correctly, the problems that result from stress can be minimized. Realistically, stress is a normal aspect of life that must be endured at some level. Additionally, a stress response can be helpful in many ways, motivating you to work, study, or increase your alertness while taking a test or giving a talk. The problem occurs when stress that exceeds a productive level interferes with your ability to think, remember, and focus on tasks. Stress that is ineffectively managed and remains too high for too long can contribute to multiple illnesses.

Those who work in the healing professions need to recognize stressors and learn the skills to cope with them. Indeed, many of the alternative and complementary therapies were developed out of the need to deal with stress in the contemporary world.

WHAT IS STRESS AND HOW DOES IT OCCUR?

Stress is a state of tension that is created when an individual responds to pressures that come from work, family, or other external sources as well as those that are internally generated from self-imposed demands, obligations, and self-criticism. In many cases stress can become a cumulative and chronic disorder if the individual does not learn to change their behavior to decrease their stress levels. Stress has the ability of adding up over time until a state of crisis is reached and symptoms appear. These symptoms may manifest themselves in the body as well as in the mind. Early symptoms of stress can be seen as irritability, anxiety, impaired concentration, mental confusion, poor judgment, frustration, and anger. As stress continues to accumulate, individuals will often develop physical symptoms. The most common physical symptoms of stress include muscle tension, headaches, low back pain, insomnia, and high blood pressure.

Stress is the response to a situation that evokes the flight-or-fight response. When your body gets stimulus from the *stressor*—the event that is perceived as stressful—that stimulus is reported to the hypothalamus. At this time, the hypothalamus gives the order to adjust the body according to the stimulus, the autonomic nerve system becomes active, and hormones increase. Since the autonomic nervous system and the hormones are being active, there will be some stimulus on the circulatory system, the respiratory organs, the digestive organs, the urinary organs, bones, muscles, and skin. There is also an effect on the metabolism of internal secretions and nerves. In nature this type of response helps animals release adrenalin and flee or attack a predator or prey. However, in an office or home setting a release of hormones and chemicals does not serve the purposes for which they were once useful. Most individuals pay a psychological and physical price when their internal balance is disrupted by a perceived threat, change, or transition and is called upon to adjust. A number of physiological changes occur, including increases in muscle tension, heart rate, and blood pressure.

Factors That Contribute to Stress

There are a number of factors that contribute to stress. It is important to note that different individuals will react differently to stress in the environment. For one individual a certain job may be invigorating and fun, for another it may be a cause of something as deadly as heart disease. In evaluating an individual in a high-stress situation we can look at:

1. *Personality.* How someone responds to stress is one of the most important factors we can analyze in looking at stress. It is commonly known that there are variations of personality, and some personality types respond very negatively to stress. If you or a patient of yours has an anxious or volatile personality, there are numerous stress management techniques to utilize that will increase the ability to cope.

2. *Home and family.* For some individuals this is the most stressful area of their lives. Many people do not find solace in their homes. They may have difficulty with their spouse, children, parents, or other family members. An individual's home life is an important element when analyzing stress levels.

3. *Current events.* Stress is not only long term but can be triggered by recent events. These events are not necessarily negative in nature. They can range from marriage to a promotion to getting a new job.

4. *Daily hassles.* The cumulative effect of incessant daily hassles is a major contributor to stress. Assess yourself and your patients for this sometimes silent, but powerful contributor to stress.

Determining Stress Levels

In addition to traits for stress and current events in an individual's life, there are other factors to determining the level of stress a certain individual is experiencing:

1. *Length of time under stress.* The longer a person has experienced a stressful situation, the greater the likelihood of resultant physical and psychological problems.

2. *Frequency of the stress.* Stress that is encountered on a weekly visit to see a parent is going to be a lot less than stress of day-to-day contact, such as we might see between a husband and wife that are having relationship problems. How often the stress is experienced makes a difference both mentally and physiologically.

3. *Degree of stress.* If the stress itself is a big event, such as a death, we can expect to see stress at very high levels over a relatively long time span. However, a smaller degree of stress over a longer period of time can result in the same types of depression and physiological concerns that we would see after extremely stressful life events. Stress is produced by both normal and unusual events as well as by both positive and negative occurrences. Just as a divorce or a low grade in school might increase stress, so might positive experiences such as an engagement or admission to graduate school. Because stress can be cumulative, one needs to monitor and regulate the number of threats (real or perceived), changes, and transitions that may be encountered in the same period of time. Stress can be more harmful when accompanied by a sense of lack of control of the events that produce stress.

FIGHT-OR-FLIGHT RESPONSE

There are two switches on your body's involuntary nervous system: one is for ordinary everyday events; the other is for emergency situations. When one switch is on, the other is off. The ordinary daily-event switch controls the normal processes of your body, such as breathing, digestion, and metabolism. The emergency switch is designed to enable you to survive in the face of life-threatening danger by triggering your body's "stress response," also known as the "fight-or-flight response." Keep in mind that your body's stress response is meant for short-term use only. If it is triggered too often, and if it stays on for too long, you can develop serious health problems. This is because when the emergency switch is triggered, powerful hormones associated with stress biochemistry, such as norepinephrine and cortisol, are secreted in your body. This occurs through a process set in motion by your reactive brain, which cues the hypothalamus and the pituitary to secrete a hormone called adrenocorticotropic (ACTH). This hormone travels in your bloodstream, and when it hits the adrenal glands sitting on top of your kidneys, adrenaline is released and another phase of the fight-or-flight response is set into motion.

The quintessential mind-body problem is that your thoughts and feelings constantly trigger your fight-or-flight response. But the hypothalamus cannot tell the difference between actual physical danger and stressful thoughts and feelings about danger. Our hypothalamus is especially sensitive to psychological cues that we are in danger. If you worry too much about your job, your relationships, or your finances, to cite some common examples, stress hormones are unnecessarily released into your bloodstream. The fight-or-flight response is constantly ongoing and is modulated by our perception of stress.

A vicious cycle results when our mind triggers a stress response, because stress biochemistry then puts our mind in a hypervigilant, or aroused, state. We then tend to become even more prone to worry because, when we look for threat, we usually can find it. This, in turn, keeps the stress hormones flowing.

How Stress Biochemistry Causes Illness

Some people have a cardiovascular response to stress biochemistry. These people are susceptible to stress-induced high blood pressure and heart disease, and the release of adrenaline and other hormones leads to a constriction in the smooth muscles lining their arterioles and blood vessels. This narrows the path that blood can flow after it is pumped from the heart, which raises blood pressure and puts strain on the heart, because it has to work harder to do its job.

Some theorists believe that certain behaviors, especially anger and rage, can contribute to the development of cardiovascular disease. Now researchers are documenting the physiology behind this theory.

Chronic stress biochemistry can also create a biochemical imbalance that weakens our immune system so that we are vulnerable to attack by cancer cells and infectious disease. Through methods such as progressive relaxation (see Glossary) and autogenic training (see Glossary), people can learn how to dilate their smooth muscles so that there is an open path for blood to flow. They can also learn how to diminish the stress response by altering stress biochemistry, thereby reducing their risk of high blood pressure as well as illnesses resulting from an

RESEARCH BOX: Correlation between Anger and Increased Platelet Aggregation

Potential relationships between increased platelet aggregability and such psychological characteristics as hostility and anger were investigated as part of a larger intervention study of the potential efficacy of stress reduction treatments. Participants performed 6-minute mental arithmetic tests under time pressure. Blood was sampled during the first minute of the task and whole-blood platelet aggregation was measured. To assess anger and hostility, the authors used Spielberger's State-Trait Anger and Anger Expression scales together with the Cook-Medley Hostility Scale. The authors found positive correlations between collagen-induced platelet aggregation and outwardly expressed anger, as measured by the Anger Expression Scale. The findings suggested that modes of anger expression may be associated with increased platelet aggregation. If confirmed by future studies, this finding could provide a mechanism for the putative connection between anger/hostility and coronary heart disease.

Source: Wenneberg, S. R., Schneider, R. H., Walton, K. G., MacLean, C. R., Levitsky, D. K., Mandarino, J. V., Waziri, R., & Wallace, R. K. (1997). Anger expression correlates with platelet aggregation. *Behavioral Medicine, 22*(4), 174–177.

impaired immune system. These methods (along with psychotherapy, if necessary, which can get to the source of habitual stress-provoking perceptual tendencies) can be a potent preventive move and treatment strategy against stress-related illnesses.

It is well worth the effort required to learn how to prevent and reverse stress-related illnesses. The chronic, undesirable, unnecessary release of stress hormones into the body is among the most dangerous of health risk factors that we can face.

We have known for a long time that too much stress can cause physical damage to the gastrointestinal tract, glandular system, skin, or cardiovascular system. But only recently have we learned that overstress actually causes physical changes in the brain. One of the most exciting medical advances of our decade has been an understanding of how overstress physically affects your brain. We now know that fatigue, aches and pains, crying spells, depression, anxiety attacks, and sleep disturbances may be related to the perception of too many stressors. When this occurs, the parts of the body affected ("weak links") respond with the manifestation of physical symptoms. Table 20-1 details some of the common weak links and the corresponding symptoms of their malfunction.

TABLE 20-1	Some Common Weak Links and the Symptoms of Their Malfunction

WEAK LINK	SYMPTOMS
Brain	Fatigue, aches and pains, crying spells, depression, anxiety attacks, sleep disturbance
Gastrointestinal tract	Ulcer, cramps and diarrhea, colitis, irritable bowel
Glandular system	Thyroid gland malfunction
Cardiovascular system	High blood pressure, heart attack, abnormal heartbeat, strokes
Skin	Itchy skin rashes
Immune system	Decreased resistance to infections and neoplasm

Hans Selye

During the 1930s, Hans Selye, a Swedish physiologist and researcher, discovered the mechanisms that link illnesses such as heart disease, high blood pressure, and other stress-related mind-body diseases. Selye conducted a number of innovative experiments on the physiology of stress. If we suffer from any one or a variety of stressful events, including injury, disease, or acute psychological stress, our body tends to respond with the same pattern of response to restore its internal equilibrium. This led Selye to discover what he called "just being sick"—a sign that our body is working hard at restoring itself. The syndrome of just being sick results from the body's nonspecific stress response to any interference with its inner harmony. If the body has to chronically struggle to do this, the syndrome of just being sick can deteriorate into disease.

Selye formulated some of his most important ideas in what he called the general adaptation syndrome (GAS). The GAS is heralded as being a cornerstone of modern behavioral medicine. Our body always seeks to maintain homeostasis or a balance of its internal environment. It makes great adaptive efforts to maintain physiological equilibrium in the face of whatever stressful changes might take place in the environment. For example, whether it is 20 degrees in the winter or 98 degrees in summer, our body seeks to maintain an internal temperature of around 98.6 degrees.

Today the most dangerous illnesses that threaten Americans, heart disease and cancer, are known to be largely "diseases of adaptation." That is, they often result from the wear and tear that the cardiovascular and immune systems go through while trying to "adapt" by maintaining a constant internal environment in the face of forces that have created disequilibrium.

GENERAL ADAPTATION SYNDROME

The GAS involves three stages: (1) the alarm reaction, (2) the stage of resistance, and (3) the stage of exhaustion. An understanding of these stages will enable us to appreciate just what is involved in stress-related illnesses. The *alarm reaction* involves the triggering of our body's emergency alert resources. Our autonomic nervous system is activated in ways that involve the release of powerful hormones such as epinephrine and norepinephrine. This is part of the stress or fight-or-flight response.

It is interesting to note here that recent mind-body research has discovered that these very same hormones play a central role in our memory. For example, in a case of physical stress, if we have a car accident, our body releases stress hormones in response to the trauma (Ursano & Fullerton, 1999). Our recollection of the accident becomes linked with the release of these hormones. When we remember the accident, we trigger the release of the hormones because our memories are tied to the condition of our mind-body at the time of the accident (Shalev, Peri, Brandes, Freedman, Orr, & Pitman, 2000). In some ways, we keep having the accident every time we remember it.

This central memory phenomenon is one of the reasons many of us tend to be imprisoned by painful experiences from our past. They continue to affect our mind-body as if they were going on now. To become free of past trauma, we have to undo the connection between our memory and the physiological conditions that were originally part of our suffering.

The *stage of resistance* represents the body's attempts to restore its inner equilibrium. Our body does what it has to do in order to overcome the stress that caused the alarm reaction and to return to the condition it was in before it happened. Our body has tremendous resources to do this. Often, mind-body symptoms such as headaches, anxiety, pain, and others can become part of the resistance stage. Unfortunately, these symptoms themselves get bound to our memory of painful events and seem to have a life of their own. They exist long after the conditions that caused them have disappeared.

The *stage of exhaustion* occurs when our body's resources for restoring the constancy of its internal environment are depleted. In the exhaustion phase, our body goes through an initial period of strain, which, if not relieved, moves further to actual physical damage and accompanying symptoms. Depending upon our unique physiological make-up, this can endanger our cardiovascular, neuromuscular, and/or immune systems.

When we reach the stage of exhaustion, we run the risk of developing the diseases of adaptation, including heart disease, high blood pressure, and cancer, among others. These illnesses are not always diseases of adaptation, but in a majority of instances they are. They result from dramatic periods of acute stress or chronic periods of extended stress at the exhaustion of the body's resources.

Effect of Negative Stress

You may have heard the often-repeated phrase that "stress is detrimental to your health." Just what does this mean? Stress is necessary for life. Stress represents any changing environment. What we mean to say is "negative stress will suppress your immune system."

Stress can be of many types. The most common are physical (accidents, strained muscles, spinal problems), emotional (fear, anxiety, depression), and chemical (drugs, pollution, food additives). Negative stress has both direct and indirect effects on the immune system. These effects are cumulative and can be compounding. The effects are usually moderated through hormones and interleukins (ILs—regulatory molecules that help orchestrate the immune response). Recent research has shown that stress will directly impact the immune system in a negative way (Stefanski & Engler, 1999; Yehuda, 1999). Initial response to an infection is an increase in IL-2 with a great cellular attack against the invader. Interleukin-2 is required for helper cell proliferation. A great number of receptors for IL-2 appear on lymphocytes, allowing for this greatly increased response. As long as IL-2 levels are high, the cellular attack phase will continue and the person is at their most viral resistant phase. Negative stress has been shown to decrease IL-2 production and also decrease the number of IL-2 receptors on lymphocytes. Other direct effects include decreased interferons, decreased NK cell activity, and lower T-cell mitogenesis.

Indirectly, stress causes the release of ACTH from the pituitary gland in the brain that signals the adrenal glands to release cortisol—anti-inflammatory hormones. These hormones will repress the lymph nodes and thymus and inhibit immune cell functions. Another pituitary hormone that is released, thyroid-stimulating hormone (TSH), causes the thyroid gland to become overactive, resulting in weight loss, nervousness, an increased demand for vitamins and minerals, and a protein deficit.

COUNTERACTING THE EFFECTS OF NEGATIVE STRESS

To counteract the effects of negative stress, you must eliminate the sources of stress to the best of your ability. Clean up your diet; stay away from fried foods, alcohol, caffeine, and overly refined foods. A nutritional approach would include B vitamins, the "antistress" vitamins. Avoid excessive use of drugs, illegal or prescription. Address any emotional problems in your life. Make sure you remain physically fit by exercising regularly and getting enough rest. Many of the alternative and complementary therapies work with the nervous system to reduce the negative effects of stress. You may want to incorporate meditation, massage, biofeedback, acupuncture, or other stress reduction techniques into your life. Your health may well depend on your ability to handle stress.

TYPES OF STRESSORS

There are at least four different categories of stressors:

1. *Physicochemical stressor.* This includes most elements in the external environment represented by nature. Examples are pollen, air pollution, tobacco, alcohol, toxic fumes, excess ultraviolet light exposure, and noise.

2. *Social stressor.* This includes the whole gamut of the social environment. Examples are divorce, difficulties raising children, and perceived social isolation.

3. *Biological stressor.* This includes bacterial, viral, surgical, and other elements in the internal environment. Examples are getting the flu and having surgery.

4. *Mental stressor.* This includes psychological conditions such as pleasantness and unpleasantness. Examples are preparing for marriage, taking exams, and caring for elderly parents.

Each stressor is closely related and works to cause the stress condition. It is probably easy to understand that you cannot discuss each type independently. Unfavorable mental states such as impatience, listlessness, frustration, emotional conflict, and nervousness as well as good mental conditions such as hope, expectation, and happiness are all examples of mental stressors.

Changes When the Body Is under Stress

What kinds of changes are there in the body when it is under stress? Certain strong stress, such as an automobile accident or a death in the family, is specific, something that we do not experience in daily life. So, when our body feels or perceives that something is wrong, in other words, when our body accepts the stimulus as a stressor, its homeostasis is disturbed. Then, our body copes with or responds to the stressor by secreting hormones through the hypothalamus and adrenal cortex system. Hormones influence internal body organization and have an effect on the immune system through white blood cells. This causes a cascade of effects that adjust the function of organs through the hypothalamus to the autonomic nerve system. This physiological change in the body is called "stress."

What is important is that the hypothalamus gives orders according to the perceived threat of the stressor. During stress, the order is given to restore the body back to its normal condition before it was affected by the stressor. No matter how much stimulation is given to the body, there is no difference in how the hypothalamus works to bring the body back to normal.

By activating the stress response and being under a stressful condition, your body responds to the stressor. It is something like developing a fever in order to make the defensive system in your body fight against an invading bacteria or virus. The stress reaction is something that happens to rally a defense. In other words, when the stress response appears, it means that your body is receiving some kind of a stress from a stressor. We can judge if the stress condition is dangerous and apt to continue or not by the degree of the stress response.

If the stress response becomes worse, your body will take some kind of an action to remove the stressor. But if there is no stress response, your body will not know that it is under some sort of stress so it will leave the stressor alone. If your body-mind perceives frequent and unrelenting stressors, the condition can result in deleterious body effects. Therefore, if your body's defensive system cannot remove the stressor by itself, you have to protect your body consciously. The stress response tells you the necessity of paying attention, while the stress reaction tells you that there is danger in your body.

Some stress responses are caused by interpreting the stressor after recognizing it. For example, some people get stomachaches before exams because of anxiety. This stress response is due to the interpretation of exams as something that they do not like or are not good at. If, however, a person perceives that the test will be composed of a simple set of questions and will have no effect on their grades, there would be decreased anxiety. In both cases, the questions and answers are the same, but the difference is that the mind perceives a bad "image" to an exam whereas a simple test does not cause anxiety.

THE STRESS SPIRAL

Because stress stems from a number of stressors, it can cause a stress spiral (see Figure 20-1). As with mental stressors, one stressor producing or worsening another stressor is a common phenomenon. And it is not rare for a stress response or an action taken to deal with a stress to ironically work as yet another stressor. This is a stress spiral.

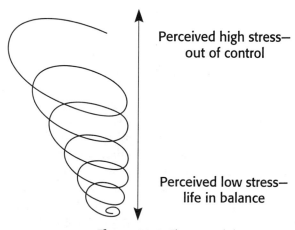

Perceived high stress—
out of control

Perceived low stress—
life in balance

Figure 20-1 The stress spiral

Role of General Adaptation Syndrome

Now why does the GAS occur in the body when stimulation is given from a stressor? As an example, consider an extremely cold situation in which body temperature drops and body function drops. The stressor, "coldness," will be noticed by the brain's hypothalamus. When that is done, the hypothalamus tries to bring back the body balance to normal using hormones and going through the autonomic nervous system giving orders to each part of the body. As a result, the body tries to fight against the cold so it can be in the best position to protect itself. That is how the shivering effect is activated.

STRESS AND ILLNESS

An individual under stress will react both mentally and physically. Both long- and short-term stress have common symptoms. They can include:

- Fatigue
- Change in relationship and sociability levels
- Change in appetite, either eating more or less
- Increased irritability and anxiety levels
- Increased alcohol, drug, or cigarette use or other self-destructive behaviors
- Body aches and pains not caused by exercise
- Change in sleeping or waking patterns
- Change in behavior or emotional patterns
- Inability to focus on tasks effectively
- Inability to concentrate
- Memory loss
- Depression

The effects of stress extend far beyond the mental level in many cases. Humans are made to tolerate stress in certain amounts and for certain lengths of time. Our bodies have the ability to repair the disturbed system of the body by the absorption of hormone and chemical surges. However, if the stress level that the body is exposed to is too strong or for a long time, the body is able to adjust properly and the symptoms will begin to appear. In these individuals, we see a manifestation of the stress in an actual physical illness. Treatment of the symptoms may provide short-term relief but is not a long-term solution. By recognizing the illness and its association with stress, it is likely that improved long-term solutions can be found, such as the individual learning stress management techniques. Table 20-2 lists some of the illnesses and diseases often related to stress.

TABLE 20-2	Illnesses and Diseases Often Related to Stress		
Immune system problems	Coronary artery disease	Amenorrhea
Anxiety	Stroke	Eating disorders
Ulcerative colitis	Headaches	Depression
Impotence	Breathing problems	Skin rashes and disorders
Fatigue	High blood pressure	Diabetes mellitus
Ulcers	Irritable bowel syndrome	Hypertension

How we experience stress is different depending on the situation. For example, an everyday stress may occur walking down the street and confronting a large, barking dog coming toward us. When we first encounter the dog, our body will begin to produce adrenaline and we will analyze what we should do in response. Our pupils will dilate as we acknowledge the potential threat and our mind tries to take in all possible information about the situation. This reaction is an important one for our survival. By having a quick reaction, an adrenalin rush, and eye dilation, we can quickly make the decision to try and appear calm as the drooling dog comes closer. Such a reaction occurs to protect the body whenever we encounter a short-span, high-stress situation. Once the owner comes out, apologizes profusely, and takes the dog in, we can get back on our walk and relax. The chemical level drops off and the body returns to normal.

Effects of Stress on the Body's Immune System

Researchers who have spent years studying the effects of stress on the body's immune system now believe they know enough to show that stress actually does have an effect on a person's health. Studies have shown that stress can alter the levels of certain biochemical markers in the body, key players in the human immune response, but only recently have research findings shown that those changes actually lead to poorer health. The alterations induced by stress are responsible for the changes in cytokine concentrations since stress hormones alter the synthesis and release of the cytokines. Research involving vaccinations for hepatitis B and for influenza showed that stress could suppress T-cell responses and lower antibody levels, two factors necessary to develop a strong immunity to these diseases (Glaser, Rabin, Chesney, Cohen, & Natelson, 1999). We also know that certain changes in lifestyle can increase a person's resistance to some infectious diseases. Most of these changes—gaining social support and companionship, maintaining a proper diet, and getting regular exercise and enough sleep—are not expensive.

Knowing this information should allow health care practitioners to focus more on the role stress plays in infections and diseases such as asthma, rheumatoid arthritis, multiple sclerosis, inflammatory bowel disease, psoriasis, and cancer.

Stress and Colds

Increasing evidence shows a relationship between a person's level of psychological stress and their susceptibility to several cold viruses. Evidence suggests that stress makes one more susceptible to colds and other forms of infection (Ben-Nathan, Lustig, & Kobiler, 1996). In one example, researchers found that events that caused stress were much more likely to precede than to follow new infections (Cohen, Line, Manuck, Rabin, Heise, & Kaplan, 1997). Those who developed a cold or infection had often felt angrier and more tense than usual, and these feelings were not signs of illness since they appeared on average four days before the physical symptoms.

RESEARCH BOX: Stress and Colds

Two-hundred seventy-six volunteers completed life stressor interviews and psychological questionnaires and provided blood and urine samples. They were then inoculated with common cold viruses and monitored for the onset of disease. Although severe acute stressful life events (less than one month long) were not associated with developing colds, severe chronic stressors (one month or longer) were associated with a substantial increase in risk of disease. This relation was attributable primarily to under- or unemployment and to enduring interpersonal difficulties with family or friends. The association between chronic stressors and susceptibility to colds could not be fully explained by differences among stressed and nonstressed persons in social network characteristics, personality, health practices, or prechallenge endocrine or immune measures.

Source: Cohen, S., Frank, E., Doyle, W. J., Skoner, D. P., Rabin, B. S., & Gwaltney, J. M., Jr. (1998). Types of stressors that increase susceptibility to the common cold in healthy adults. *Health Psychology, 17*(3), 214–223.

Stress and Skin Disease

Stress can be detrimental to every organ of the body. Skin diseases related to stress include psoriasis and eczema. Likewise, conscious attention to symptoms can often awaken us to the need to do something to alleviate the condition. In the following instance mindfulness meditation was used to counteract stress-related skin lesions.

RESEARCH BOX: Mindfulness Meditation to Reduce Stress

This study tested the hypothesis that stress reduction methods based on mindfulness meditation can positively influence the rate at which psoriasis clears in patients undergoing phototherapy or photochemotherapy treatment. Thirty-seven patients with psoriasis about to undergo ultraviolet phototherapy (UVB) or photochemotherapy (PUVA) were randomly assigned to one of two conditions: a mindfulness meditation-based stress reduction intervention guided by audiotaped instructions during light treatments or a control condition consisting of the light treatments alone with no taped instructions. Psoriasis status was assessed in three ways: direct inspection by unblinded clinic nurses, direct inspection by physicians blinded to the patient's study condition (tape or no tape), and blinded physician evaluation of photographs of psoriasis lesions. Four sequential indicators of skin status were monitored during the study: a first-response point, a turning point, a halfway point, and a clearing point. Cox-proportional hazards regression analysis showed that subjects in the tape groups reached the halfway point ($p = 0.013$) and the clearing point ($p = 0.033$) significantly more rapidly than those in the no-tape condition for both UVB and PUVA treatments. The conclusion is that a brief mindfulness meditation-based stress reduction intervention delivered by audiotape during ultraviolet light therapy can increase the rate of resolution of psoriatic lesions in patients with psoriasis.

Source: Kabat-Zinn, J., Wheeler, E., Light, T., Skillings, A., Scharf, M. J., Cropley, T. G., Hosmer, D., & Bernhard, J. D. (1998). Influence of a mindfulness meditation-based stress reduction intervention on rates of skin clearing in patients with moderate to severe psoriasis undergoing phototherapy (UVB) and photochemotherapy (PUVA). *Psychosomatic Medicine, 60*(5), 625–632.

Stress and Heart Disease

The link between heart disease and stress has been documented. What many people still do not know, however, is that this ailment, like so many others, can be helped and in some cases reversed by use of stress reduction techniques.

RESEARCH BOX: Transcendental Meditation and
Heart Disease

Twenty-one patients with documented coronary artery disease were
tested at baseline by exercise tolerance testing and assigned to either
stress reduction using the transcendental meditation (TM) program or
to a wait-list control. After eight months, the TM group had a 14.7%
increase in exercise tolerance, an 11.7% increase in maximal workload,
an 18% delay in onset of ST-segment depression, and significant reductions in rate-pressure product at 3 and 6 minutes and at maximal exercise
compared with the control group.

Source: Zamarra, J. W., Schneider, R. H., Besseghini, I., Robinson, D. K., & Salerno, J. W.
(1996). Usefulness of the transcendental meditation program in the treatment of patients
with coronary artery disease. *American Journal of Cardiology, 77*(10), 867–870.

STRESS MANAGEMENT

Stress management is largely a learnable skill. Another perspective of stress is
that it is a "false alarm," that is, the erroneous activation of the "danger alarm"
system of the brain. Try to visualize it as a big red fire alarm inside the head. This
is a system we are all born with and it is a good thing to have. However, the biological purpose of this system is to help prepare us for dealing with real, physical
danger. When the danger alarm is activated, it produces a physiological response
called the fight-or-flight response, which helps us to fight danger or flee it.

When you are in real, immediate physical danger, it is appropriate to feel afraid.
Getting your body charged up with adrenaline may well help to keep you alive.
However, most of the time, when we feel stress, there is no immediate danger, so
it is a false alarm. The fire alarm is sounding, but there is no fire! So how do you
learn to manage stress? There are basically two main ways:

1. Learn how to turn off the alarm system through various relaxation
   methods.

2. Learn how to not turn it on inadvertently in the first place.

Relaxation methods work on the idea that you cannot be relaxed and uptight at
the same time. Basically, anything you do that is the opposite of what the danger
alarm system does will tend to shut it off. Some examples include:

■ *Deep breathing.* Taking deep, slow breaths rather than the shallow, fast
  breathing we feel when we are stressed. This really works physiologically
  to help shut off the danger alarm.

■ *Muscular relaxation.* Tensing and relaxing various muscle groups can work wonders. Try your neck and shoulders, your shoulder blades, your forehead and eyes, tensing these groups for a few seconds, then relaxing them. You can also combine this with deep breathing by inhaling while you tense, then exhaling when you relax the muscles. There are more sophisticated versions of these muscular methods, like the shower of relaxation and progressive relaxation.

■ *Visualization.* Imagining a very peaceful scene, like lying on the beach, being out in a fishing boat on a lake, or being in a mountain cabin. It can be a real or imaginary place. Try to invoke all your senses as you imagine being in this very peaceful, relaxing place. What do you see? What sounds are there? Imagine the sensations of touch, temperature, or smell. For example, you might imagine the sun on your skin, the cool breeze on your forehead, the salt tang of the ocean, or the grit of the sand.

■ *Note taking.* If you are an analytical person, you may want to jot down a list of options and alternatives. Sometimes writing and organizing several different choices help to put the situation into perspective.

Try all these methods and see which works better for you. Some people do better with muscular methods, others with visualization. All these can be learned quite readily and often work very well.

In the long run, however, it is better to learn how to avoid getting too much stress in the first place. So how do you do that? For example, for some it is in the visualization method. Thinking peaceful thoughts makes you feel relaxed. In imagining a peaceful place, you have also distracted yourself from whatever thoughts you were having before. This points out the basic premise of cognitive/behavioral psychology that our feelings and behaviors are largely caused by our own thoughts. This is oversimplified, because there are many feedback loops that make the connection between thoughts, feelings, and behaviors. But the simple version of the cognitive theory is that peaceful thoughts cause relaxation and stressful thoughts cause stress. In other words, the reason we get stressed out is not what is happening to us and not what happened in the past (at least not directly), but rather, how we are thinking about what is happening. Past experience does influence us strongly, but the medium of that influence is beliefs or thoughts. For example, if you were abused as a child, you might have developed the belief that you are worthless. It is this belief today that is making you feel depressed, not the fact of the abuse itself. This is a powerful concept because it means we can overcome many of the bad experiences from the past. It means we have power over ourselves, so we do not have to be victims of past or present circumstances.

Learn to Change Anxiety to Concern

The best way to manage stress is to learn to change anxiety to concern. Concern means you are motivated to take care of real problems in your life, but your danger alarm system is not erroneously activated. Changing your feelings is largely a matter of learning to identify and change the upsetting thoughts that are the immediate and proximate cause of upset emotions.

Tolerance to Stress

The tolerance to stress is how strong you are against the condition when you are under stress. In the same condition, some people lose heart and some people may become ill. This differs because the tolerance to stress differs from one person to another. The factors that depend on your tolerance to stress include:

1. Stress recognition ability is whether or not you know the stress when it is there. Even under stressful conditions, being careless about it makes it easy to bear it (or rather, not even realize its existence). This differs between personality types as well as physical constitution. A robust man may not mind a little dizziness. On the other hand, a sudden illness of a usually healthy person may cause anxiety.

2. Stress avoidance ability is whether you dodge stress easily or not. For example, someone used to being continually directed by others does not feel too stressed by somebody's selfish action.

3. Fundamental stressor-dealing ability is how you can get rid of or diminish the stressors, the cause of stress. Being able to take good measures against stressors is as good as being strong against stressful situations.

4. Stress conversion ability is being able to reconsider the meaning of the stressor and to use the stressor as a chance to improve yourself.

5. Stressor experience is the amount of experience with various stressors. Sometimes, seeing the same stressor makes you used to it, making the situation less stressful. On the other hand, sometimes this weakens your tolerance.

6. Stress capacity is how much stress you can contain in yourself. If the stress level is within your limits of the capacity, you may not even feel the stressor as stress.

The strength of stress tolerance is not only different between people, but can also change in one person as well, depending on the time and the circumstance. Mainly, personality, physique, environment, and condition affect the strength of tolerance to stress.

STRESS CAPACITY

Stress capacity means how much stress you can hold in. If the level of the stress is within the range of the stress capacity, you will not feel it as stress. Therefore, one who has a small stress capacity will be less able to bear any small stress and might complain or become sick. Those with a large stress capacity often do not recognize minimal stressors and hence have a lowered stress response and are less inclined to get sick.

Stress capacity is not the same for everyone and it varies with an individual over time, each person's mental condition, physical condition, and the specific situation. The stress capacity may be large when you are in a good mood but become smaller when you are sick.

INCREASING STRESS TOLERANCE

Be joyful as you realize there are even more things you can do to increase your capacity to tolerate the inevitable stresses of life. A few of these are:

- Exercise regularly.
- Eat right.
- Get enough sleep.
- Do not overuse intoxicants.
- Do not smoke.
- Take routine work breaks.
- Make a concern list.
- Prioritize values.
- Periodically evaluate relationships and commitments.
- Do occasional career, life, and financial planning.
- Talk out problems with a trusted friend.

Coping Statements

Learning how to manage your feelings and behaviors takes work and practice. However, one simple way to get started is to develop "coping statements" to counter upsetting thoughts. Coping statements are somewhat like affirmations, but they are not necessarily positive ideas. Rather, they are realistic or reality based. Coping statements are usually challenges to specific upsetting thoughts, although you can use them any time.

The idea here is to stop yourself whenever you feel upset, anxious, worried, depressed, angry, guilty, ashamed, frustrated, and so on. You can also use undesired urges or behavior, like procrastination, smoking, drinking, or drugs as a cue to start the process. Catch yourself, and then try to observe what thoughts are running through your mind. Take a sheet of paper and divide it in half. On the left side of the sheet, write whatever thoughts you have observed. On the right side, write options for dealing with the problems.

Once you have identified the offending thoughts, just try changing them. As you get into this more, you will probably want to learn how to dispute or evaluate your thoughts on several levels, but the simple form of this exercise is to change the thoughts in any way that helps you feel or behave differently. Keep trying different alternatives until you find one that works for you.

Behavioral Psychology

Recent developments in behavioral psychology promise the possibility of a new drug-free approach to the problem of stress management. Behavioral psychologists have long treated autonomic responses—counterconditioning anxiety, phobias, and other psychological conditions—that are characterized by increased autonomic arousal. The sweaty hands, dry mouth, cold feet, tense muscles, and accelerated heart rate of the fearful airline flyer and anxious dental patients are familiar physiological manifestations of the anxiety response.

Counterconditioning procedures not only reduce the subjective experience of what the psychologist calls anxiety or stress but also modify its physiological manifestations. When the patient learns to reduce his anxiety, he is also learning to lower his blood pressure, slow down his heart rate, reduce the tensions in his muscles, increase the blood flow to his extremities, and in other ways control the activity of his autonomic nervous system.

It was with the realization that these behavioral procedures produced physiological side effects with important implications for physical medicine that attention to anxiety and stress turned from neurosis to psychosomatic. Many, if not all, stress-related and psychophysiological disorders involve autonomically innervated organs, and consequently many psychosomatic disorders have been demonstrated to be amenable to stress-reducing behavioral procedures. Biofeedback, hypnosis, deep-muscle relaxation, and other methods have been used to treat migraine headaches, muscle spasms, essential hypertension, premature ventricular contractions (PVCs), angina, spastic colon, Raynaud's syndrome, sympathetic reflex dystrophy, and many other physical disorders associated with sustained autonomic arousal.

Stress control continues to take on new importance as more studies validate that disease processes such as diabetes, arteriosclerosis, cardiovascular diseases, and other physical disorders might be manifestations, to the point of end-organ pathology, of chronic sustained autonomic activity.

STRESS AND EXERCISE

A regular exercise routine can have one of the best influences on reducing physical stress. Exercise can be as short as 10 minutes a day. Everybody can use a brief brisk walk during a busy day. Other forms of short exercise can be riding your bike to work or parking your car further away from your classroom or office and walking the extra distance. Not taking the elevator but walking the stairs is another fit-in exercise in a busy day. The more you can release your stress through brief exercise on a busy day, the better. Other health-minded changes for dealing with stress include meditation, swimming, rowing, aerobics, yoga, massage therapy, and diaphragmatic breathing. Obviously, a better diet that limits fried and fatty food will make the body stronger and make it easier to cope with stress. However, all of these physical changes need to be done simultaneously and consistently. Just doing exercise and still eating fatty food will not necessarily increase a person's physical threshold for dealing with stress.

Using Tai Chi to Combat Stress

People use a variety of alternative strategies to deal with stress. In the story that follows, Martha tells how tai chi made a difference in her life.

HEALING STORY: Using Tai Chi for Stress Reduction

Martha has been taking tai chi in a class twice a week for six months now. Friday morning, this last week, was the morning the teacher chose to do multiple forms. This experience of multiple forms in a row, with a period of standing chi gung in between, takes Martha deeper and deeper into what tai chi has to offer. She can feel her body loosen with each successive move and become deeply relaxed. Her body becomes more open and quiet and grounded with each passing form.

Martha finds it interesting how this tai chi experience takes her deeper into the body, expanding and opening the tissues down to the bone. There is nothing else in her life that produces the same result in body or spirit. If she doesn't do tai chi for a few days she feels noticeably more stiff and less mobile—a slow but inexorable contraction of her body, like a net being drawn tighter and tighter around her, restricting her movements. This is all reversed after a session of tai chi. It feels like a nurturing breeze is coursing through her body and the pulse of life which is her heartbeat is moving through every part of her body, similar to how a piece of music, when played softly with passion will allow you to hang on every note until

(Continued on next page)

the last one, which lingers in the air and expands the seconds after the actual note has played? According to Martha, tai chi expands that last second that is opened up in the music, one can live there, look around at life from that expanded vista and feel connected to the life around you with more than a surface connection. It is as if you are joined and have a perception of a level of reality that is not ordinary and is touching the pulse of life more directly.

At this level, the body and spirit are not separate. But the violence done to our bodies, which we accommodate to on a daily basis, closes our spirits and tightens our bodies and obscures the connection between our bodies, our spirits, and ultimately ourselves.

Observations and Insights

Think back to the last time you took a long vacation and remember how it felt. How long did that feeling last when you got back into your daily life? Three days? A week? Our state of being can become pinched or contracted just through the demands of everyday life. Unless we take the time to get in touch and bring relaxation back into our bodies and consciousness, we often remain contracted and stressed. The tissues of our body can and do change their shape, and shorten causing actual physical constriction. For Martha, tai chi reversed that. An exercise such as tai chi has the ability to transport you to the state of being you experience when very relaxed. It can provide a path for a return to the natural, balanced, and opened state that is how we were meant to live, free from the constricting reactivity that many generate in order to cope with the events of their lives. People like Martha are grateful when they discover a modality like tai chi, and can use it as an avenue to relieve life stresses.

COPING WITH STRESS

When people recognize stress, they try to get rid of it in some way. There are a lot of ways to cope with stressors, and people will use them differently depending on each person's personality and situation. As the stress response becomes greater, those ways of coping with stress become more necessary and important.

Taking Care of Yourself

Taking care of yourself starts with recognizing the unhealthy ways of dealing with stress (for example, drinking too much alcohol or eating unhealthful foods).

You can then try a healthier approach. You can reduce the negative effects of stress on your life by following these recommendations:

- Exercise for 30 minutes at least three times a week.
- Recognize the things that upset you. When something is increasing your stress, ask yourself, "Is there anything I can do to change the situation?" If there is, figure out what you can do. If there is not, find ways to accept this lack of control.
- Develop healthy methods for relaxation; for example, talk with supportive people, listen to music, watch movies, and take walks.
- Learn to use relaxation techniques, such as mental imaging, diaphragmatic breathing, and progressive muscle relaxation. Information is available in books, seminars, and via the Internet.
- Get adequate, regular amounts of rest and sleep (6 to 10 hours a night).
- Eat three to six small, balanced meals a day.
- Avoid caffeinated beverages and alcohol.
- Drink four to eight glasses of water a day.
- Use positive thoughts and humor to overcome negative thoughts.
- Identify ways you think yourself into higher levels of stress, including catastrophizing (making mountains out of mole hills), overgeneralizing (jumping to conclusions), dichotomous thinking (right-wrong, good-bad), and perfectionist thinking ("I'm no good unless I'm perfect"). Then find ways to nudge yourself out of these mental ruts.
- Seek professional help for dealing with especially stressful events in your life.

There is hope. If you learn how to manage your stress, you will be taking action to make your life longer and more enjoyable. The body must have an outlet for stress. You should either find ways to let the tension out of your body or cut down on the things that cause the tension. The best ways to deal with stress are to recognize the problem, find the causes, and find ways to stop the stress.

SUMMARY

Throughout recorded history people have dealt with stress. However, with the advent of the scientific, technological age, stress has grown exponentially. Researchers have documented the relationship between the perception of too much stress and the development of illness and disease. Once conscious recognition of this relationship exists, people can work to build coping skills that alleviate or prevent stress from harming their body-mind. A host of alternative therapies can be used to combat stress.

ASK YOURSELF

1. What are the psychological events that can trigger the stress response?

2. What are some physiological events that result in bodily manifestations of stress?

3. What are some different personality types and how do they react differently to stress?

4. What are at least three alternative therapies that can help people adjust to stress?

REFERENCES

Ben-Nathan, D., Lustig, S., & Kobiler, D. (1996). Cold stress-induced neuroinvasiveness of attenuated arboviruses is not solely mediated by corticosterone. *Archives of Virology, 141*(7), 1221–1229.

Calderon, R., Jr., Schneider, R. H., Alexander, C. N., Myers, H. F., Nidich, S. I., & Haney, C. (1999). Stress, stress reduction and hypercholesterolemia in African Americans: A review. *Ethnicity and Disease, 9*(3), 451–462.

Cohen, S., Line, S., Manuck, S. B., Rabin, B. S., Heise, E. R., & Kaplan, J. R. (1997). Chronic social stress, social status, and susceptibility to upper respiratory infections in nonhuman primates. *Psychosomatic Medicine, 59*(3), 213–221.

Glaser, R., Rabin, B., Chesney, M., Cohen, S., & Natelson, B. (1999). Stress-induced immunomodulation: Implications for infectious diseases? *Journal of the American Medical Association, 281*(24), 2268–2270.

Greenberg, P. E., Sisitsky, T., Kessler, R. C., Finkelstein, S. N., Berndt, E. R., Davidson, J. R., Ballenger, J. C., & Fyer, A. J. (1999). The economic burden of anxiety disorders in the 1990s. *Journal of Clinical Psychiatry, 60*(7), 427–435.

Grossarth-Maticek, R., Eysenck, H. J., Boyle, G. J., Heeb, J., Costa, S. D., & Diel, I. J. (2000). Interaction of psychosocial and physical risk factors in the causation of mammary cancer, and its prevention through psychological methods of treatment. *Journal of Clinical Psychology, 56*(1), 33–50.

Harenstam, A., Theorell, T., & Kaijser, L. (2000). Coping with anger-provoking situations, psychosocial working conditions, and ECG-detected signs of coronary heart disease. *Journal of Occupational Health Psychology, 5*(1), 191–203.

Kiecolt-Glaser, J. K., & Glaser, R. (1999). Psychoneuroimmunology and cancer: Fact or fiction? *European Journal of Cancer, 35*(11), 1603–1607.

Preville, M., Potvin, L., & Boyer, R. (1998). Psychological distress and use of ambulatory medical services in the Quebec Medicare system. *Health Services Research, 33*(2, Pt. 1), 275–286.

Shain, M. (1999). The role of the workplace in the production and containment of health costs: The case of stress-related disorders. *International Journal of Health Care Quality Assurance Incorporating Leadership in Health Services, 12*(2/3), i–vii.

Shalev, A. Y., Peri, T., Brandes, D., Freedman, S., Orr, S. P., & Pitman, R. K. (2000). Auditory startle response in trauma survivors with posttraumatic stress disorder: A prospective study. *American Journal of Psychiatry, 157*(2), 255–261.

Stefanski, V., & Engler, H. (1999). Social stress, dominance and blood cellular immunity. *Journal of Neuroimmunology, 94*(1/2), 144–152.

Ursano, R. J., & Fullerton, C. S. (1999). Posttraumatic stress disorder: Cerebellar regulation of psychological, interpersonal, and biological responses to trauma? *Psychiatry, 62*(4), 325–328.

Yehuda, R. (1999). Linking the neuroendocrinology of post-traumatic stress disorder with recent neuroanatomic findings. *Seminars in Clinical Neuropsychiatry, 4*(4), 256–265.

Bolstering the Immune System

Chapter Objectives

- Learn about the effect of the mind, body, and emotions on the immune system.
- Review the physiological concepts of the immune system.
- Recognize how conscious awareness of emotions and behaviors is related to the development of lifestyle changes that can enhance the immune system.
- Build knowledge about how regular exercise and healthy nutrition contribute to a stronger immune system.
- Develop new skills to incorporate joy, optimism, and hope into your psychological defense system.

INTRODUCTION

It is natural for a chapter on bolstering the immune system to follow a chapter on stress since stress is one of the key elements that impact the immune system. In the previous chapter stress theories, effects, and management techniques were discussed. Many of those concepts are likewise related to the immune system. This chapter builds upon the last one as some of the methodologies interrelate to both combat stress and build the immune system. Physical exercise, healthy nutrition, and an optimistic mind set, all of which are under our personal control, are essential ingredients in bolstering the immune system. An individual can use many of the alternative and complementary therapies to become increasingly conscious of as well as strengthen their body, mind, and spirit.

In the past decade, the concept of the "immune system" has achieved nationwide attention. Many people fear their "immune system is weak" and seek treatment options to enhance it. In some ways, this is an exciting sociological development for at last the general population has recognized the importance of self-care. Now it is possible for everyone to use natural medicine—food, herbs, homeopathic remedies, hydrotherapy, and lifestyle changes—to boost their immune system. The fact is that thousands of people are beginning to recognize that their bodies have built-in defense mechanisms and want to do what they can to support and improve these intrinsic protective devices.

Not everyone shares the same definition of the immune system. In medical terminology, the immune response is defined as the reaction of the body to substances perceived as foreign or as a threat. Fever, inflammation, and pain are common symptoms when this immune response is in action.

OUR IMMUNE ARMY

With the emergence of antibiotic-resistant bacteria along with the everyday virus exposures, it is clear that we must bolster our immune system so that it can defend us. This important internal "army" is able to destroy bacteria, viruses, fungi, and cancer cells effectively when it is working at peak efficiency. Unfortunately, due to poor nutrition, stress, and environmental toxins, for many people, their immune system is failing at its job.

Until recently our immune system was not well understood. With the introduction of the human immunodeficiency virus (HIV) the study of immunology has advanced dramatically. We are beginning to realize how intricately all the body systems are connected. Even our nervous system is hard wired into our immune system. With this knowledge we are aware of the importance of our thoughts and feelings. Loneliness is now recognized as a major predictor of disease due to its immune suppressing action. Laughter and feelings of satisfaction increase and enhance the actions of our immune cells, making our internal army more effective (Vanderhaeghe, 1999).

The intestine is surrounded by powerful immune factors that ward off invaders such as fungi, bacteria, and parasites that enter the body via our food. The increased incidence of parasitic infections may be due to the poor function of the immune system.

The skin is the largest immune organ, protecting us when it is intact and excreting immune agents that fight bacteria when it is wounded. All of the entrances to the body—eyes, nose, mouth, vagina, and anus—contain potent immune factors in their secretions to fight invaders and halt them from entering the body.

HOW THE IMMUNE SYSTEM WORKS

The immune system is composed of many interdependent cell types that collectively protect the body from bacterial, parasitic, fungal, and viral infections and the growth of tumor cells. Many of these cell types have specialized functions. The cells of the immune system can engulf bacteria, kill parasites or tumor cells, or kill viral-infected cells. Often, these cells depend on the T-helper subset for activation signals in the form of secretions formally known as cytokines, lymphokines, or more specifically interleukins.

Organs of the Immune System

There are four primary organs of the immune defense system:

- ◼ *Bone marrow.* All the cells of the immune system are initially derived from the bone marrow. They form through a process called hematopoiesis. During hematopoiesis, bone marrow–derived stem cells differentiate into either mature cells of the immune system or precursors of cells that migrate out of the bone marrow to continue their maturation elsewhere. The bone marrow produces B cells, natural killer cells, granulocytes, and immature thymocytes, in addition to red blood cells and platelets.

- ◼ *Thymus.* The function of the thymus is to produce mature T cells. Immature thymocytes, also known as prothymocytes, leave the bone marrow and migrate into the thymus. Through a remarkable maturation process sometimes referred to as thymic education, T cells that are beneficial to the immune system are spared, while those T cells that might evoke a detrimental autoimmune response are eliminated. The mature T cells are then released into the bloodstream.

- ◼ *Spleen.* The spleen is an immunological filter of the blood. It is made up of B cells, T cells, macrophages, dendritic cells, natural killer cells, and red blood cells. In addition to capturing foreign materials (antigens) from the blood that passes through the spleen, migratory macrophages and dendritic cells bring antigens to the spleen via the bloodstream. An immune response is initiated when the macrophage or dendritic cells present the antigen to the appropriate B or T cells. This organ can be thought of as an immunological conference center. In the spleen, B cells become activated and produce large amounts of antibody. Also, old red blood cells are destroyed in the spleen.

- ◼ *Lymph nodes.* The lymph nodes function as an immunological filter for the bodily fluid known as lymph. Lymph nodes are found throughout the body. Composed mostly of T cells, B cells, dendritic cells, and macrophages, the nodes drain fluid from most of our tissues. Antigens are filtered out of the lymph in the lymph node before returning the lymph to the circulation. In a similar fashion as the spleen, the macrophages and dendritic cells that capture antigens present these foreign materials to T and B cells, consequently initiating an immune response.

Cells of the Immune System

There are six primary types of cells comprising the immune system:

- ◼ *T cells.* T cells are the generals in our immune arsenal. The "T" in T cell stands for thymus derived. They include helper T cells, cytotoxic T cells, and suppressor T cells. Helper T cells excrete proteins, or cytokines, that regulate immune function. There are two types of helper T cells: T helper 1 cells and T helper 2 cells. When these two types of cells and their cytokines are in balance, we are healthy. When we are sick with cancer or infectious diseases such as hepatitis C, herpes, HIV, tuberculosis, colds, and flu, our T helper 1 cells are suppressed. With allergies, autoimmune disorders, including rheumatoid arthritis, lupus, and multiple sclerosis (MS), and inflammatory conditions such as osteoarthritis and fibromyalgia, we know that our T helper 2 cells are overactive and secreting too many inflammatory immune factors.

T lymphocytes are usually divided into two major subsets that are functionally and phenotypically (identifiably) different. The T helper subset, also called the CD4+ T cell, is a pertinent coordinator of immune regulation. The main function of the T helper cell is to augment or potentiate immune responses by the secretion of specialized factors that activate other white blood cells to fight off infection.

Another important type of T cell is called the T killer/suppressor subset or CD8+ T cell. These cells are important in directly killing certain tumor cells, viral-infected cells, and sometimes parasites. The CD8+ T cells are also important in downregulation of TH2 immune responses. Both types of T cells can be found throughout the body. They often depend on the secondary lymphoid organs (the lymph nodes and spleen) as sites where activation occurs, but they are also found in other tissues of the body, most conspicuously the liver, lung, blood, and intestinal and reproductive tracts.

■ *Natural killer cells.* Natural killer cells, often referred to as NK cells, are similar to the killer T cell subset (CD8+ T cells). They function as effector cells that directly kill certain tumors such as melanomas, lymphomas, and viral-infected cells, most notably herpes and cytomegalovirus-infected cells. The NK cells, unlike the CD8+ (killer) T cells, kill their targets without a prior "conference" in the lymphoid organs. However, NK cells that have been activated by secretions from CD4+ T cells will kill their tumor or viral-infected targets more effectively.

■ *B cells.* The major function of B lymphocytes is the production of antibodies in response to foreign proteins of bacteria and viruses. Antibodies are specialized proteins that specifically recognize and bind to one particular protein. Antibody production and binding to a foreign substance or antigen often are critical as a means of signaling other cells to engulf, kill, or remove that substance from the body.

■ *Granulocytes or polymorphonuclear leukocytes.* Another group of white blood cells is collectively referred to as granulocytes or polymorphonuclear (PMN) leukocytes. Granulocytes are composed of three cell types identified as neutrophils, eosinophils, and basophils, based on their staining characteristics with certain dyes. These cells are predominantly important in the removal of bacteria and parasites from the body. They engulf these foreign bodies and degrade them using their powerful enzymes.

■ *Macrophages.* Macrophages are important in the regulation of immune responses. They are often referred to as scavengers or antigen-presenting cells (APCs) because they pick up and ingest foreign materials and present these antigens to other cells of the immune system such as T cells and B cells. This is one of the important first steps in the initiation of an immune response. Stimulated macrophages exhibit increased levels of phagocytosis and are also secretory.

■ *Dendritic cells.* Another cell type, addressed only recently, is the dendritic cell. Dendritic cells, which also originate in the bone marrow, function as APCs. In fact, the dendritic cells are more efficient APCs than macrophages. These cells are usually found in the structural compartment of the lymphoid organs such as the thymus, lymph nodes, and spleen. However, they are also found in the bloodstream and other tissues of the body. It is believed that they capture antigen or bring it to the lymphoid organs where an immune response is initiated. Unfortunately, one reason we know so little about dendritic cells is that they are extremely hard to isolate, which is often a prerequisite for the study of the functional qualities of specific cell types.

The Immune Response

An immune response to foreign antigen requires the presence of an APC (usually either a macrophage or dendritic cell) in combination with a B cell or T cell. When an APC presents an antigen on its cell surface to a B cell, the B cell is signaled to proliferate and produce antibodies that specifically bind to that antigen. If the antibodies bind to antigens on bacteria or parasites, they act as a signal for macrophages to engulf (phagocytose) and kill them. Another important function of antibodies is to initiate the "complement destruction cascade." When antibodies bind to cells or bacteria, serum proteins called complement bind to the immobilized antibodies and destroy the bacteria by creating holes in them. Antibodies can also signal NK cells and macrophages to kill viral- or bacterial-infected cells.

If the APC presents the antigen to T cells, the T cells become activated. Activated T cells proliferate and become secretory in the case of CD4+ T cells, or, if they are CD8+ T cells, they become activated to kill target cells that specifically express the antigen presented by the APC. The production of antibodies and the activity of CD8+ killer T cells are highly regulated by the CD4+ helper T cell subset. The CD4+ T cells provide growth factors or signals to these cells that signal them to proliferate and function more efficiently.

BODY-MIND PHYSIOLOGY AND NEUROPEPTIDES

Research in the 1980s uncovered ubiquitous neuropeptide-receptor distribution in brain structures associated with emotional processing and throughout many organ systems (Pert, Ruff, Weber, & Herkenham, 1985; Ostrowski, Burke, Rice, Pert, & Pert, 1987; Algiati, Quirion, Bowen, & Pert, 1982). These findings supported neuropeptides as biochemical substrates of emotion and the neuropeptide-receptor network as a parasynaptic system crossing traditional brain-body boundaries. The medical relevance of these findings was affirmed by psycho-neuroimmunology research: Neuropeptides help to regulate immunocyte trafficking, there is bidirectional communication between nervous and immune system components, immunocytes produce neuropeptides, and nerve cells produce immune-associated cytokines. In the past decade, animal and human research demonstrating relationships between behavior and neuropeptide-mediated regulation of immune functions has strengthened the concept of a unified psychosomatic network. Research on emotional expression or disclosure in healthy human subjects as well as in cancer and HIV-positive patients has shown significant positive correlations with clinically relevant immune functions and/or positive health outcomes. Psychosocial interventions emphasizing emotional expression or active coping have evidenced survival benefits in breast cancer and melanoma. In other words, people who emote in psychosocial sessions, either during group support sessions or with friends and family, tend to have longer survival times. These findings suggest that emotional expression generates balance in the neuropeptide-receptor network and a functional healing system. Emotional expression is also a marker for psychospiritual vitalization, and further research should evaluate links between energy-based models of health and neuropeptide-receptor-based models under the rubric of an informational paradigm (Pert, Dreher, & Ruff, 1998).

Immunity and Stress

During the last 10–20 years it has become clear that the immune system not only protects the individual against potentially harmful intruders but also interacts with both the nervous and endocrine systems. Today we know that immune competent cells have receptors for hormones and neurotransmitters and also produce neurotransmitters and that cytokine receptors are expressed in certain areas of the brain. Furthermore, in many animal models immune suppression has been induced by classical conditioning. In vitro (test tube) and vivo studies have shown signs of reduced immunity in individuals during acute and chronic stress. Some studies have also indicated that chronic stress may increase the risk of infections and cancer. On the other hand, various psychotherapeutic techniques appear to strengthen the immune system.

In many immunological diseases, we know that psychological factors are important. Moreover, serious life events prior to onset of disease are reported more frequently by seronegative than by seropositive rheumatoid arthritis patients. For example, prospective studies have shown that psychotherapeutic intervention can reduce disability in rheumatoid arthritis patients, but disease activity is diminished only rarely (Kjeldsen-Kragh, 1996).

A long-term mystery in medicine has been the nature of the relationship between physical illness and the mind. In this instance, the mind is meant to include feelings, thoughts, behavior, and attitude. Great advances have been made in the study and understanding of the immune system, which consists of a complex organ or network that defends the body against microorganisms and other invaders. Researchers have learned much about its relationship to the central nervous system (CNS), whose major component is the brain and spinal cord.

The nervous and endocrine systems modulate the immune system functions through releasing neurotransmitters, neuropeptides, and endocrine hormones as they regulate the other physiological functions. The immune system in turn communicates with the nervous and endocrine systems through secreting immunocompetent substances, certokines and neurotransmitters. It has been found that the inhibition of acetylcholine (ACh) biosynthesis in the CNS causes the enhancement of the humoral immune response. By contrast, the inhibition of acetyl-cholinesterase (AChE) activity in the CNS results in the suppression of the immune response. It seems that ACh in the brain plays an immunoinhibitory role. It is suggested that there is a functional connection present between the ACh of the brain and the immune system. These results provide evidence for the bidirectional information exchange network between the monoamine neurotransmitters and the immune system (Qui, Peng, & Wang, 1996).

LEARNING AND MEMORY

The immune system may also, like the CNS, have the capacity to "learn." This means learning occurs when there is a more useful response when something is exposed to a stimulus the second time. Such a thing happens, in part, as a result of memory. This can be seen when white blood cells are exposed to an infecting agent the second time. They are more effective at fighting off the infection. The reason this information is important is that if indeed the immune system and CNS can learn, then we can teach them to behave or respond to events in new ways.

Conditioned Response

One kind of learning is called conditioning. Conditioning is a phenomenon made popular by the work of Pavlov in 1906 and 1927 that may provide insight into the pathways of communication between the brain and possibly any organ system of the body. Conditioning allows one to separate the afferent from the efferent circuits. That is, signals from the immune system (IS) to the CNS (IS → CNS) can be effectively separated from signals from the CNS to the immune system (CNS → IS). This permits one to study each pathway individually. Simple, single association trial models to condition fever, NK cell, and cytotoxic lymphocyte (CTL) activities have been developed to evaluate the pathways. Thus, conditioning can be used to train the brain to activate the immune system and other organ systems participating in the response. During the course of the conditioned response, presumably, the CNS, via the hypothalamus, integrates in a cohesive orderly fashion all input and output signals and coordinates the responses made by the brain to the organ systems. In one experiment (Hiramoto, Rogers, Demissie, Hsueh, & Hiramoto, 1997), mice were repeatedly exposed to the smell of camphor while injected with a substance that caused their cells to develop material important in fighting cancer. When they were finally exposed to the camphor without the injection, the activity of the cancer cells increased anyway.

RESEARCH BOX: Immune Processes Can Affect Behavioral Functioning

Evidence is presented that the immune system can affect central nervous system functioning, leading to changes in learning. In this study immune complex disease was induced in rats and their behavior was tested using a maze. Significant differences in behavior were found between the animals with high disease activity and those with low disease activity and the nondisease controls. These changes were most likely due to the immune response. This provides a model by which immunological processes can cause neuropsychiatric manifestations in autoimmune diseases like lupus as well as shows that immune processes can affect behavior.

Source: Hoffman, S. A., Shucard, D. W., & Harbeck, R. J. (1998). The immune system can affect learning: Chronic immune complex disease in a rat model. *Journal of Neuroimmunology, 86*(2), 163–170.

Psychedelic Drugs and the Immune System

Some events can boost the immune system (as indicated by levels of salivary immunoglobulin A). Some instances of spontaneous remission and mystical experiences seem to share a similar cluster of thoughts, feelings, moods, perceptions, and behaviors. Entheogens (psychedelic drugs used in a religious context) can also produce mystical experiences (peak experiences, states of unitive consciousness, intense primary religious experiences) with the same cluster of effects. When this happens, it is also possible that such entheogen-induced mystical experiences strengthen the immune system (Roberts, 1999). Some theorize that spontaneous remissions occur more frequently under such conditions and contend that entheogen-induced mystical experiences influence the immune system in ways we do not yet fully understand. Thus, here is yet another frontier open to investigation of the potential ways to enhance our marvelous immune system.

JOY, OPTIMISM, AND HOPE

Attitude affects behavior. Together, behavior and attitude affect the immune system. Research studies have shown that our remarkable immune system can be boosted by such things as faith, friendship, humor, hope, and joy.

For one thing, we now have evidence that faith may make you healthier. Researchers found that older adults who attended religious services once a week or more had lower levels of interleukin-6, an immune system protein linked to some autoimmune diseases, cancer, and heart disease, than nonchurchgoers (Koenig, Cohen, George, Hays, Larson, & Blazer, 1997).

Even going out with friends can boost your spirits and your defenses. A 1997 study of 276 people conducted at Carnegie Mellon University in Pittsburgh found that those who had a variety of social relationships were better able to fend off colds and had 20% greater immune function than more introverted people.

Imagery, a relaxation technique that, like daydreaming, involves allowing images to drift through your mind, may heighten immune response to disease (see Figure 21-1). In some studies the subjects have increased T-cell and white blood cell count. In others, there was a rise in NK cell activity. In a study of women who had completed treatment for breast cancer, the women who used imagery therapy did not have any significant changes in their immune function, but they did report less stress, more vigor, and an improved quality of life (Richardson, Post-White, Grimm, Moye, Singletary, & Justice, 1997). Although imagery reduced stress and improved quality of life, both imagery and support improved coping, attitudes, and perception of support. The clinical implications of these changes warrant further testing.

SENSE	IMAGERY
Visual	See the dark blue sky
Auditory	Hear the babbling brook
Kinesthetic	Feel yourself floating on a cloud
Gustatory	Taste the tartness of a freshly cut lemon
Olfactory	Smell the salt air at the ocean

Figure 21-1 Incorporating all five senses into imagery

RESEARCH BOX: Optimism and Strengthened Immunity

This study explored prospectively the effects of dispositional and situational optimism on mood ($N = 90$) and immune changes ($N = 50$) among law students in their first semester of study. Optimism was associated with better mood, higher numbers of helper T cells, and higher NK cell cytotoxicity. Avoidance coping partially accounted for the relationship between optimism and mood. Among the immune parameters, mood partially accounted for the optimism–helper T cell relationship, and perceived stress partially accounted for the optimism-cytotoxicity relationship. Individual differences in expectancies, appraisal, and mood may be important in understanding psychological and immune responses to stress. The law students who began their first semester optimistic about the experience had more helper T cells midsemester, which can amplify the immune response, and more powerful NK cells. The reason? They experience events such as their grueling first year as less stressful than their more pessimistic classmates. This research establishes the possibility that a person's outlook and mood when stressed might affect responses to common immune challenges such as exposure to cold viruses.

Source: Segerstrom, S. C., Taylor, S. E., Kemeny, M. E., & Fahey, J. L. (1998). Optimism is associated with mood, coping, and immune change in response to stress. *Journal of Personality and Social Psychology, 74*(6), 1646–1655.

Having a positive outlook when under stress can make you and your immune system feel high.

PHYSICAL EXERCISE

Along with conscious awareness, stress management, positive attitude enhancement, and a healthy diet, regular exercise plays a key role in our health. Physical activity enhances the immune system and helps control obesity, a risk factor for some cancers. It may also play a role in reducing a woman's risk of breast cancer (Rockhill, Willett, Hunter, Manson, Hankinson, & Colditz, 1999).

Another investigation studied the types and prevalence of conventional and alternative therapies used by women in four ethnic groups (Latino, white, black, and Chinese) diagnosed with breast cancer from 1990–1992 in San Francisco, CA, and explored factors influencing the choices of their therapies (Lee, Lin, Wrensch, Adler, & Eisenberg, 2000). Findings were that half of the women used at

RESEARCH BOX: Relationship of Physical Exercise to Breast Cancer

Although several studies have suggested that physical activity is associated with a decreased risk of breast cancer, such a decrease has not been found consistently, perhaps because physical activity has been assessed in different ways and for restricted periods. Few studies have assessed the risk of breast cancer in relation to lifetime physical activity. Data from a population-based, case-control study, including 918 case subjects (aged 20–54 years) and 918 age-matched population control subjects, were examined for associations between breast cancer risk and physical activity at ages 10–12 years and 13–15 years, lifetime recreational activity, and title of longest held job.

Women who were more active than their peers at ages 10–12 years had a lower risk of breast cancer [odds ratio (OR) = 0.68; 95% confidence interval (CI) = 0.49–0.94]. Women who had ever engaged in recreational physical activity had a reduced risk of breast cancer compared with inactive women (OR = 0.70; 95% CI = 0.56–0.88). Neither very early recreational activity (before age 20 years) nor recent activity (last 5 years) was associated with a greater reduction in risk than recreational activity in the intermediate period. Furthermore, women who started recreational activities after age 20 years and women who started earlier and continued their activities throughout adult life experienced a similar reduction in risk. Lean women, that is, women with a body mass index (weight in kilograms/meters squared) less than 21.8 kg/m^2, appeared to have a lower risk associated with recreational physical activity than women with a body mass index greater than 24.5 kg/m^2 [OR = 0.57 (95% CI = 0.40–0.82) and OR = 0.92 (95% CI = 0.65–1.29), respectively].

Findings support the hypothesis that recreational physical activity is associated with a decreased risk of breast cancer. Physical activity in early or recent life does not appear to be associated with additional beneficial effects.

Source: Verloop, J., Rookus, M. A., van der Kooy, K., & van Leeuwen, F. E. (2000). Physical activity and breast cancer risk in women aged 20–54 years. *Journal of the National Cancer Institute, 92*(2), 128–135.

least one type of alternative therapy, and about one-third used two types; most therapies were used for a duration of less than six months. Both the alternative therapies used and factors influencing the choice of therapy varied by ethnicity. Blacks most often used spiritual healing (36%), Chinese most often used herbal remedies (22%), and Latino women most often used dietary therapies (30%) and spiritual healing (26%). Among whites, 35% used dietary methods and 21% used physical methods, such as massage and acupuncture. In general, women who had a higher educational level or income, were of younger age, had private insurance, and exercised or attended support groups were more likely to use alternative therapies. About half of the women using alternative therapies reported discussing this use with their physicians. More than 90% of the subjects found the therapies helpful and would recommend them to their friends. The conclusion was that given the high prevalence of alternative therapies used in San Francisco by the four ethnic groups and the relatively poor communication between patients and doctors, physicians who treat patients with breast cancer should initiate dialogues on this topic to better understand patients' choices with regard to treatment options.

The U.S. Surgeon General's Office recommends that children and adults get at least 30 minutes of accumulated physical activity a day. Unfortunately, when it comes to actually doing the physical exercise, most of us fall into three groups:

- Those who do nothing
- Those who do the same thing over and over
- Those who wonder what they should do

Doing something physical is better than doing nothing. If you are among those stuck in a rut, you may increase your tolerance for exercise by varying what you do. For those already motivated but wondering how to make aerobic progress, the answer is to vary the intensity and the duration of your exercise and take time for recovery.

Swimming, skiing, biking, running, and even gardening result in aerobic exercise benefits, including reduced incidence of heart disease, high blood pressure, and certain cancers and relief from depression, anxiety, and stress. Besides those physiological benefits, routine exercise prevents you from becoming among those millions who number among the flabby and fat from muscle disuse atrophy.

Beginning an Exercise Program

To get you or your client active, here are a few basics. If you are just starting an aerobic exercise program, go easy and build slowly (see Figure 21-2). Beginning too fast and hard sets you up for injuries. As a general guideline, in the beginning it is a good idea not to up your training mileage or your effort by any more than 5% every two weeks. In the beginning, for at least four to eight weeks, everything you do should be at an easy, conversational pace (if it is difficult to talk easily, the pace is probably too hard).

How much exercise you do is up to you. The goal to build up to and keep healthy is to exercise five to six days a week for a minimum of 30 minutes each session. However, two to three workouts a week will do (especially if your goals are less athletic—lose a few pounds, reduce stress, reduce your risk of heart

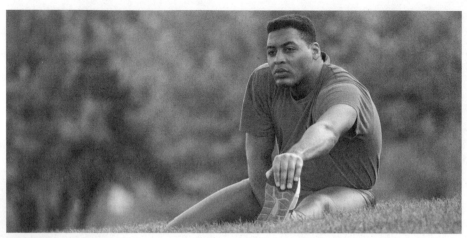

Figure 21-2 When beginning a new exercise program, it is important to start slowly, and to stretch both before and after exercise. (Photo courtesy of Photodisc.)

disease). The real key to exercise is not pushing to accomplish 8 hours this week, it's about being consistent over the next twenty years.

Aerobic Fitness

There are two components to aerobic fitness: the cardiovascular (oxygen delivery by the heart and lungs) and the peripheral (oxygen uptake—accomplished by finer nuances like muscle capillary and mitochondrial enzyme metabolism). For example, to be a faster swimmer you must hone the peripheral components specific to swimming, and the only way to do that is to swim. If you just want to condition your heart, lungs, and a broad range of muscles, then kayak, mountain bike, in-line skate, run, or jump rope. Your heart does not know whether you are bicycling or running, it only knows how fast it is beating.

Maintaining is one thing, but building muscle is another. Most exercise programs advise how many calories you burn, but do not consider advancing aerobic fitness. Most people exercise at the same pace for the same time all the time, not too hard, but not too easy. The problem with this is that your body has adapted. You are not really causing any additional demands that require the body to grow. So it is unlikely that you will make additional aerobic improvements. You may think you are pushing the parameters, but you are not. If you want to get down to the serious business of improving your cardiovascular capability, you need to focus on two things: the length of your workouts and their intensity.

LENGTH OF WORKOUT

Keep it simple. Running the same 30-minute loop every day will keep you in shape, but it will not make you a better runner. The physiology is complex, but basically your ability to run faster relies on two things: your body's ability to draw in oxygen and deliver it to the working muscles and the ability of those working muscles to use that oxygen for energy, thus preventing them from seizing up and the run coming to an abrupt end. In general, going hard (intensity) improves the delivery system. Going long (duration) at a comfortable conversational pace improves the oxygen extraction system. If you normally run 30 minutes a day, to improve the extraction system, try an hour-plus run one to two days a week instead. Generally, on the long days try to double the time, remembering that the emphasis is on duration.

HEALING STORY: Healing through Exercise

Katie was a first-year student in a professional program. Her fall semester classes were difficult and life seemed increasingly stressful. She heard from a friend that running made a big difference in her life, but Katie lived in a neighborhood that was unsafe to run. She decided that, like her friend, exercise might make a difference and help to decrease the stress, so she joined a nearby spa. As it turned out, it just seemed too much trouble to take her clothes to the spa and exercise before school and she felt too tired to make the trip after she got home in the late afternoons. Consequently, she rarely got there and felt that she had wasted her money. She heard from another friend that regular exercise on a treadmill made a huge difference to her, so Katie asked her parents for a treadmill as a Christmas gift. It got installed in her apartment during semester break and when school resumed in snowy January, Katie began the new semester with a new exercise regimen in her very own apartment.

Katie began the first week walking at a 3-mile/hour pace for half a mile about four days a week. She used the time to watch television news on study breaks. Gradually she increased both her pace and her distance to 3.8 miles an hour doing a combination of fast walking and jogging for 4 miles. Within weeks she felt remarkably better and even enjoyed her studies more. By semester's end her grades, physical stamina, body tone, and general overall attitude had measurably improved.

Observations and Insights

It is not always increasing study time and intensity that improves grades. A balanced regimen of physical, mental, and spiritual activities is necessary for actualized living. Most exercise regimens will pay off in rewards of weight balancing, mental attitude improvement, and increased daily productivity.

INTENSITY OF WORKOUT

Though long, slow distance is important, intensity is really the crux of aerobic advancement, To improve, you will have to work hard. For the serious recreational athlete this means effort that brings your heart rate up to 90–95% of its maximum. You can gauge this with a heart rate monitor. It should be hard enough so you do not want to talk. And if you have to talk, your sentences are two words long. That is the intensity you are looking for.

How you add this intensity to your routine is up to you. There are near-limitless variations on the theme. Most people will prosper with one or two intense workouts a week with the rest of the week comprising easier, recovery workouts. Sometimes try a change and go hiking or kayaking. Here you might alternate 100 meters of easy paddling with 100-meter hard bursts. Pay attention to the fact that there needs to be a fairly long recovery time in each of the exercise sequences. Some experts recommend a 1:1 effort-to-recovery ratio (hard for 3 minutes, easy for 3 minutes; hard for 30 seconds, easy for 30 seconds).

You want to focus on maintaining good form and technique because you are actually developing neuromuscular patterns by maintaining your form and quitting before that form deteriorates. Good form and technique are key. And as you move through the program, remember that aerobic gains come easy in the beginning and then they slow down. Eventually you will have to do more and more work for less and less gain. The fitter you get, the harder you have to work.

SAMPLE PROGRAMS

It is important to note that you do not have to spend an entire hour on exercise for it to be effective. If you plan what you do, 30 minutes is enough. There are dozens of different kinds of exercise programs, but in this chapter we focus on two as a sample of the possibilities. Tables 21-1 and 21-2 give some examples of simple, easy-to-follow routines for adequate exercise in 30 minutes or less.

Recovery Phase

More is not always better. To maximize results, you have to give your body a break. Not doing so can cause problems. The problems range from sprains and torn ligaments to actual immune suppression and resultant illnesses.

VIGOROUS EXERCISE AND IMMUNE SUPPRESSION

Many immune functions are stimulated by moderate physical activity. However, more vigorous effort and periods of heavy training suppress various immune response parameters. Cellular infiltration of the active muscle is accompanied by phagocyte activation, suppressed NK cell function, impaired lymphocyte proliferation, decreased in vitro immunoglobulin production, proinflammatory

---

TABLE 21-1 **Twenty-Minute Running Plan**

- Warm up: 5 minutes of easy running or fast walking
- Warm up: 5 minutes of stretching and bending
- Run: 3 minutes
- Jog: 2 minutes
- Run: 1 minute
- Jog: 4 minutes
- Cool down: 5 minutes walking

TABLE 21-2 **Swimming**

Ease into this workout, warming up as you go. Take 10 seconds rest between each swim. You can do this all freestyle, but using different strokes works more muscles and makes being in the water more fun.

- Warm up: slow strokes, stretching and reaching as you stroke
- Swim: 200 meters freestyle
- Swim: 100 meters backstroke
- Swim: 200 meters freestyle
- Swim: 100 meters breast stroke
- Swim: 100 meters freestyle
- Swim: 100 meters individual medley
- Swim: 200 meters freestyle
- Cool down: 200 meters; go easy, concentrate on stretching out, relaxing, and slowing the breaths

---

eicosanoid release, cytokine cascade activation, and altered expression of cytokine receptors. Examples of overexercise include deliberate heavy training; single bouts of fatiguing, submaximal work; repeated bouts of intense exercise; and ultralong distance athletic events. In young adults, age, environment, and light physical training do not change immune response parameters. Vigorous exercise probably induces subclinical muscle injury and an associated inflammatory response. Heavy exercise may be a useful experimental model for developing more effective treatments for sepsis (Shepard & Shek, 1996).

In essence the immune system is enhanced during moderate and severe exercise, and only intense long-duration, heavy-intensity exercise is followed by immune suppression. The latter include suppressed concentration of lymphocytes, suppressed NK cells, lymphokine-activated killer cytotoxicity, and secretory IgA in mucosa. Whether or not the "open window" in the immune system occurs is dependent on the intensity and duration of exercise. One reason for the "overtraining effect" seen in elite athletes could be that this window of opportunity for

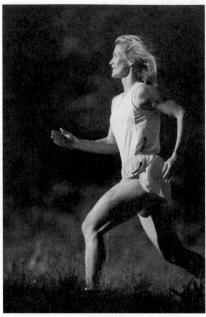

Figure 21-3 Regular physical activity coupled with proper nutrition and adequate sleep promotes health. (Photo courtesy of Photodisc.)

RESEARCH BOX: Vigorous Exercise and Immune Suppression

There is an increased risk of infections in athletes undertaking prolonged, strenuous exercise. There is also some evidence that cells of the immune system are less able to mount a defense against infections after such exercise. The level of plasma glutamine, an important fuel for cells of the immune system, is decreased in athletes after endurance exercise; this may be partly responsible for the apparent immune suppression that occurs in these individuals. Researchers monitored levels of infection in more than 200 runners and rowers. The levels of infection were lowest in middle-distance runners and highest in runners after a full or ultramarathon and in elite rowers after intensive training. In this study, athletes participating in different types of exercise consumed two drinks containing either glutamine (group G) or placebo (group P) immediately after and 2 hours after exercise. They subsequently completed questionnaires ($n = 151$) about the incidence of infections during the seven days following the exercise. The percentage of athletes reporting no infections was considerably higher in the experimental group G (81%, $n = 72$) than in the control group P (49%, $n = 79$, $p < 0.001$).

Source: Castell, L. M., Poortmans, J. R., & Newsholme, E. A. (1996). Does glutamine have a role in reducing infections in athletes? *European Journal of Applied Physiology,* *73*(5), 488–490.

pathogens is longer and the degree of immune suppression more pronounced (Pedersen, Rohde, & Zacho, 1996).

For protection against immune suppression, average athletes may take the antioxidant vitamins C and E. Glucosamine sulfate is helpful in reducing inflammation and is often used to rebuild or strengthen connective tissue (Mornhinweg, 2000). Top-level athletes sometimes receive immunoglobulin preparations (Shepard, 1996).

Make It Fun

Once you are aware that overworking can be a hazard, you will most likely moderate and move into a balanced program. You will have a better chance of success if you mix it up, try new things, and keep your program interesting. The exercise you choose is up to you. But keep in mind that bringing large muscle groups into play taxes the heart and burns calories more effectively. For example, kayaking works the abdominal and back muscles. You may want to try some combinations such as running in the spring and fall, swimming in the summer, and cross-country skiing in the winter. This way you keep it interesting while rotating emphasis on different muscle groups. Mix up your program, do different things, play with it, then it will be more fun and you will be more apt to do it. Find an activity you enjoy and vary your exercise routine to keep it fresh and fun. The key is to choose a program that meets your needs and then exercise regularly.

HEALING NUTRITION

The third element in the triad of attitude, exercise, and nutrition is healthy eating. Perhaps in no other realm has there been so many advances in such a short time as in the arena of nutrition. We now know for certain that "we are what we eat," and never before in history have we had so many choices of foods. Without knowledge of good nutrition, it is easy to get more than enough calories but difficult to get the nutrients necessary for building a strong immune system. Armed with information about what your body needs, you will be better able to fight infections and chronic disease.

A Basic Plan

One of the best ways to protect the body against disease is to have a strong immune system. Some ways to help the immune system include eating a balanced diet rich in organic fruits and vegetables, adding vitamins A, C, E, and B complex to the diet, and getting plenty of rest. A healthy diet includes energy components, protein, fiber, and thousands of other macro- and microvitamins and microminerals. There are several basic patterns anyone can follow to enhance the immune system and increase health in general. A diet rich in fruits and vegetables can help protect your immune system, keep bones strong, have regular elimination patterns, reduce risk of heart disease and cancer, and maintain body weight during the aging process. To begin a basic plan, simply eat right.

- Appetite often declines with age, but many nutritional needs increase, so the quality of each portion becomes more important. Make certain the diet includes five daily servings of fruits and vegetables plus generous portions of whole grains, beans, and dairy products. A sample breakfast would be raisin bran with skim milk, orange juice, whole wheat toast with jam, and a piece of fruit. For lunch, try a salad with sliced vegetables, whole wheat pita bread, and skim milk. For dinner, eat a 3-ounce chicken breast, brown rice, broccoli, a whole wheat roll, and low-fat frozen yogurt with fresh strawberries.

- Eat whole grains, green leafy vegetables, seafood, lean meats, and moderate amounts of vegetable oils to get vitamins and minerals.

- Strengthen bones by drinking milk and eating cheese and yogurt for calcium. Milk also has vitamin D. If you get little direct sunlight, be sure your daily supplement gives you vitamin D, which helps your body absorb calcium more effectively. The primary problem with milk, however, is that it is a double-edged sword. It has the calcium but also has hormones and chemicals that may be toxic to the body. Some humans lack the proper digestive enzymes, and for them, milk and dairy products can cause allergies and/or chronic disease. An excellent source of calcium is seaweed and most other green plants. The Institute of Medicine of the National Academy of Sciences recommends that people ages 51–70 get 400 IU of calcium per day and people over 70 get 600 IU per day.

- Develop regular elimination habits. Try to eat 20–35 grams (g) of fiber a day to keep your digestive system active and healthy. Good fiber sources are fruits and vegetables, oats, beans, and wheat-bran cereals. Here is what it takes to reach 25 g of fiber: a bowl of raisin bran (5 g), an apple (3 g), a banana (2 g), a fig (2 g), a bowl of lentil soup (5 g), a slice of whole wheat bread (2 g), a half-cup serving of peas (2 g), and two raw carrots (4 g).

- Consider your vision. Eat citrus fruits, tomatoes, and orange, yellow, and green vegetables to get the antioxidant power of vitamin C and the carotenoids. Cataract formation is just one of the damaging effects of oxidation in the body. Macular degeneration, a disease of old age, may be prevented by long-term intake of sufficient quantities of green and yellow vegetables.

■ Reduce your risk of heart disease and cancer. Limit saturated fats by limiting your intake of fatty meats, cheeses, butter, and partially hydrogenated fats (trans fatty acids) found in many margarines and commercial baked goods; focus on getting fruits and vegetables. Get nutrients such as vitamin B_6, potassium, and folate. An analysis of more than 200 studies shows that a diet high in fruits and vegetables cuts your cancer risk in half.

■ Maintain your body weight. It is harder to keep off the pounds as we age because our muscle tissue tends to decline and, with it, our ability to use all the energy in foods. Our bodies store that energy as fat, and that can hasten the onset of diabetes, heart disease, arthritis, and other problems.

Herbs as Immune Boosting Foods

Modern pharmaceutical drugs are designed to knock down the body's inflammatory response or to decrease pain. For the most part they are the medical treatment of choice. It makes sense, then, to be thoughtful when we discuss the immune system and when we explore ways to treat or to strengthen it. From an allopathic, or treat-the-symptom, point of view, herbs that directly decrease inflammation, such as willow bark, may be considered "immune system herbs." Goldenseal and Oregon grape, with their antibacterial action, could also arguably be labeled immune herbs. However, to many, treating the immune system is synonymous with strengthening what some have traditionally called the "vital force"—a complex, multifaceted pillar of good health (Starbuck, 1998). Some plants cross the line between food and medicine and can therefore be used routinely in establishing the first tenet of a healthy immune system—good nutrition.

There are hundreds of healing herbs. The following represents a few.

FLAX

Flax (*Linum usitatissimum*) is one of the cross-over plants. The flax plant produces a small, oily, nut-brown seed rich in omega-3 fatty acids. These fatty acids are essential to human life. In recent years it has become increasingly clear that polyunsaturated fatty acids are key in both producing prostaglandins, which, in turn, influence immune function (like T cells) and in modulating inflammatory/immune response. The eicosanoids (e.g., prostaglandins and thromboxane) regulate, in fact, many cell functions and play critical roles in wide-ranging activities, including various immune and inflammatory functions. In addition, they play a role in heart function, hormone production, brain activity, as well as the making of healthy skin, hair, and cell membranes throughout the body. Recent research has shown that essential fatty acids (EFAs) may even play an important role in getting a good night's sleep. Because foods in many American diets—such as meat, dairy products, sweets, and packaged and fast foods—are low in EFAs, many people are deficient in the fundamental constituents needed for a healthy immune system.

Freshly pressed flaxseed oil is an excellent source of omega-3 fatty acids. The oil is a pale yellow color, pleasant, almost bland, in taste. Substituting flax oil for butter or other oils on vegetables or over rice or supplementing with flax oil capsules is an excellent way to support your immune system. However, do not cook with or heat flax oil; the beneficial fats are quickly destroyed at high temperatures and the flash point is very low. It is also important to pay attention to how you feel when taking flax in any form, as some are allergic to this plant (Starbuck, 1998).

DHA, IMMUNITY, AND INFLAMMATION

Also powerful is a sea-vegetable source docosahexaenoic acid (or DHA), which has shown immune benefits in reference to cancer (colon and liver), multiple sclerosis, and other diseases of inflammation—rheumatoid arthritis, asthma, inflammatory bowel disease (such as ulcerative colitis and Crohn's disease), and inflammatory skin disorders.

TEA

Green tea (*Camellia sinensis*) is another botanical that is both a food (or, more accurately, a beverage) and a medicine for the immune system. Green tea and black tea are both derived from the same plant; however, black tea is fermented, a process that causes the plant to lose some of the medicinal compounds present in green tea. Among these are polyphenols, compounds with great antioxidative and anticancer properties.

Studies show that men who regularly consumed green tea have a reduced risk of colon cancer, compared with men who were not green tea drinkers (Yang, Liao, Kim, Yurkow, & Yang, 1998). The rate for rectal and pancreatic cancers was also reduced among the green tea drinking men (Ji, Chow, Hsing, McLaughlin, Dai, Gao, Blot, & Fraumeni, 1997). Moreover, research shows that women can also reap the benefits of green tea. A recent Japanese study found that the consumption of green tea correlated with a decreased risk of recurrence of stage I and stage II breast cancer in women (Murray, 1997). Green tea has also been found to reduce the incidence of ultraviolet-B-radiation-induced skin tumors in mice (Liu, 1998).

Herbs as Medicine

For some, supporting the immune system with good nutrition, digestion, elimination, and a positive mental outlook is all that is required to live a healthy, illness-free life. Unfortunately, not all of us are that lucky. Viruses, bacteria, accidents, vulnerabilities, and life circumstances intervene, causing sickness, even when we have taken the best care of ourselves. In these instances, herbal medicine can again offer potent immune support, stimulating and enhancing our innate healing mechanisms.

In the history of herbalism, women prepared food and healing potions. Women generally practiced herbalism on a day-to-day basis, as well as took care of the ills of other members of the family or tribal unit. However, throughout history, men were the ones who compiled the remedies and wrote them down, which is why nearly all the herbals are named and recorded by men. Herbs come from a vast array of sources that include plants, flowers, fruits, seeds, nuts, bark, and roots and have been used in healing since people first began caring for one another.

ECHINACEA

Echinacea is one example of a healing herb. Many are aware of echinacea's value in helping us to prevent or treat colds and flu. Taking echinacea at the onset of a cold can prevent it from lasting more than a day or so (and can reduce severity).

Much has been written about echinacea, and theories about its appropriate therapeutic use abound. In the last 10 years, herbal practitioners have most commonly held that echinacea was best used in the early stages of acute illness and, then, for short periods of time only. The theory has been that echinacea is an immune system stimulator and, therefore, should not be used for long periods, since perpetually stimulating the immune system can be harmful. Some suggest that echinacea, as an immune stimulator, might be dangerous in autoimmune conditions or in illnesses where the immune system is severely taxed, such as AIDS, tuberculosis, and leukemia.

Bone (1997), a British-trained herbalist who now works in Australia, suggests that echinacea might best be viewed as an immunomodulator, rather than as an immunostimulant. In contrast to a stimulator, which simply turns on or pushes a system, a modulator adjusts and regulates a bodily function, allowing it to work at its best. As a modulator, echinacea acts to enhance and balance overall immune function, in fact "toning down" inappropriate immune responses. Native Americans, and later the Eclectics, who practiced herbal medicine in the United States in the late nineteenth and early twentieth centuries, used echinacea to treat all manner of chronic diseases, including tuberculosis, diabetes, and chronic bronchitis. Echinacea is one of today's most widely consumed herbs and perhaps has a capacity for healing of which we are not yet aware.

ASTRAGALUS

Astragalus is another herb that can enhance overall immune function. The plant's medicine comes from the root of *Astragalus membranaceus,* part of the pea family, native to northeast China. The genus *Astragalus* is a large plant group, containing over 2000 species. Infamous locoweed, a toxic plant found in the American West, belongs to the *Astragalus* genus. Only *A. membranaceus* and *A. mongholicus* have been used and studied as medicine (Foster, 1996).

In China, astragalus has been considered a tonic herb for over 2000 years. It has been used to treat lassitude, debility, colds, and viral and bacterial illness. Some practitioners find astragalus to be of great benefit in reducing patient susceptibility to wintertime viral conditions, such as colds, flu, sinusitis, and sore throat. Chinese scientists have studied astragalus for its benefit in supporting the immune system of patients receiving chemotherapy and radiation treatments for cancer. As these medical treatments work to kill cancer, they put a great strain on the immune system, lowering white cell and T-helper cell counts significantly. Astragalus is helpful in restoring healthy cell numbers and cell activity (Chu, Wong, & Mavligit, 1998).

Table 21-3 outlines the health benefits of some additional healing herbs.

Some Foods Harm

We are born with certain immune cells that act quickly to destroy any offending agent. These include macrophages and NK cells. Macrophages are like pac-man cells devouring any foreign or abnormal looking cells, bacteria, fungi, and more. Natural killer cells go after cancer cells and virus-infected cells. Sugar consumption seriously hampers these two immune cells. As little as one teaspoon of sugar can inhibit our NK cells and macrophages for up to six hours, leaving us unprotected against viruses and cancer. While sugar is toxic to the immune system, fruits and vegetables are healing.

Other harmful foods include the vast assortment of carbonated soda pops. Not only is there no benefit in the artificial coloring, but the carbonated potassium has the ability to pull the calcium out of the bones. This is not good for either the young or the old. Additionally, we do not yet have enough data to support the contention, but some believe that the large amounts of artificial sweeteners used are deleterious to health. Aspartame (Nutrasweet) converts to formic acid at 110°F. Formic acid destroys nerve tissue and is implicated in many chronic neurological diseases.

Fuel for the Immune Cells

We must provide our immune system with the fuel to fight its never-ending battles. Seven to 10 half-cup servings of fruits and vegetables per day are the min-

TABLE 21-3 Healing Herbs

NAME	ORIGIN	BENEFITS
Camellia sinensis (green tea)	Long cultivated in China, now popular worldwide	• Contains high amounts of polyphenols—protective multifunctional antioxidants • Slows the formation of damaged cells
Crataegus oxacantha (hawthorn)	A spiny tree or shrub native to Europe; often grown as a hedge plant	• Normalizes blood pressure and cholesterol levels • Improves coronary circulation
Curcuma longa (turmeric)	Herb or spice with origins in southern Asia, used as a seasoning	• Tones liver and gallbladder • Normalizes cholesterol • Soothes redness and swelling
Ginkgo biloba (GBE)	Comes from a tree that can live for up to 1000 years	• Regulates oxygen/glucose usage • Stabilizes critical membranes • Enhances blood circulation to the brain
Panax ginseng (Oriental ginseng)	Small perennial plant, widely cultivated in the Far East	• Enhances intellectual performance • Strengthens heart muscle • Enhances male sexual vitality
Zingiber officinale (ginger)	Fleshy and aromatic root used in cooking and healing for centuries	• Soothes the gastrointestinal tract • Exerts an antinausea action • Strengthens smooth muscle
Lavender	From ancient Greece to modern times, among the most widely cultivated and used	• Potent topical antiseptic, may even ward off infections and viruses • Aroma used to evoke relaxation

imum requirements to ensure optimal levels of vitamins, minerals, and plant nutrients. Eliminating the bad fats in margarine, some oils, shortenings, and lard will also help enhance immunity. Organic foods should be chosen whenever possible to ensure that we limit our consumption of pesticides and fungicides, which are known to inhibit the action of immune cells.

NUTRIENTS TO ENHANCE IMMUNITY

Vitamins C, E, A, and B complex, reduced L-glutathione, selenium, zinc, magnesium, coenzyme Q10, and DHEA have immune-enhancing actions. Zinc is known to increase the size of the thymus gland, the powerhouse of one's immune system, and improve T-cell function. Both coenzyme Q10 and selenium have been proven to protect against cancer. Reduced L-glutathione is the most potent detoxifier, eliminating environmental pollutants from the body rapidly, thereby protecting the immune system. Magnesium is involved in over 200 enzymatic reactions in the body. Deficiency of this important mineral is common, due to the consumption of caffeinated drinks, which cause magnesium to be excreted. Vitamin B_6 is required for maintaining hormone levels and a healthy immune and nervous system. Vitamin B_6 should be taken along with a B complex to ensure the full complement of B vitamins are present. Vitamins C, E, and A are important antioxidants that enhance our immune system and protect us from infections and neutralizing cell-damaging free radicals. DHEA is our mother hormone, in charge of regulating all the hormones in the body. It is known as the antiaging hormone. As we age, DHEA levels decline and many degenerative diseases are associated with low DHEA levels. Plant sterols and sterolins are precursors to DHEA. This means that the body will take the plant fats and make DHEA from them. It is always better if we can rely on our body to make what we require and this is true with DHEA (Vanderhaeghe, 1999).

Nutrition Cautions

As with anything we do, we must have balance. That is to say, there is little merit in extremes. In nutrition that translates to beware of food fads, unwarranted, unsubstantiated claims about a product, and any new product that sounds too good to be true. Look for evidence-based reports that validate the merits of the product.

Imbalance in the Immune System

Although research on the role of single nutrients in immune function is extensive, this is not the case for multiple nutrients and subsequent nutrient-nutrient interactions. Imbalance of more than one nutrient has interactive effects on immunocompetence. Availability of one nutrient may impair or enhance the action of another in the immune system, as reported for nutrients such as vitamin E and selenium, vitamin E and vitamin A, zinc and copper, and dietary fatty acids and vitamin A. Nutrient-nutrient interactions may negatively affect immune function. For example, excess calcium interferes with leukocyte function by displacing magnesium ions, thereby reducing cell adhesion (Kubena & McMurray, 1996).

Malnutrition and the Immune System

Nutrition is a critical determinant of immune responses and malnutrition is the most common cause of immunodeficiency worldwide. Protein-energy malnutrition is associated with a significant impairment of cell-mediated immunity, phagocyte function, complement system, secretory immunoglobulin A antibody concentrations, and cytokine production. Deficiency of single nutrients also results in altered immune responses: This is observed even when the deficiency state is relatively mild. Of the micronutrients, zinc, selenium, iron, copper, vitamins A, C, E, and B_6, and folic acid have important influences on immune responses. Overnutrition and obesity also reduce immunity. Low-birth-weight infants have a prolonged impairment of cell-mediated immunity that can be partly restored by providing extra amounts of dietary zinc. In the elderly, impaired immunity can be enhanced by modest amounts of a combination of micronutrients. This information has considerable practical and public health significance (Chandra, 1997). Malnutrition also frequently contributes to the immunocompromise seen in hospitalized patients while nutritional support corrects malnutrition and can reverse the associated immunocompromise. Developing an understanding of nutritional needs and the role of nutrition in immune function is essential to prevention and treatment of nutrition-related immunocompromise, both inside and outside the hospital. Current research is defining the role of specific nutrients in immune function. Recent evidence also suggests that the route (enteral versus parenteral) of providing nutritional support can affect immune competence (Krenitsky, 1996).

Stress Reduction Is Essential to Immune Health

Poor nutrition, coupled with too much stress, is a recipe for illness. When we are under stress, our body sends out the stress hormone cortisol. This hormone then causes a proinflammatory immune factor called interleukin-6 to be excreted. Interleukin-6 is involved in the exacerbation of autoimmune disorders and other inflammatory conditions such as fibromyalgia and osteoarthritis. The human immunodeficiency virus uses interleukin-6 to replicate itself. This powerful inflammatory immune factor is also involved in pulling calcium from bone into the blood, causing osteoporosis. Sterols and sterolins effectively reduce cortisol and subsequently interleukin-6, alleviating symptoms associated with these diseases. Knowing this cortisol–interleukin-6 connection, stress reduction is of paramount importance to the health of our immune system.

Eliminate the stressors that you have control over and learn how to better handle those that you do not. We can improve our immune function rapidly by adopting good nutrition and stress-reducing behaviors; including plant nutrients, vitamins, and minerals in our diet; and eliminating many of the toxins we are exposed to daily. Relying on our immune system to fight off bacteria, viruses, candida albicans and parasites is just what Mother Nature ordered.

SUMMARY

Immune health can be boosted by a number of factors that are under our control. Attitude toward life, physical exercise, and what and how we eat can make or break our intricate immune system. When we are young, a foul disposition and poor lifestyle behaviors may seemingly not be detrimental, but as we age, those bad qualities catch up with us with resultant ill health and an early demise. Consequently, for a healthy immune system and good quality of life, act consciously:

- ■ Eat a balanced diet rich in organic fruits, vegetables, nuts, and seeds. Eliminate the bad fats—margarine and processed oils. Choose fish and free-range eggs over red meat and add plenty of yogurt or kefir to your diet. Sugar and alcohol both cause immune dysfunction; avoid them.

- ■ Reduce stress in any way possible—it is extremely damaging to one's immune health.

- ■ Add vitamins A, C, E, and B complex, along with the minerals magnesium, selenium, zinc, L-glutathione, and coenzyme Q10.

- ■ Add the plant nutrients sterols and sterolins. They are essential for modulating (balancing) the immune system, enhancing it if it is underactive and reducing it when it is overstimulated. Include carotenoids such as lycopene, known to protect against cancer, and bioflavonoids, which are powerful antioxidants that help eliminate toxins.

- ■ Walk, walk, walk! Exercise is a good way to relieve stress and enhance oxygen flow, improving the immune system.

- ■ Get plenty of sleep. Rest gives time for the body to regenerate.

Our collective knowledge about the immune system—how it works, what foods help it to maintain itself, and what medicines help it to heal—is a fascinating area of study. There is much to be learned from history and much to look forward to in future research and exploration. Anticipate great changes and a powerful role for healers in this essential health arena.

ASK YOURSELF

1. Can you give a brief overview of the physiological concepts in the immune system?
2. How does healthy nutrition relate to a strong immune system?
3. Name at least one alternative food that is a good source of calcium?
4. What group of women tried alternative therapies for their breast cancer? What were the therapies?
5. What is an effective exercise program to boost the immune system?

REFERENCES

Algiati, V., Quirion, R., Bowen, W. D., & Pert, C. B. (1982). Characterization of type 2 opiate receptors. *Life Science, 31*(16–17), 1675–1678.

Bone, K. (1997). Echinacea: When should it be used? *Alternative Medicine Review, 2*(2), 87–93.

Chandra, R. K. (1997). Nutrition and the immune system: An introduction. *American Journal of Clinical Nutrition, 66*(2), 460S–463S.

Chu, D. T., Wong, W. L., Mavligit, G. M. (1998 March 25). Immunotherapy with Chinese medicinal herbs. *Journal of Clinical and Laboratory Immunolology,* (3), 119–123.

Foster, S. (1996). Bundle up with botanicals. *Better Nutrition, 58*(11), 64–71.

Hiramoto, R. N., Rogers, C. F., Demissie, S., Hsueh, C. M., Hiramoto, N. S., Lorden, J. F., & Ghanta, V. K. (1997). Psychoneuroendocrine immunology: Site of recognition, learning and memory in the immune system and the brain. *International Journal of Neuroscience, 92*(3/4), 259–285.

Kjeldsen-Kragh, J. (1996). The influence of psychological factors on the immune system and immunological diseases. *Tidsskrift for den Norske Laegeforening, 116*(26), 3102–3170.

Koenig, H. G., Cohen, H. J., George, L. K., Hays, J. C., Larson, D. B., & Blazer, D. G. (1997). Attendance at religious services, interleukin-6, and other biological parameters of immune function in older adults. *International Journal of Psychiatry in Medicine, 27*(3), 233–250.

Krenitsky, J. (1996). Nutrition and the immune system. AACN *Clinical Issues, 66*(3), 359–369.

Kubena, K. S., & McMurray, D. N. (1996). Nutrition and the immune system: A review of nutrient-nutrient interactions. *Journal of the American Dietetic Association, 96*(11), 1156–1164; quiz 1165–6.

Lee, M. M., Lin, S. S., Wrensch, M. R., Adler, S. R., & Eisenberg, D. Alternative therapies used by women with breast cancer in four ethnic populations. *Journal of the National Cancer Institute, 92*(1), 42–47.

Liu, Q., et al. (1998). Effect of green tea of p52 mutation in ultraviolet B radiation-induced mouse skin tumors. *Carcinogenesis, 19*(7), 1257–1262.

Mornhinweg, G. (2000), Glucosamine sulfate. *Holistic Nursing Update, 1*(2), 16.

Murray, M. (1997). Botanical monograph—green tea. *American Journal of Natural Medicine, 4*(5), 18–19.

Ostrowski, N. L., Burke, T. R. Jr., Rice, K. C., Pert, A., & Pert, C. B. (1987). The pattern of [3H] cyclofoxy retention in rat brain after in vivo injection corresponds to the in vitro opiate receptor distribution. *Brain Research, 402*(2), 275–286.

Pedersen, B. K., Rohde, T., & Zacho, M. (1996). Immunity in athletes. *Journal of Sports Medicine and Physical Fitness, 36*(4), 236–245.

Pert, C. B., Dreher, H. E., & Ruff, M. R. (1998). The psychosomatic network: Foundations of mind-body medicine. *Alternative Therapy Health Medicine, 15*(2), 30–41.

Pert, C. B., Ruff, M. R., Welier, R. J., & Herkenham, M. (1985). Neuropeptides and their receptors: A psychosomatic network. *Journal of Immunology, 135*(a Supplement), 820–826.

Qiu, Y., Peng, Y., & Wang, J. (1996). Immunoregulatory role of neurotransmitters. *Advances in Neuroimmunology, 6*(3), 223–231.

Richardson, M. A., Post-White, J., Grimm, E. A., Moye, L. A., Singletary, S. E., & Justice, B. (1997). Coping, life attitudes, and immune responses to imagery and group support after breast cancer treatment. *Alternative Therapy Health Medicine, 3*(5), 62–70.

Roberts, T. B. (1999). Do entheogen-induced mystical experiences boost the immune system? Psychedelics, peak experiences, and wellness. *Advances in Mind Body Medicine, 15*(2), 139–147.

Rockhill, B., Willett, W. C., Hunter, D. J., Manson, J. E., Hankinson, S. E., & Colditz, G. A. (1999). A prospective study of recreational physical activity and breast cancer risk. *Archives of Internal Medicine, 159*(19), 2290–2296.

Shepard, R. J., & Shek, P. N. (1996). Impact of physical activity and sport on the immune system. *Reviews of Environmental Health, 11*(3), 133–147.

Starbuck, J. (1998). Team up with natural immmune boosters! *Better Nutrition, 60*(11), 44–51.

Vanderhaeghe, L. (1999). Rev up your immune system to prevent disease. *Total Health, 21*(3), 30–31.

PART VI

Healing Resources and Support Networks

Alternative and Complementary Health Care Resources

Chapter Objectives

- Become knowledgeable about where to get information from various organizations, associations, and educational institutes.
- Discover Internet sites for on-line libraries.
- Learn about "virtual" sites for on-line information.
- Recognize that attending specialty conferences may add to your knowledge base.
- Learn how support groups may be helpful.

INTRODUCTION

We live in an era of knowledge explosion. Never in the history of humankind has there been such a proliferation of information on science and technology. This new knowledge base coupled with the growing realization of the interconnectedness of body, mind, and spirit has resulted in new ways of being and doing. Part of that new way is the advent of alternative and complementary therapies that augment our rich history of traditional medicine. Western medicine, which grew out of Egyptian, Greek, and European heritages, is coupled with Indian and Asian methods, and is offering new options and possibilities. The body of this book has been about the what, where, when, why, and how these therapies interface with conventional health care. This chapter details the specifics of how to locate many of the resources discussed in the text.

ASSOCIATIONS, ORGANIZATIONS, AND EDUCATIONAL INSTITUTIONS

There are hundreds of organizations, associations, and educational institutions that provide information on complementary and alternative medicine. This area of health care is rapidly proliferating with new modalities and philosophies, and their corresponding organizations are developing faster than for any other health arena. Consequently, the associations covered here are not all inclusive. In addition, many associations are mobile in their developmental stages and thus may

437

have changed their telephone number or address since the publication of this book or a URL address or other locator information may have changed or been deleted. Internet searches should be conducted by association, keyword, and/or topic.

Acupuncture and Chinese Medicine

American Association of Oriental Medicine
433 Front St.
Catasaugua, PA 18032
(919) 787-5181
E-mail: aoml@aol.com
Web site: http://www.aaom.org

Provides referrals to acupuncturists in your area.

American College of Acupuncture and Chinese Medicine
1010 Wayne Ave., #1270
Silver Spring, MD 20910

There are about 40 colleges. To locate them write to the address above. To find the colleges accreditation status, write to the Accreditation Commission of Acupuncture and Oriental Medicine at the above address.
    Offers information and referrals to licensed acupuncturists and Oriental medical doctors.

American Foundation of Traditional Chinese Medicine
505 Beach St.
San Francisco, CA 94133
(415) 776-0502
E-mail: aftcm@earthlink.net

Write to request information on Chinese medicine or referrals to acupuncturists or Oriental medical doctors in your area and large cities near your area. The foundation is nonprofit, and donations are requested to help defray costs.

National Acupuncture and Oriental Medicine Alliance
14637 Starr Rd. SE
Olalla, WA 98359
(206) 851-6896
(206) 851-6883 (fax)
Web site: http://www.healthy.netlnaoma

The national professional membership association founded in 1993 to represent the diversity of practitioners of acupuncture and Oriental medicine in the United States. Professional referrals available at the web site.

Internet

http://www.acupuncture.com

Aromatherapy

American Alliance of Aromatherapy
P.O. Box 7309
Depoe Bay, OR 97341
(800) 809-9850
(800) 809-9808 (fax)
Web site: http://www.healthy.net/aaoa

A nonprofit organization and resource center that allows aromatherapy practitioners, educators, manufacturers, retailers, and consumers to share valuable knowledge, encourage education, and promote ethical and equitable business practices. Offers subscriptions to the International Journal of Aromatherapy *and the* American Alliance of Aromatherapy News Quarterly.

Aromatherapy for Health Professionals
R.J. Buckle Associates
P.O Box 868
Hunter, NY 12442
(518) 263-4402
(518) 263-4031 (fax)
E-mail: rjbuckle@delphi.com

Offers courses in aromatherapy throughout the country.

National Association for Holistic Aromatherapy
219 Carl St.
San Francisco CA 94117–3804
(415) 564-6785

Internet

http://www.healthy.net/aromatherapy

Ayurvedic Medicine

Ayurvedic Institute
11311 Menual NE, Suite A
Albuquerque, NM 87112
(505) 291-9698
Web site: http://www.ayurveda.com

Trains the general public and health professionals in all aspects of Ayurveda. Correspondence course, newsletter, and mail order sale of Ayurvedic remedies.

College of Maharishi Ayur-Veda Health Center
P.O. Box 282
Fairfield, IA 52556
(515) 472-8477
(800) 248-9050 (for referrals)
E-mail: theraj@lisco.net
Web site: http://www.theraj.com

Provides information on Ayurvedic medicine to the general public and offers referrals to health centers that offer Ayurvedic methods for the prevention and treatment of a wide range of health conditions.

Internet

http://www.ayurvedic.com

Biofeedback

Association for Applied Psychophysiology and Biofeedback
10200 West 44th Ave.
Wheat Ridge, CO 80033
(303) 422-8436
E-mail: aapb@resourcecenter.com
Web site: http://www.aapb.org

Send a self-addressed, stamped envelope to receive information, a list of publications, and contacts in your state for obtaining referrals.

Biofeedback Certification Institute of America
10200 West 44th Ave., Suite 304
Wheat Ridge, CO 80033–2840
(303) 420-2902

Bodywork, Massage, and Acupressure

Acupressure Institute
1533 Shattuck Ave.
Berkeley, CA 94709
(800) 442-2232 (outside California)
(510) 845-1059 (inside California)
E-mail: info@acupressure.com
Web site: http://www.acupressure.com

Provides trainings in acupressure and Oriental bodywork as well as books, audiotapes, CDs, and videos on acupressure.

Alexander Technique International
1692 Massachusetts Ave.
Cambridge, MA 02138
(617) 497-2242
Web site: http.//www.ati-net.com

American Society for the Alexander Technique
P. O. Box 60008
Florence, MA 01062
(413) 584-2359
(800) 473-0620
Offers teacher listings, workshops, classes, and options for teacher training.

American Massage Therapy Association
820 Davis St., Suite 100
Evanston, IL 60201–4444
(847) 864-0123
(847) 864-1178 (fax)
Web site: http://www.amtamassage.org
Offers referrals of certified massage therapists throughout the United States. Call the main office for the number of the AMTA chapter in your state, and your state chapter will provide referrals in your area based on zip code.

American Oriental Bodywork Therapy Association
AOBTA National Headquarters
Glendale Executive Campus, Suite 510
1000 White Horse Rd.
Voorhees, NJ 08043
(609) 782-1616
(609) 782-1653 (fax)
E-mail: ShinnAOBTA@aol.com
Web site: http://www.healthy.net/aobta
Provides information, practitioner directory, and referrals.

American Polarity Therapy Association
2888 Bluff St., Suite 149
Boulder, CO 80301
(303) 545-2080
(303) 545-2161 (fax)
E-mail: satvahq@aol.com
Web site: http://www.polaritytherapy.org
Provides referrals to practitioners and information about trainings.

Associated Bodywork and Massage Professionals
28677 Buffalo Park Rd.
Evergreen, CO 80439–7347
(800) 458-ABMP (2267)
E-mail: expectmore@abmp.com
Web site: http://www.abmp.com

A professional membership association that provides practitioners with services and information. Devoted to promoting ethical practices, protecting the rights of practitioners, and educating the public as to the benefits of massage, bodywork, and somatic therapies. On-line referrals to massage and bodywork professionals available on Web site.

Feldenkrais Guild
524 Ellsworth St. SW
P.O. Box 489
Albany, OR 97321–0143
(800) 775-2118
(541) 926-0981
(541) 926-0572 (fax)
E-mail: website@feldenkrais.com
Web site: http://www.feldenkrais.com

Provides information on the Feldenkrais method.

Hakomi Institute
P.O. Box 1873
Boulder, CO 80306
(888) 421-6699
E-mail: institute@hakomi.com
Web site: http://www.hakomi.com

The Hakomi method of body-centered therapy is the integrated use of mindfulness, the body, and nonviolence in psychotherapy that originated in the mid-1970s by the internationally renowned therapist and author Ron Kurtz and members of his training staff. Contact the institute for trainings, workshops, and nationwide referrals.

Hellerwork International
406 Berry St.
Mount Shasta, CA 96067
(916) 926-2500
(800) 392-3900
(916) 926-6839 (fax)
E-mail: Hellerwork@aol.com
Web site: http://www.hellerwork.com

Provides information on trainings in Hellerwork and referrals to certified practitioners.

International Institute of Reflexology
P.O. Box 12642
St. Petersburg, FL 33733
(813) 343-4811
E-mail: ftreflex@concentrix.net

Offers a worldwide referral service for qualified reflexology practitioners and trainings in the Ingham method of reflexology.

International Massage Association
3000 Connecticut Ave. NW, Suite 308
Washington, DC 20008
(202) 387-6555
Web site: http://www.imagroup.com

North American Society of Teachers of the Alexander Technique
3010 Hennepin Ave. S, Suite 10
Minneapolis, MN 55408
(800) 473-0620
(612) 822-7224 (fax)
E-mail: nastat@ix.netcom.com
Web site: http://www.prarienet.org/alexandertech/nastatl.html

Provides information on the Alexander technique or a list of practitioners in your area.

Rolf Institute
205 Canyon Blvd.
Boulder, CO 80302
(303) 449-5903
(303) 449-5978 (fax)
(800) 530-8875
E-mail: rolfinst@rolforg
Web site: http://www.rolf.org

Provides information on Rolfing (structural integration) and referrals to certified practitioners.

Rosen Method Professional Association, referrals only
800-893-2622

Trager Institute
21 Locust Ave.
Mill Valley, CA 94941
(415) 388-2688

Upledger Institute (Craniosacral Therapy)
1211 Prosperity Farms Rd.
Palm Beach Gardens, FL 33410
(407) 622-4334
(800) 233-5880
E-mail: upledger@upledger.com
Web site: http://www.upledger.com

Offers referrals to qualified practitioners of craniosacral therapy in your area. Contact the Upledger Foundation, (407) 624-3888, about their community outreach programs (Share Care) to teach basic craniosacral techniques to the lay public.

Chiropractic

American Chiropractic Association
1701 Clarendon Blvd.
Arlington, VA 22209
(703) 276-8800
Web site: http://wuw.amerchiro.org

International Chiropractors Association
1110 North Glebe Rd., Suite l000
Arlington, VA 22201
(800) 423-4690
Web site: http://www.chiropractic.org

Energy Work

Bio-Electro-Magnetics Institute
2490 W. Moana Lane
Reno, NV 89509–3936
(702) 827-9099

Information on products, services, repairs, and conferences of magnet therapy.

Colorado Center for Healing Touch
12477 W. Cedar Dr.
Lakewood, CO 88828
(303) 989-0581
E-mail: ccheal@aol.com
Web site: www.healingtouch.com

Offers sources of individual practitioners, literature, and ongoing courses.

Healing Touch International
12477 W. Cedar Dr., Suite 202
Lakewood, CO 80228
(303) 989-7982
(303) 980-8683 (fax)
E-mail: htiheal@aol.com
Web site: www.healing touch.net

Offers ongoing classes in the United States and abroad from beginning to certification in healing touch.

Nurse Healers Professional Associates
1211 Locust St.
Philadelphia, PA 19107
(215) 545-8079
(215) 545-8107 (fax)
E-mail: nhpa@nursecominc.com
Web site: http://www.therapeutic-touch.org

(Primarily focuses on therapeutic touch.) Nurse Healers, the procedure's leading advocacy group, offers a list of its roughly 1500 members but recommends checking the individual practitioner's background. If you are offered therapeutic touch at a health care facility, you might want to ask whether the organization follows Nurse Healers' policies and procedures.

Reiki Alliance
P.O. Box 41
Cataldo, ID 83810
(208) 682-3535

Rubenfeld Synergy Center
115 Waverly Place
New York, NY 10011
(800)747-6897
Web site: http://www.members.aol.com/rubenfeld/synergy/index.html

Nurse Healers Professional Associates International
11250 Roger Bacon Dr., Suite 8
Reston, VA 20190
(703) 234-4149
Web site: http://www.therapeutic-touch.org

Environmental Medicine

American Academy of Environmental Medicine
American Financial Center
7701 East Kellogg, Suite 625
Wichita, KS 67207–1705
(316) 684-5500
(316) 684-5709
E-mail: aaem@swbell.net
Web site: http://www.healthy.net/aaem

Provides physician referral in your geographic area and reading list of relevant literature or on-line referral database of AAEM members at Web site.

Human Ecology Action League
P.O. Box 49126
Atlanta, GA 30359–1126
(404) 248-1898
E-mail: HEALN@tnl@aol.com
Web site: http://www.members.aol.com/HEALNatnl/index.html

Support organization for sufferers of environmental illness, including food and chemical sensitivity. Provides information on self-management as well as referrals to practitioners.

Internet

http://www.healthy.net/environmentalmedicine

Flower Essence

Flower Essence Society
P.O. Box 1769
Nevada City, CA 95959
(530) 265-9163
Web site: http://www.floweressence.com

Guided Imagery

Academy for Guided Imagery
P.O. Box 2070
Mill Valley, CA 94942
(800) 726-2070
E-mail: agll996@aol.com
Web site: http://www.healthy.net/agi

The academy offers seminars in interactive guided imagery for the lay public and advanced training programs for licensed health practitioners. Referrals are available on their Web site for professionals certified in the practice of interactive guided imagery.

Herbal Medicine

American Botanical Council
P.O. Box 201660
Austin, TX 78720–1660
(512) 331-8868
(512) 331-1924 (fax)
E-mail: abc@herbalgram.org
Web site: http://www.herbalgram.org

Publishes the quarterly journal HerbalGram, *the English translation of the German Commission E Reports on botanical medicine. Also available are books on herbs, ethnobotany, and botanic medicine.*

American Herbalist Guild
P.O. Box 70
Roosevelt, UT 84066
(435) 722-8434
(435) 722-8452 (fax)
E-mail: ahgoffice@earthlink.net
Web site: http://www.healthy.net/herbalist

Founded in 1989 as a nonprofit, educational organization to represent the goals and voices of herbalists. The only peer review organization for professional herbalists specializing in the medicinal use of plants. Membership consists of professionals, general members (including students), and benefactors.

Herb Research Foundation
1007 Pearl St., Suite 200
Boulder, CO 80302
(303) 449-2265
E-mail: info@herbs.org
Web site: http://www.herbs.org

Provides research material on herbs to consumers, pharmacists, physicians, scientists, and industry.

Internet

http://www.herbalism.com

Holistic Medicine

American Holistic Health Association
P.O. Box 17400
Anaheim, CA 92817
(714) 779-6152
E-mail: ahha@healthy.net
Web site: http://www.ahha.org

Publishes and distributes literature on holistic medicine and provides interviews and public service announcements on TV and radio on the holistic approach to health.

American Holistic Medical Association
6728 Old McLean Village Dr.
McLean, VA 22101–3906
(703) 556-9728
(703) 556-8729 (fax)
E-mail: HolistMed@aol.com
Web site: http://www.ahmaholistic.com

Provides referral list of member physicians organized by state and booklets, including How to Choose a Holistic Physician, What to Do When Facing an Illness, *and* Ten Most Asked Questions about Holistic Medicine and Holism.

American Holistic Veterinary Medical Association
2218 Old Emmorton Rd.
Bel Air, MD 21015
(410) 569-0795
(410) 569-2346 (fax)
E-mail: AHJMA@compuserve.com

Publishes and distributes literature, holds annual and regional conferences, and provides information to consumers.

American Preventive Medical Association
459 Walker Rd.
Great Falls, VA 22066
(703) 759-0662
(703) 759-6711 (fax)
E-mail: apma@healthy.net
Web site: http://www.apma.net

A nonprofit health care advocacy organization whose mission is to ensure the existence of a health care system in which practitioners can practice in good conscience with the well-being of the patient foremost in their minds and without fear of recrimination. Encourages public and professional education in alternative medicine and lobbies for the development of a health care system that gives patients a wide range of therapies.

Holistic Dentists Association
P.O. Box 5007
Durango, CO 81301
Web site: holisticdental.org

Publishes and distributes literature, holds annual and regional conferences, and provides information to consumers.

Mind/ Body Medical Institute
Beth Israel Deaconess Medical Center, Division of Behavioral Medicine
100 Francis St., Suite 1A
Boston, MA 02215
(617) 632-9525

Holistic Nursing

American Holistic Nurses Association
P.O. Box 2130
Flagstaff, AZ 86003–2130
(520) 526-2196
(800) 278-AHNA
(520) 526-2752 (fax)
E-mail: ahna-flag@flaglink.com
Web site: http://www.ahna.org

Founded in 1980 by a group of nurses, AHNA is dedicated to bringing the concepts of holism to every arena of nursing practice. A 501(c)3 nonprofit educational organization whose international membership is open to nurses and others interested in holistically oriented health care practices. Among its objectives, AHNA supports the education of nurses, allied health practitioners, and general public on health-related issues.

Holistic Alliance of Professional Practitioners, Entrepreneurs, and Networkers
P.O. Box 665
Black Mountain, NC 28711
(888) 8HA-PPEN
Web site: http://www.happen.org

Offers ongoing courses in transformational pathways.

Holistic Nursing Certification Corporation
P.O. Box 845
Clarksville, AZ 86324
(877) 284-0998
E-mail: Simpson@Sedona.net

Offers the ongoing education and examination process for becoming certified as a holistic nurse.

Nightingale Institute for Health and the Environment
P.O. Box 412
Burlington, VT 05402
(802) 846-1680
Web site: tni@together.net

Nurses Certificate Program in AMMA Therapy
New York College for Wholistic Health Education & Research
6801 Jericho Turnpike, Suite 300
Syosset, NY 11791–4413
(800) 922-7337, ext. 206
E-mail: MBHolz@nycollege.eduHome
Web site: http://www.nycollege.edu

Nurses Certificate Program in Imagery
Beyond Ordinary Nursing
P.O. Box 8177
Foster City, CA 94404
(605) 570-6157
E-mail: members.aol.com/NCPII/

Seeds and Bridges
Center for Holistic Nursing Education
P.O. Box 307
Shutesbury, MA 01072–0307
E-mail: cphn@seedsandbridges.com

Offers ongoing courses in holistic nursing education.

Homeopathy

American Association of Homeopathic Pharmacists
1441 West Smith Rd.
Ferndale, WA 98248
(800) 478-0421

American Institute of Homeopathy
801 N. Fairfax St., Suite 306
Alexandria, VA 22314
(703) 246-9501
Web site: http://www.healthy.net/aih

A trade association whose membership comprises medical and osteopathic physicians and dentists. Dedicated to the promotion and improvement of homeopathic medicine and the dissemi-

nation of pertinent medical knowledge. Established in 1844, one year after the death of home-opathy's German-born founder, Samuel Hahnemann, the AIH is the oldest national medical professional organization in the United States.

British Institute of Homeopathy (U.S.)
PMB 423
520 Washington Blvd.
Marina del Rey, CA 90292
(310) 306-5408
(310) 827-5766 (fax)
E-mail: bihus@thegrid.net

Provides information and home study courses on homeopathy.

Homeopathic Academy of Naturopathic Physicians
12132 S.E. Foster Place
Portland, OR 97266
(503) 761-3298
(503) 762-1929 (fax)
E-mail: hanp@igc.apc.org
Web site: http://www.healthy.netthanp

A professional association of naturopathic physicians certified in homeopathy.

Homeopathic Educational Services
2124 Kittredge St.
Berkeley, CA 94704
(510) 649-0294
E-mail: mail@homeopathic.com
Web site: http://www.homeopathic.com

Provides a catalogue of homeopathic books, tapes, videos, and software.

National Center for Homeopathy
801 N. Fairfax St., Suite 306
Alexandria, VA 22314
(703) 548-7790
(703) 548-7792 (fax)
E-mail: nchinfo@igc.apc.org
Web site: http://www.homeopathic.org

Offers referrals to physicians and other licensed health practitioners who practice homeopathy and publishes a Directory of Homeopathic Practitioners *that lists practitioners, study groups, and pharmacies throughout the United States and Canada. Provides courses for lay-people and professionals and sponsors study groups throughout the United States.*

Internet

http://www.homeopathic.net

Hypnosis

American Board of Hypnotherapy
16842 Von Kannan Ave., Suite 475
Irvine, CA 92606
(800) 872-9996
Web site: http://www.hypnosis.com

American Society of Clinical Hypnosis
33 W. Grand Ave., Suite 402
Chicago, IL 60610
(312) 645-9810
Web site: http://www.asch.net

International Medical and Dental Hypnotherapy Association
4110 Edgeland, Suite 800
Royal Oak, MI 48073
(248) 549-5594

National Guild of Hypnotists
P.O. Box 308
Merrimack, NH 03054
(603) 429-9438
E-mail: ngh@ngh.net

Light Therapy

Environmental Health & Light Research Institute
16057 Tampa Palms Blvd., Suite 227
Tampa, FL 33647
(800) 544-4878

Society for Light Treatment & Biological Rhythms
10200 W. 44th Ave., Suite 304
Wheat Ridge, CO 80033–2840
(303) 424-3697

Mental Health and Psychology

Association of Humanistic Psychology
45 Franklin St., Suite 315
San Francisco, CA 94102
(415) 864-8850
E-mail: ahpoffice@aol.com
Web site: http://www.ahpweb.org

An international community of diverse people dedicated to the exploration and healing of the human mind, body, and soul and to building a society that advances the ability to choose, grow, and create. Membership is open to all.

Association for Transpersonal Psychology
P.O. Box 3049
Stanford, CA 94309
(650) 327-2066
E-mail: atp@igc.apc.org
Web site: http://www.igc.org/atp

Based on observations and practices from many cultures, the transpersonal perspective is informed by modern psychology, the humanities, and human sciences as well as contemporary spiritual disciplines and the wisdom traditions. This organization has activities and publications for those wanting to develop personal, professional, and educational interests in transpersonal psychology.

Mind/Body Medicine

Center for the Improvement of Human Functioning
3100 North Hillside Ave.
Wichita, KS 67219–3904
(316) 682-3100
E-mail: staff@brightspot.org
Web site: www.brightspot.org

Offers clinical services, diagnostic testing, educational classes, conferences, and seminars on alternative approaches to healing.

Center for Mind/Body Medicine
5225 Connecticut Ave. NW, Suite 414
Washington, DC 20015
(202) 966-7338
(202) 966-2589 (fax)
E-mail: cmbm@ids2.idsonline.com
Web site: http://www.healthy.net/cmbm

A nonprofit, educational organization dedicated to reviving the spirit and transforming the practice of medicine. The center is actively involved in demonstrating the cost-effectiveness and universal appropriateness of mind/body medicine as well as making it a shaping force in the current debate on health care reform.

Chopra Center for Well-Being
7630 Fay Ave.
La Jolla, CA 92037
(619) 551-7788
(619) 551-9570 (fax)
E-mail: info@chopra.com
Web site: http:Hwww.chopra.com

A healing center where guests experience a full range of natural therapies, learn techniques for personal development, and participate in classes in mind/body medicine and healthy living. The mission is to provide guests with a life-changing experience and then show them how to transform their daily lives by applying the knowledge and insights they have gained.

Life Sciences Institute of Mind/Body Health
2955 SW Wanamaker Dr.
Topeka, KS 66614
(785) 271-8686
E-mail: lifesci@cjnetworks.com
Web site: http://www.healthy.net/univ/profess/schools/edu/Isi

Focuses on providing clinical services and research in mind/body medicine.

Mind-Body Medical Institute
Beth Israel Deaconess Medical Center
110 Francis St., Suite 1A
Boston, MA 02215
(617) 632-9530
(617) 632-7383 (fax)
E-mail: mbclinic@west.bidmc.harvard.edu
Web site: http://www.med.harvard.edu/programs/mindbody

Uses yoga, meditation, and stress reduction as part of its treatment program.

Stress Reduction and Relaxation Program
University of Massachusetts Memorial Health Care
55 Lake Ave. North
Worcester, MA 01655
(508) 856-2656
E-mail: stress.reduction@banyan.ummed.edu

The oldest and largest hospital-based, outpatient stress reduction clinic in the country, this pioneering center uses intensive training in mindfulness meditation and yoga to help patients work with their own stress, pain, and illnesses more effectively. The program consists of an eight-week course taken to complement existing treatment. Patients are referred for stress-related conditions such as heart disease, cancer, chronic pain, gastrointestinal problems, anxiety, fatigue, or insomnia.

Internet

http://www.mind-body.com

Music Therapy

American Music Therapy Association
8455 Colesville Rd., Suite 1000
Silver Spring, MD 20910
(301) 589-3300
Web site: http://www.musictherapy.org.

Naturopathic Medicine

American Association of Naturopathic Physicians
601 Valley St., Suite 105
Seattle, WA 98109
(206) 298-0126
(206) 298-0129 (fax)
(206) 298-0125 (referrals)
E-mail: 74602.3715@compuserve.com
Web site: http://w-ww.naturopathic.org

Provides a directory of naturopathic physicians and offers referrals to a nationwide network of accredited or licensed practitioners. On-line directory available at http://www.healthy.net/referrals.

American Naturopathic Medical Association
P.O. Box 96273
Las Vegas, NV 89193
(702) 897-7053
Web site: http://www.anma.com.

Bastyr University College of Naturopathic Medicine
14500 Juanita Dr. N.E.
Kenmore, WA 98028–4966
(425) 823-1300
Web site: http://www.bastyr.edu

Internet

http://www.naturopathy.com

Neuro-Linguistic Programming

Dynamic Learning Center
P.O. Box 1112
Ben Lomond, CA 95005
(408) 336-3457, 336-5854

NLP Comprehensive
2897 Valmont Rd.
Boulder, CO 80301
(303) 442-1102

Western States Training Associates
2290 East 4500 South, Suite 120
Salt Lake City, UT 84117
(801) 278-1022, 278-1088

Nutritional Medicine

American College for Advancement in Medicine
23121 Verdugo Dr., #204
Laguna Hills, CA 92653
(714) 583-7666
(714) 455-9679 (fax)
E-mail: acam@acam.org
Web site: http://www.acam.org

Provides a global directory of physicians who have trained in nutritional and preventative medicine. Also has an extensive list of books and articles on nutritional medicine.

American Dietetic Association
216 West Jackson Blvd.
Chicago, IL 60606
(312) 899-0040
Web site: http://www.eatright.org

Council for Responsible Nutrition
1300 19th St., N.W., Suite 310
Washington, DC 20036–1609
(202) 872-1488

(202) 872-9594 (fax)
E-mail: webmaster@crnusa.org
Web site: http://www.crnusa.org

A trade association representing more than 80 companies in the nutritional supplements and ingredients industry. Members are dedicated to enhancing the public's health through improved nutrition, including the appropriate use of nutritional supplements.

International Society for Orthomolecular Medicine
16 Florence Ave.
Toronto, Ontario, Canada M2N IE9
(416) 733-2117
E-mail: centre@orthomed.org
Web site: http://www.orthomed.org

Internet

http://www.nutritionsite.com
http://www.healthy.net/SupplementBenefits http://www.healthy.netNitaminSafety

Qigong

Qigong Institute
561 Berkeley Ave.
Menlo Park, CA 94026
E-mail: qigonginstitute@healthy.net
Web site: http://www.healthy.net/qigonginstitute

A 501(c)(3) nonprofit organization that promotes medical qigong via education, research, and clinical studies, to improve health care by integrating qigong and Western medicine. It also makes available information on qigong, especially as developed in China, to medical practitioners, scientists, the public, and policymakers.

Internet

http://www.healthy.net/qigong

Spiritual Psychology/Psychospiritual Integration

Association of Transpersonal Psychology
P.O. Box 3049
Stanford, CA 94309
(415) 327-2066
E-mail: atp@igc.apc.org
Web site: http://www.lgc.apc.org/atp

Esalen Institute
Highway 1
Big Sur, CA 93920–9616
(408) 667-3000
(408) 667-2724 (fax)
Web site: http://www.esalen.org

A center for exploring work in the humanities and sciences that promotes human values and potentials. The institute sponsors, encourages, and attempts evaluation of work in these areas, both inside and outside its organizational framework, through public seminars, residential work-study programs, invitational conferences, research, and semiautonomous projects.

Eupsychia Institute
P.O. Box 3090
Austin, TX 78764
(512) 327-2795
(512) 327-6043 (fax)
E-mail: jacquelinesmall@aol.com
Web site: www.eupsychia.com

Eupsychia offers training and healing programs throughout the country for both health professionals and lay public. In an environment of loving support and heartfelt company, Eupsychia is committed to the process of self-discovery and a shift to higher, more integrated ways of living and serving.

HeartNet International
P.O. Box 159
Boynton Beach, FL 33425
(561) 733-2733
(561) 733-5757 (fax)
E-mail: heartnet@aol.com
Web site: http://www.heart-net.com

Presents programs to increase people's quality of life, efficiency, and productivity. The workshops create an environment that reduces stress and allows for the development of higher personal mastery, management, and power in individuals, groups, businesses, and organizations. The staff combines diverse cultural experience with expertise in the fields of medicine, psychology, philosophy, business, finance, and computers to produce world-class educational and humanitarian programs.

Omega Institute for Holistic Studies
Lake Drive Rd. 2, Box 377
Rhinebeck, NY 12572
(914) 266-4301
Web site: http:Homega-inst.org

Through workshops and retreats, brings in teachers and facilitators to help participants explore and embrace new ideas in a peaceful, vegetarian environment.

Psychosynthesis International
P.O. Box 279
Ojai, CA 93024
(805) 646-7041
(805) 646-9338 (fax)
E-mail: psi@west.net
Web site: http://www.healthy.net/psi

Available to students, teachers, ministers, nuns, psychiatrists, psychologists, doctors, home-makers, businesspeople, and other individuals interested in healing and spirituality, its mission is to facilitate awareness, personal healing, and educate on the mental, emotional, physical, and spiritual levels.

Spiritual Emergence Network (SEN)
E-mail: sen@cruzio.com
Web site: http://Helfi.com/sen

Offers information and referral service for an international population and connects those in transformational crisis with educated and compassionate helpers.

Internet

http://www.bodymindspirit.com

Vegetarianism

American Vegan Society
P.O. Box H
Malaga, NJ 08328
(609) 694-2887

Association of Vegetarian Dietitians & Nutrition Educators
3674 Cronk Rd.
Montour Falls, NY 14865
(607) 535-6089

International and American Associations of Clinical Nutritionists
5200 Keller Springs Rd., Suite 102
Dallas, TX 75248
(972) 250-2829

North American Vegetarian Society
P.O. Box 72
Dolgeville, NY 13329
(518) 568-7970

Vegan Action
P.O. Box 4353
Berkeley, CA 94704
(510) 654-6297

Vegetarian Education Network
P.O. Box 3347
West Chester, PA 19381
(717) 529-8638

Vegetarian Resource Center
P.O. Box 38–1068
Cambridge, MA 02238
(617) 625-3790

Vegetarian Resource Group
P.O. Box 1463
Baltimore, MD 21203
(410) 366-8343

Women's Health

Phillips Publishing
7811 Montrose Road
Potomac, MD 20854
(800) 211-8561

Publishes Health Wisdom for Women, *a provocative monthly newsletter focusing on natural healing alternatives and the role the emotions play in health.*

Mind/Body Health Sciences
393 Dixon Rd.
Boulder, CO 80302
(303) 440-8460
(303) 440-7580 (fax)

Offers a free annual publication featuring Joan Borysenko's lecture and workshop itinerary and information on A Gathering of Women's weekend spiritual retreats. Includes books, audiotapes, and videos, plus a select offering of healing music, art, and meditation tapes for adults and children.

Natural Woman Institute
(888) 489-6626

Through a program of outreach and education for women and physicians, this organization supports a greater understanding of plant-derived hormones for women at midlife and the importance of hormonal balance in keeping healthy, active, and vital. A database of updated doctor referrals is maintained as well as compounding pharmacies providing natural hormones.

Yoga

International Association of Yoga Therapists
109 Hillside Ave.
Mill Valley, CA 94941
(415) 383-4587

A nonprofit organization focusing on education and research in yoga and yoga therapy.

ON-LINE LIBRARIES AND JOURNALS

Information gathering that can require hours of research and travel can now be accessed in minutes through a system of "universal libraries" located on-line. A number of different organizations, from a network of public universities to the Library of Congress, are becoming increasingly available. While some libraries want to make their collections available in a digitized form, others are taking a much larger view. They envision a day when all recorded human knowledge can be searched, retrieved, and studied on-line. In the future there will be an exponentially larger, global body of information, including a host of newly digitized collections of text, sound, and images. It will also change the way you search for information. Now most people use the Web to browse using strings of words. In the future we will be able to search by posing semantic queries by adding topics and concepts.

Some on-line libraries offering information on complementary and alternative medicine are:

Health World Online—abundant online holistic health information including free medline searches: www.healthy.net

Internet Public Library: www.ipl.org

Library of Congress: www.lcweb.loc.gov

National Center for Complementary and Alternative Medicine: www.Alt med.od.nih.gov

National Library of Medicine: www.ncbi.nlm.nih.gov/PubMed

Thomas, legislative information: http://thomas.loc.gov

Conducting Internet Searches on Alternative Medicine Subjects

MEDLINE uses a "keyword" indexing system called MESH (Medical Subject Headings) to access information. To search for a subject on MEDLINE, you may enter your own term, or you may select from the MESH keyword list of approximately 18,000 terms. Currently, there are 23 main headings in MEDLINE under the term *alternative medicine*. More specific terms are listed under those main headings. For example, *meditation* is a more specific term under the heading *relaxation techniques*.

Many alternative medicine terms are not yet included in MESH. Although many articles relating to alternative medicine from conventionally focused peer-reviewed journals are in MEDLINE, researchers may have difficulty finding them.

The U.S. National Library of Medicine (NLM) is aware of the increasing interest in alternative medicine and the need for adequate MESH terms. The Office of Alternative Medicine (OAM) is working with NLM to review the current terms, making suggestions for new terms and improving the indexing for alternative medicine. Currently, more than 30,000 citations can be retrieved by searching under the term *alternative medicine*.

The main headings in MEDLINE under the term "alternative medicine" are:

Acupuncture	Mental healing
Anthroposophy	Moxibustion
Biofeedback	Music therapy
Chiropractic	Naturopathy
Color therapy	Organotherapy
Diet fads	Radiesthesia
Eclecticism	Reflexotherapy
Electric stimulation therapy	Rejuvenation
Homeopathy	Relaxation techniques
Kinesiology, applied	Therapeutic touch
Massage	Tissue therapy
Medicine, traditional	

ALTERNATIVE MEDICINE JOURNALS CURRENTLY IN MEDLINE

The NLM procedure for reviewing and accepting journals of current interest is appropriately rigorous. Not all journals concerning alternative medicine are indexed on MEDLINE. For example, MEDLINE only indexes 3 of the 16 journals available on chiropractic. Some of the journals relating to alternative medicine indexed in MEDLINE are:

Acupuncture and Electro-Therapeutics Research

Alternative Therapies in Health and Medicine

American Journal of Chinese Medicine

Biofeedback and Self-Regulation

Chen Tzu Yen Chui (Acupuncture Research)

Chinese Medical Journal

Chung-Hua I Hsueh Tsa Chih (Chinese Medical Journal)

Chung-Kuo Chung Hsi I Chieh Ho Tsa Chih

Chung-Kuo Chung Yao Tsa Chih (China Journal of Chinese Materia Medica)

Holistic Nursing Practice

Journal of Holistic Nursing

Journal of Manipulative and Physiological Therapeutics

Journal of Natural Products

Journal of Traditional Chinese Medicine

Planta Medica

Additional journals are:

Advances: The Journal of Mind-Body Health

Alternative and Complementary Therapies

Commercial Internet Sites

New information is appearing daily on the Internet. Much of this information can be found at specific Internet sites. All of the national Internet servers, such as America Online, Yahoo, and Excite offer numerous health connections. Many of these sites are not associated with organizations and associations but are "virtual" sites. That is, they have no buildings or street addresses; rather they exist solely on the Internet. At these sites information is posted and exchanged. In addition to their Internet address, many of the sites have telephone numbers where one can call to order the books and/or products offered from the site and an E-mail contact address to solicit more information or ask questions. In some instances the virtual sites are linked with organizations or associations. Some of the more popular sites are becoming well known and offer advice and information to millions of people. These include but are not limited to the sites listed in Table 22-1.

Browsers in the Internet marketplace will find that the quality of information is very diverse. Some sites offer depth of data, with credentials to back them up.

TABLE 22-1   Commercial Internet Health Sites

INTERNET ADDRESS	SITE FEATURES
www.Adoctorinyourhouse.com	Video, medical updates, chats, and support groups with physicians and celebrities. An on-line community for those seeking advice, inspiration, and empowerment
www.WebMD.com	
www.drKoop.com	Associated with the former Surgeon General and is known for innovative support groups.
www.AllHealth.com	
www.AmericasDoctor.com	
www.InteliHealth.com	Has on-line questions and answers with Johns Hopkins doctors.
www.Med-help.com	
www.onhealth.com	
www.PlanetRx.com	Offers detailed, relevant answers to pharmaceutical questions such as drug actions and interactions.
www.Americasdoctor.com	Wait in line for your turn to ask the doctor a question.
www.Yourhealth.com	Moderated by a qualified nutritionist who answers questions.
http://1HealthyUniverse	Source for the latest news and information in the field of holistic, alternative, complementary, and integrative medicine. This site's goal is to provide holistic and self-care approaches for promoting optimal wellness and overcoming disease.
Mothernature.com	Offers a health library, shopping, and information about natural products, pet supplies, cosmetics, and a variety of general merchandise.

Others display nice site designs but have thin content. The explosion of Internet sites is both valuable and dangerous. It is wonderful to have an encyclopedia of information at our fingertips. However, consumers must be wary of seeking and following advice from a virtual source without some provider/client face-to-face interaction. Practitioners and clients alike will be prudent to exercise the follow cautions:

- ■ Seek information from several sources.
- ■ Trust only information that is attributed and validated.
- ■ Question the sites billing themselves as the sole source on a topic.
- ■ Do not be misled by a long list of links; they do not signify endorsement.

- Find out if a site is professionally managed and has content reviewed by experts.
- Ensure that all clinical information carries a date, since medical knowledge is evolving.
- Advertising and sponsorship messages should be separate from editorial content.
- Avoid on-line practitioners who diagnose or treat without an examination.

CONFERENCES

Alternative and complementary care conferences are happening all over the nation. At these conferences participants link up with other like-minded people, attend keynote and workshop sessions, and spend time in exhibit areas that feature products and specialty books. Oftentimes attendance at a conference opens doors to other modalities or philosophies the participant had not previously considered because of lack of exposure. Interested people can find the location of conferences by reading newsletters or tapping into a particular organization's Web site.

SUPPORT GROUPS

Very often attendance at a local, regional, or national conference will lead to joining a special interest support group. Just as the range of alternative and complementary therapies are expanding, so are the numbers and kinds of support groups. For example, people with fibromyalgia are finding that spending time with others who have the same condition not only lends emotional support but also offers an environment for sharing of information about new methods of therapy that may not yet be publicly available.

SUMMARY

Alternative and complementary therapies are the fastest growing segment of the health care arena. Organizations, associations, and educational institutes are proliferating as the need for support of specialty groups evolves. Coinciding with the development of this new phase of health care delivery is the advent of the Internet and all its specialty sites. Many sites can be easily accessed to find leading-edge information on the topic of interest. Attending specialty conferences and support groups adds one more layer of ways to increase your knowledge and appreciation of the myriad available resources.

ASK YOURSELF

1. Are there one or more organizations that fit within the framework of my practice?
2. Should I take the time to access some of the above information to add to my body of knowledge?
3. Can any of my patients be referred to one or more of the organizations listed here?
4. Is it possible that my agency or organization could be listed in a resource section or have a Web address?

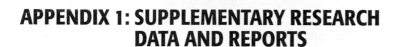

APPENDIX 1: SUPPLEMENTARY RESEARCH DATA AND REPORTS

The material is this area includes supplemental research studies and reports of some of the modalities featured in Chapters 6–13. They are categorized according to the same nine categories used in the modalities chapters.

HEALING PHILOSOPHIES

Kinds of Patients Who Use Alternative Practitioners

This study compares the social and health characteristics of patients of five kinds of practitioners: family physicians (used as a baseline group), chiropractors, acupuncturists/traditional Chinese medicine doctors, naturopaths, and Reiki practitioners. The data were gathered in a large Canadian city during the period 1994–1995. Face-to-face interviews were conducted with 300 patients (60 from each type of treatment group). While the most striking social and health differences occur between patients of family physicians and the patients of alternative practitioners, significant differences are also evident between the different groups of alternative patients. Reiki patients, for example, have a higher level of education and are more likely to be in managerial or professional positions than other alternative patients. The profiles presented here indicate that users of alternative care should not be regarded as a homogeneous population. The findings also show that almost all alternative patients also consult family physicians. The pattern revealed is one of multiple use: Patients choose the kind of practitioner they believe can best help their particular problem.

Source: Kelner, M., & Wellman, B. (1997). Who seeks alternative health care? A profile of the users of five modes of treatment. *Journal of Alternative and Complementary Medicine, 3*(2), 127–140.

MENTAL THERAPIES

Music Therapy and Parkinson's Disease

This was a prospective study conducted to evaluate the effects of music therapy (MT) in the neurorehabilitation of patients with Parkinson's disease (PD), a common degenerative disorder involving movement and emotional impairment. Sixteen PD patients took part in 13 weekly sessions of MT each lasting 2 hours. At the beginning and at the end of the session, every two weeks, the patients were evaluated by a neurologist, who assessed PD severity, emotional functions with Happiness Measures (HM), and quality of life using the Parkinson's Disease Quality of Life Questionnaire (PDQL). After every session a significant improvement in motor function, particularly in relation to hypokinesia, was observed both in the overall and in the pre-post session evaluations. The changes confirmed an improving effect of MT on emotional functions, activities of daily living, and quality of life. In conclusion, active MT, operating at a multisensorial level, stimulates motor, affective, and behavioral functions. Finally, we propose active MT as a new method to include in PD rehabilitation programs.

Source: Pacchetti, C., Aglieri, R., Mancini, F., Martignoni, E., & Nappi, G. (1998). Active music therapy and Parkinson's disease: methods. *Functional Neurology, 27*(3), 57–67.

Music Therapy and Alzheimer's Disease

Music therapy is known to have healing and relaxing effects. These effects appear to be mediated by release of neurotransmitters and neuohormones. This study was done to assess the effect of a music therapy intervention on concentrations of melatonin, norepinephrine, epinephrine, serotonin, and prolactin in the blood of 20 male inpatients with Alzheimer's disease. Melatonin concentration in serum increased significantly after music therapy and was found to increase further at six weeks follow-up. The conclusion from this study is that music therapy may contribute to patients' relaxation.

Source: Kumar, A., Tims, F., Cruess, D., Mintzer, M., Ironson, G., Loewenstein, D., Cattan, R., Fernandez, J. B., Eisdorfer, C., & Kumar, M. (1999). Music therapy increases serum melatonin levels in patients with Alzheimer's disease. *Alternative Therapies, 5*(6), 49–57.

TOUCH THERAPIES AND BODYWORK

Effects of Massage on Asthma

Thirty-two children with asthma (sixteen 4- to 8-year-olds and sixteen 9- to 14-year-olds) were randomly assigned to receive either massage therapy or relaxation therapy. The children's parents were taught to provide one therapy or the other for 20 minutes before bedtime each night for 30 days. The younger children who received massage therapy showed an immediate decrease in behavioral anxiety and cortisol levels after massage. Also, their attitude toward asthma and their peak air flow and other pulmonary functions improved over the course of the study. The older children who received massage therapy reported lower anxiety after the massage. Their attitude toward asthma also improved over the study, but only one measure of pulmonary function (forced expiratory flow 25%– 75%) improved. The reason for the smaller therapeutic benefit in the older children is unknown; however, it appears that daily massage improves airway caliber and control of asthma.

Source: Field, T., Henteleff, T., Hernandez-Reif, M., Martinez, E., Mavunda, K., Kuhn, C., & Schanberg, S. (1998). Children with asthma have improved pulmonary functions after massage therapy. *Journal of Pediatrics, 132*(5), 854–858.

Effects of Massage on Cystic Fibrosis

This study measured the effects of parents giving massage therapy to their children with cystic fibrosis to reduce anxiety in parents and their children and to improve the children's mood and peak air flow readings. Twenty children (5–12 years old) with cystic fibrosis and their parents were randomly assigned to a massage therapy or a reading control group. Parents in the treatment group were instructed and asked to conduct a 20-minute child massage every night at bedtime for one month. Parents in the reading control group were instructed to read with their child for 20 minutes a night for one month. On days 1 and 30, parents and children answered questions relating to present anxiety levels, and children answered questions relating to mood, and their peak air flow was measured. Following the first and last massage session, children and parents reported reduced anxiety. Mood and peak air flow readings also improved for children in the massage therapy group. These findings suggest that

(Continued on next page)

parents may reduce anxiety levels by massaging their children with cystic fibrosis and their children may benefit from receiving massage by having less anxiety and improved mood, which in turn may facilitate breathing.

Source: Hernandez-Reif, M., Field, T., Krasnegor, J., Martinez, E., Schwartzman, M., & Mavunda, K. (1999). Children with cystic fibrosis benefit from massage therapy. *Journal of Pediatric Psychology, 24*(2), 175–181.

Effects of Massage on Burn Patients

Twenty-eight adult patients with burns were randomly assigned before debridement to either a massage therapy group or a standard treatment control group. State anxiety and cortisol levels decreased, and behavior ratings of state, activity, vocalizations, and anxiety improved after the massage therapy sessions on the first and last days of treatment. Longer term effects were also significantly better for the massage therapy group, including decreases in depression and anger and decreased pain on the McGill Pain Questionnaire, Present Pain Intensity Scale, and Visual Analogue Scale. Although the underlying mechanisms are not known, these data suggest that debridement sessions were less painful after the massage therapy sessions due to a reduction in anxiety and the clinical course was probably enhanced as the result of a reduction in pain, anger, and depression.

Source: Field, T., Peck, M., Krugman, S., Tuchel, T., Schanberg, S., Kuhn, C., & Burman, I. (1998). Burn injuries benefit from massage therapy. *Journal of Burn Care Rehabilitation, 19*(3), 241–244.

ENERGETIC THERAPIES

Therapeutic Touch with Psychiatric Patients

Seven hospitalized adolescent psychiatric patients who received a total of 31 therapeutic touch treatments over two two-week periods were interviewed about their experience. Findings from the interviews were categorized within two overarching themes—the therapeutic relationship and the body-mind connection. The study participants enjoyed the therapeutic touch, and in fact, they wanted more of it. This research shows the possibility of therapeutic touch as an intervention with adolescent psychiatric patients if all care is taken to obtain their consent and to provide them with a safe environment for touch therapy.

Source: Hughes, P. P., Meize-Grochowski, R., & Harris, C. N. (1996). Therapeutic touch with adolescent psychiatric patients. *Journal of Holistic Nursing, 47*(1), 6–23.

Therapeutic Touch and the Immune System

The specific aim of this experimental design study was to evaluate the effectiveness of therapeutic touch in reducing the adverse immunological effects of stress in a sample of highly stressed students. Long-term goals are to develop methods by which a variety of stress reduction techniques can be tested for efficacy. Healthy medical and nursing students who were taking professional board examinations received therapeutic touch, and subjects who did not had significantly different levels of immunoglobulin A and M (IgA, IgM); CD25 (mitogen-stimulated T-lymphocyte function) and IgG levels differed in the expected direction between the two groups, but the differences were not statistically significant. Apoptosis (programmed cell death) was significantly different between the two groups. The small sample size requires cautious interpretation of the results. This was a pilot study designed to provide evidence to show that further study of therapeutic touch as an intervention that may be useful in reducing the adverse immunological consequences of anxiety related to stress in otherwise healthy students is warranted. Change in immune function related to anxiety and the relief of anxiety can be measured. Subsequent power analysis suggests sample sizes of 90 subjects per group are required to confirm the conclusions.

Source: Olson, M., Sneed, N., LaVia, M., Virella, G., Bonadonna, R., & Michel, Y. (1997). Stress-induced immunosuppression and therapeutic touch. *Alternative Therapies in Health and Medicine, 47*(2), 68–74.

EASTERN THERAPIES

Acupuncture for Pain Relief during Childbirth

There are few studies on acupuncture in childbirth despite the generally established analgesic effect of acupuncture treatment. The analgesic effect of acupuncture during childbirth was assessed by comparing the need for other pain treatments (epidural analgesia using bupivacaine, pudendal nerve block, intramuscular meperidine, nitrous oxide/oxygen, intracutaneous sterile water injections) in 90 women given acupuncture (acupuncture group) with that in 90 women not given acupuncture (control group). The results were that 52 women (58%) in the acupuncture group and 13 (14%) in the control group managed their deliveries without further pain treatment ($p < 0.001$). The groups were similar with respect to age, pariety, duration of delivery, use of oxytocine, and incidence of Cesarean section. Acupuncture treatment was found to have no major side effects, and 85 women (94%) given acupuncture reported that they would reconsider acupuncture in future deliveries. The conclusion of this study is that acupuncture reduces the need for other methods of analgesia in childbirth.

Source: Ternov, K., Nilsson, M., Lofberg, L., Algotsson, L., & Akeson, J. (1998). Acupuncture for pain relief during childbirth. *Acupuncture Electrotherapy Research, 23*(1), 19–26.

Acupuncture in Recurrent Lower Urinary Tract Infection

This study evaluated the effectiveness of acupuncture in the prevention of recurrent lower urinary tract infection (UTI) in adult women. The design was a controlled clinical trial with three arms: an acupuncture group, a sham-acupuncture group, and an untreated control group. Sixty-seven adult women with a history of recurrent lower UTI were followed for six months in an acupuncture clinic in Bergen, Norway. Eighty-five percent were free of lower UTI during the six-month observation period in the acupuncture group, compared with 58% in the sham group ($p < 0.05$), and 36% in the control group ($p < 0.01$). There were half as many episodes of lower UTI per person-half-year in the acupuncture group as in the sham group and a third as many as in the control group ($p < 0.05$). The conclusion is that acupuncture seems a worthwhile alternative in the prevention of recurring lower UTI in women.

Source: Aune, A., Alraek, T., LiHua, H., & Baerheim, A. (1998). Acupuncture in the prophylaxis of recurrent lower urinary tract infection in adult women. *Scandinavian Journal of Primary Health Care, 23*(1), 37–39.

Acupuncture for Treatment of Diabetic Neuropathy

Forty-six diabetic patients with chronic painful peripheral neuropathy were treated with acupuncture analgesia to determine its efficacy and long-term effectiveness. Twenty-nine (63%) patients were already on standard medical treatment for painful neuropathy. Patients initially received up to six courses of classical acupuncture analgesia over a period of 10 weeks using traditional Chinese medicine acupuncture points. Forty-four patients completed the study with 34 (77%) showing significant improvement in their primary and/or secondary symptoms ($p < 0.01$). These patients were followed for a period of 18–52 weeks with 67% able to stop or reduce their medications significantly. During the follow-up period only 8 (24%) patients required further acupuncture treatment. Although 34 (77%) patients noted significant improvement in their symptoms, only 7 (21%) noted that their symptoms cleared completely. All the patients but one finished the full course of acupuncture treatment without reported or observed side effects. There were no significant changes either in the peripheral neurological examination scores, or hemoglobin levels during the course of treatment. These data suggest that acupuncture is a safe and effective therapy for the long-term management of painful diabetic neuropathy, although its mechanism of action remains speculative.

Source: Abuaisha, B. B., Costanzi, J. B., & Boulton, A. J. (1998). Acupuncture for the treatment of chronic painful peripheral diabetic neuropathy: A long-term study. *Diabetes Research and Clinical Practice, 39*(2), 115–121.

Use of Acupuncture in Dentistry

The objective of this study was to review the scientific validity of published papers on the efficacy of acupuncture in dentistry based on predefined methodological criteria. A literature search performed by the Royal Society of Medicine and the University Library, Copenhagen, Denmark, was able to identify 74 papers written in English, German, Danish, Swedish, Norwegian, Italian, French, and Russian published between 1966 and 1996. The search words were: *acupuncture* and *electro-acupuncture, randomized controlled trials (RCT), dental pain, postoperative dental pain, pain relieving in dentistry,* and *dental analgesia.* Among the 74 listed papers, 48 papers were reviewed in the following

(Continued on next page)

languages: English, Danish, Swedish, Norwegian, and German. Fifteen papers were excluded because they were written in French, Italian, or Russian; 11 papers were excluded because the abstract clearly indicated the paper was not an RCT or the paper was of a general nature without relevance to acupuncture. To assess the methodological quality of the included papers, all papers were scored on the basis of predefined criteria. A total of 92 points could be achieved, and on the basis of this scale papers were rated as excellent (85%–100%), good (70%–84%), fair (60%–69%), and bad (<60%). Fifteen out of 48 papers met the inclusion criteria. Only one study met the criteria with more than 85%. Five studies met the criteria with 70%–84%. Three studies met the criteria with 60%–69%. Six studies did not meet the criteria. Acupuncture in 11 out of 15 studies proved effective in the treatment of tempero-mandibular dysfunction (TMD) and as analgesia. Four studies showed no effect of acupuncture. The conclusion of this study is that the value of acupuncture as an analgesic must be questioned. The effect of acupuncture in treating TMD and facial pain seems real and acupuncture could be a valuable alternative to orthodox treatment.

Source: Rosted, P. (1998). The use of acupuncture in dentistry: A review of the scientific validity of published papers. *Oral Disease, 39*(2), 100–104.

Acupuncture Utilization in Taiwan

The objective of this study was to examine the prevalence of acupuncture utilization in Taiwan by people over 20 years of age. Stratified cluster sampling was used to randomly select 20 villages and neighborhoods (townships), a total of 8280 people, from northern, central, southern, and eastern Taiwan. A structured questionnaire was used to collect information during home visits. A total of 5805 questionnaires were valid for use in the study. The complete rate of home visits was 70.1%; 73.2% of those interviewed recognized acupuncture as one of the common therapeutic methods used in traditional Chinese medicine, whereas only 12.4% had received acupuncture treatment. Typical interviewees who had received acupuncture treatment were generally ethnic, from southern Fukien, and aged from 30 to 39 years; 58.3% of the 716 interviewees had received acupuncture treatment from licensed practitioners, while the remainder were treated by nonlicensed practitioners. The response rate to the questionnaire was high (70.1%). However, the percentage of people who had received acupuncture treatment was only

12.4%, while many people (73.2%) were familiar with it. Approximately 40% of those who received acupuncture treatment did so from non-licensed practitioners. This may reveal either a lack of awareness by the public or a lack of public protection of health and safety.

Source: Chou, P., Lai, M. Y., Chung, C., Chen, J. M., & Chen, C. F. (1998). Acupuncture utilization in Taiwan. *Chung Hua I Hsueh Tsa Chih (Taipei), 39*(2), 151–158.

Acupuncture and the Opioid System

Researchers investigated the effectiveness of acupuncture in childhood migraine in 22 children with migraine, randomly divided into two groups: a true acupuncture group (12 children) and a placebo acupuncture group (10 children). Ten healthy children served as a control group. Opioid activity in blood plasma was assayed by two methods: (1) determination of total (panopioid) activity with an opiate radioreceptor assay and (2) determination of beta-endorphin-like immunoreactivity by radioimmunoassay. The true acupuncture treatment led to significant clinical reduction in both migraine frequency and intensity. At the beginning of the study, significantly greater panopioid activity was evident in plasma of the control group than in plasma of the migraine group. The true acupuncture group showed a gradual increase in the panopioid activity in plasma, which correlated with the clinical improvement. After the tenth treatment, the values of opioid activity of the true acupuncture group were similar to those of the control group, whereas the plasma of the placebo acupuncture group exhibited insignificant changes in plasma panopioid activity. In addition, a significant increase in beta-endorphin levels was observed in the migraine patients who were treated in the true acupuncture group as compared with the values before treatment or with the values of the placebo acupuncture group. The results suggest that acupuncture may be an effective treatment in children with migraine headaches and that it leads to an increase in activity of the opioidergic system.

Source: Pintov, S., Lahat, E., Alstein, M., Vogel, Z., & Barg, J. (1997). Acupuncture and the opioid system: Implications in management of migraine. *Pediatric Neurology, 17*(2), 129–133.

Traditional Chinese Medicine

China is the only country in the world where Western medicine and traditional medicine are practiced alongside each other at every level of the health care system. Traditional Chinese medicine has a unique theoretical and practical approach to the treatment of disease, which has developed over thousands of years. Traditional treatments include herbal remedies, acupuncture, acupressure and massage, and moxibustion. They account for around 40% of all health care delivered in China. The current government policy of expansion of traditional facilities and manpower is being questioned because many hospitals using traditional Chinese medicine are already underutilized and depend on government subsidies for survival. Research priorities include randomized controlled trials of common treatments and analysis of the active agents in herbal remedies. As more studies show the clinical effectiveness of traditional Chinese medicine, an integrated approach to disease using a combination of Western medicine and traditional approaches becomes a possibility for the future.

Source: Hesketh, T., & Zhu, W. X. (1997). Health in China. Traditional Chinese medicine: One country, two systems. *BMJ: British Medical Association,* 315(7100), 115–117.

Factors Influencing Patients' Choice of Traditional Chinese Medicine

This study investigated the different factors influencing patients' choice of traditional Chinese medicine or modern Western medicine, applying Andersen's health service utilization model to analyze the basic demographic, enabling, and need factors related to the choice of clinics by patients who use a two-method treatment (i.e., both Chinese medicine and Western medicine). Systemic sampling was done and a structured questionnaire survey was carried out among patients from the outpatient departments of 13 teaching hospitals accepting reimbursement by Labor Medical Insurance in Taiwan. The total number of valid respondents was 549. Of them, 181 (33%) were visiting Western medicine clinics and 368 (67%) visiting Chinese medicine clinics. There were 279 (51%) males and 270 (49%) females, whose age distribution was in the range from 16 to 87 years old, with a mean of 42.7 years. Under univariate analysis, the significant variables ($p < 0.05$) related to visiting the two types of clinics were applicability of medical insurance, bed rest from discomfort in recent years, the amount of discomfort from this disease episode, respiratory disease, circulatory disease, endocrine or metabolic disease, and sense organ and skin disorders. By logistic regression analysis, the significant variables ($p < 0.05$) related to visiting the two types of clinics were religion, bed rest during the past year, discomfort associated with the episode, respiratory disease, and endocrine or metabolic diseases. Patients with folk-religion beliefs or respiratory diseases favored Chinese medicine; patients with illness requiring bed rest in the past year, who experienced discomfort in this episode, or who suffered from endocrine or metabolic diseases were likely to visit Western medicine clinics.

Source: Kang, J. T., Chen, C. F., & Chou, P. (1996). Factors related to the choice between traditional Chinese medicine and modern Western medicine among patients with two-method treatment. *Chung Hua I Hsueh Tsa Chih (Taipei)*, *57*(6), 405–412.

Potential for Traditional Chinese Medicine in Urology

There are several other alternative medicines apart from vitamins and minerals that the clinician should be aware of because they have grown in popularity in other fields of medicine. In time, these therapies should impact the arena of urologic oncology. Traditional Chinese medicine, which includes acupuncture, is an area that has received some attention. The theory behind it can be quite daunting because it is so different from the theory behind Western medical science. In addition, exactly how acupuncture can be applied to a patient and its potential use in prostate cancer need to be addressed. Other herbal therapies for the patient experiencing symptoms related to a localized cancer diagnosis also need to be evaluated. St John's wort for depression and kava for anxiety are two examples of herbal alternatives that some prostate patients are inquiring about. Finally, ginkgo biloba, recognized for its use in memory stimulation, has received attention in the media for erectile dysfunction, but there is a dearth of evidence in this area, and the information that already exists can be misleading until further studies are conducted. Also, it is imperative that additional studies be performed in all of the above subjects as they relate to prostate cancer, but a general survey on alternative medicine use in urologic diseases is needed before an adequate review of the most popular therapies can be published.

Source: Moyad, M. A., Hathaway, S., & Ni, H. S. (1999). Traditional Chinese medicine, acupuncture, and other alternative medicines for prostate cancer: An introduction and the need for more research. *Seminars in Urological Oncology*, *17*(2), 103–110.

Traditional Chinese Medicine and Acute Viral Myocarditis

To investigate the combination therapy of Western and traditional Chinese medicine on treatment of acute viral myocarditis, 48 patients were randomly divided into two groups. The first group consisted of 30 patients receiving the combination therapy of Western and traditional Chinese medicine, including *Astragalus membranaceus,* taurine, coenzyme Q10, and antiarrhythmics, while the second group consisted of 18 patients receiving the conventional therapy, including glucose-insulin-potassium (GIK), coenzyme Q10, and antiarrhythmics. The efficacy of combination therapy of Western and traditional Chinese medicine was better than that of conventional therapy in improving the clinical manifestation, and controlling the premature beats. The conclusion was that the combination therapy of Western and traditional Chinese medicine was an effective method in treating acute viral myocarditis.

Source: Gu, W., Yang, Y. Z., & He, M. X. (1996). A study on combination therapy of Western and traditional Chinese medicine of acute viral myocarditis. *Chung Kuo Chung Hsi I Chieh Ho Tsa Chih, 17*(12), 713–716.

Use of Tai Chi for Rheumatoid Arthritis Patients

The good news about using tai chi as a therapeutic exercise is that it does not seem to have any adverse effects. In studies of patients with osteo and rheumatoid arthritis, investigators discovered that, unlike certain other types of exercise, tai chi did not make joints more tender and increase the number of swollen or damaged joints. Nor did it cause any further bone deterioration. There are also reports of less joint tenderness and swelling and greater hand grip strength.

Source: Kirsteins, A., Dietz, F., & Hwang, S. M. (1991). Evaluating the safety and potential use of a weight bearing exercise, tai chi chuan, for rheumatoid arthritis patients. *American Journal of Physical and Medical Rehabilitation, 70*(3), 136.

MISCELLANEOUS THERAPIES

Hydrotherapy for Chronic Low Back Pain

Sixty subjects with chronic low back pain (LBP) were sequentially allocated to either hydrotherapy treatment or land treatment groups in order of presentation. Subjects acted as their own controls for a period of three weeks, after which they attended their respective group sessions twice weekly for six weeks. Twenty-eight subjects from each group attended all treatment and assessment sessions. Results indicated that both groups improved significantly in functional ability and in decreasing pain levels. Thoracolumbar mobility did not improve significantly in either group. Overall there was no significant difference found between the two types of treatment, although results should be viewed as encouraging for advocates of both hydrotherapy and land-based exercise as a treatment for chronic LBP.

Source: Sjogren, T., Long, N., Storay, I., & Smith, J. (1997). Group hydrotherapy versus group land-based treatment for chronic low back pain. *Physiotherapy Research International, 46*(4), 212–222.

Delivery in Birthing Pools

The use of birthing pools during labor is increasing in the United Kingdom. This is without good scientific evidence of their efficacy or safety. To further investigate the value and safety of intrapartum hydrotherapy, an historical cohort study was performed in a District General Hospital in Liverpool. The study group consisted of 100 women of low obstetric risk who used the birthing pool at some stage during their labors and the control group consisted of 100 women who were matched in terms of age, parity, and obstetric history but labored and delivered in air. The main outcome measures were operative delivery rates, duration of labor, analgesic requirements, perineal trauma, and Apgar scores at 1 and 5 minutes. The results showed that nulliparas who used the birthing pool had significantly reduced operative delivery rates, a shorter second stage of labor, reduced analgesic requirements, and a lower incidence of perineal trauma. In multiparas there were significant reductions in analgesic requirements.

Source: Aird, I. A., Luckas, M. J., Buckett, W. M., & Bousfield, P. (1997). Effects of intrapartum hydrotherapy on labour related parameters. *Australian and New Zealand Journal of Obstetrics and Gynaecology, 46*(2), 137–142.

Effects of Hydrotherapy on Pressure Ulcer Healing

Pressure ulcers are a prevalent and potentially serious medical problem encountered in both the medical and rehabilitation settings. Because the progress of rehabilitation is often interrupted by the presence of pressure ulcers, the efficient care of these wounds is of great interest to the rehabilitation team. Patients in two acute care facilities with Stage III or IV pressure ulcers were identified and consented to participate in the study contained herein. All wounds were mechanically debrided of necrotic tissue, and then the patients were randomly assigned to the conservative treatment group (A; $n = 18$) or the conservative treatment plus whirlpool group (B; $n = 24$). Conservative treatment included measures to maximize pressure relief and wound care with wet-to-wet dressings using normal saline. The dressings were changed twice daily and when they became soiled. Whirlpool was administered for 20 minutes per day in group B patients. Only those patients whose ulcers were followed up for 2 or more weeks were included in the study. Ulcers were then measured by a physician who was blinded as to the treatment groups. Ulcer dimension changes over time were compared between groups. The results indicate that the conservative treatment plus whirlpool group improved at a significantly faster rate than did the conservative treatment only group ($p < 0.05$).

Source: Burke, D. T., Ho, C. H., Saucier, M. A., & Stewart, G. (1998). Effects of hydrotherapy on pressure ulcer healing. *American Journal of Physical Medicine and Rehabilitation, 46*(5), 394–398.

Whirlpool Therapy on Postoperative Pain and Surgical Wound Healing

Postoperatively, patients who have major abdominal surgery experience pain because of increased tension on muscles and tissues at the abdominal incision site. Also, pain is due to trapped anesthesia gases in the intestines. These postoperative events can cause increased anxiety and stress resulting in poor pain management and altered tissue regeneration. An intervention such as whirlpool therapy can enhance relaxation and promote pain relief and normal wound healing. The purpose of this study was to examine the effects of whirlpool therapy on pain and surgical wound healing in adults having major abdominal surgery. Sixty-three subjects (43 female and 20 male), ages 25–60, participated in a quasi-experimental study of repeated measures of pain and surgical wound assessments over a three-day period. Statistical tests for repeated measures revealed that the experimental group response to verbal pain was not significant. However, it did reveal that observable pain behaviors using the Pain Rating Scale (PRS) were significant for three consecutive days. Also, statistical tests for repeated measures of wound healing revealed less signs of surgical wound inflammation in the experimental group over a three-day period. It was concluded that the intervention of whirlpool therapy promoted some degree of comfort and positive signs of wound healing.

Source: Juv'e Meeker, B. (1998). Whirlpool therapy on postoperative pain and surgical wound healing: an exploration. *Patient Education and Counseling, 46*(1), 39–48.

Patient Characteristics and Practice Patterns of Physicians Using Homeopathy

The use of homeopathy is growing in the United States, but little is known about practice patterns of physicians using homeopathy and the patients who seek homeopathic care. Data for consecutive patient visits to 27 doctors of medicine and doctors of osteopathy using homeopathy in 1992 were collected and compared with the National Ambulatory Medical Care Survey of 1990. Patients seen by the homeopathic physicians were younger, more affluent, and more likely to present with long-term complaints. Physicians using homeopathic medicine surveyed spent more time with their patients, ordered fewer tests, and prescribed fewer pharmaceutical medications than physicians practicing conventional medicine. While definite conclusions cannot be made based on this survey, the study documented that the use of diagnostic testing and conventional medications by physicians who use homeopathy to treat common chronic conditions is well below that of conventional primary care physicians. These findings, if associated with comparable clinical outcomes, suggest a potential for substantial cost savings. Further studies documenting outcomes, cost benefits, physician decision making, and patient satisfaction will be required to further explore this subject.

Source: Jacobs, J., Chapman, E. H., & Crothers, D. (1998). Patient characteristics and practice patterns of physicians using homeopathy. *Archives of Family Medicine, 350*(6), 537–540.

An Overview of Homeopathy Evidence

Forty percent of general practitioners in the Netherlands practice homeopathy. With over 100 homeopathic medical schools, homeopathy is
practiced in India along with conventional Western medicine in government clinics. In Britain, 42% of general practitioners refer patients to
homeopaths. Two recent meta-analyses of homeopathy both indicate
that there is enough evidence to show that homeopathy has added
effects over placebo. Against this evidence is a backdrop of considerable
scientific scepticism. Homeopathic remedies are diluted substances;
some are so diluted that statistically there are no molecules present to
explain their proposed biological effects (ultrahigh dilutions, or UHDs).
Without knowledge of the evidence, most scientists would reject UHD
effects because of their intrinsic implausibility in the light of our current
scientific understanding. The objective of this article is to critically
review the major pieces of evidence on UHD effects and suggest how
the scientific community should respond to its challenge. Such evidence has been conducted on a diverse range of assays: immunologic,
physiological, behavioral, biochemical, and clinical in the form of trials
of homeopathic remedies. Evidence of UHD effects has attracted the
attention of physicists who have speculated on their physical mechanisms. Included is a critique of several experiments that form the
Benveniste affair, which was sparked by a publication in *Nature* that
advocated the existence of UHD effects of anti-immunoglobulin E (IgE)
on human basophils and is the paradigm example of how a controversial
phenomenon can split the scientific community. It is argued that if the
phenomenon was uncontroversial, the evidence suffices to show that
UHD effects exist. However, given that the observations contradict well-
established theory, normal science has to be abandoned and scientists
need to decide for themselves what the likelihood of UHD effects are.
Bayesian analysis describes how scientists ought rationally to change
their prior beliefs in the light of evidence. Theories by Kuhn and Lakatos
indicate that whether UHD effects are proved or not depends on the
beliefs and behaviors of scientists in their communities. This article
argues that there is as yet insufficient evidence to drive rational scientists
to a consensus over UHD effects, even if they possessed knowledge of all
the evidence. The difficulty in publishing high-quality UHD research in
conventional journals prevents a fair assessment of UHD effects. Given
that the existence of UHD effects would revolutionize science and
medicine, and given the considerable empirical evidence of them, the
philosophies of science tell us that possible UHD effects warrant serious

investigation by conventional scientists and serious attention in scientific journals.

Source: Vallance, A. K. (1998). Can biological activity be maintained at ultra-high dilution? An overview of homeopathy, evidence, and Bayesian philosophy. *Journal of Alternative and Complementary Medicine, 350*(1), 49–76.

Use of and Satisfaction with Homeopathy in a Patient Population

This study describes a survey of new clients entering care with nine practicing classical homeopaths in the Los Angeles metropolitan area between January 1994 and July 1995. Participants completed a self-administered questionnaire before undergoing diagnosis by the homeopath. Follow-up interviews were conducted by phone one month after diagnosis and face to face four months after diagnosis, along with a self-administered questionnaire before the final interview. A total of 104 participants entered the study; 77 completed all data collection. Clients sought homeopathic care for a wide array of largely chronic conditions. Respiratory, gastrointestinal, and female reproductive problems were the most common primary complaints. Most clients were highly educated but had limited knowledge about homeopathy before entering treatment. Approximately 80% reported earlier, unsuccessful attempts to get relief from mainstream care. Four months after treatment, general measures of health status showed improvement, and only 29% of participants reported no improvement for the primary complaint leading to treatment. Satisfaction with homeopathic treatment was high regardless of outcome. Three outcome measures of perceived change—overall health status, primary condition for which treatment was sought, and outlook on life—were predicted by different combinations of study variables. Homeopathy does not divert people from seeking mainstream care. The use of alternative modes of care such as homeopathy can be understood as attractive and satisfying to educated individuals with chronic problems.

Source: Goldstein, M. S., & Glik, D. (1998). Use of and satisfaction with homeopathy in a patient population. *Alternative Therapies in Health and Medicine, 4*(2), 60–65.

Homeopathic and Psychiatric Perspectives on Grief

This review describes the homeopathic analysis of grief and common remedies corresponding to this reaction. Homeopathic descriptions of grief are compared with contemporary psychiatric criteria. Each homeopathic rubric (i.e., symptom) is identified on the basis of a computerized repertory search, grouped according to body systems, and compared with a current set of operational criteria derived from the psychiatric literature. The major homeopathic remedies for grief were identified. One hundred four rubrics for grief were found incorporating mental and physical symptoms as well as physical disease. Homeopathic phenomenology of grief was closely matched with its current psychiatric definition. A close correspondence was seen between psychiatry and homeopathy, even though each has a differing heritage and temporal origin. The correspondence of a later descriptive system (i.e., psychiatry) to an earlier, independently derived system (i.e., homeopathy) confers validation to both systems' description of the grief response. The similarities and differences between homeopathic and psychiatric descriptions of grief have been noted. Similar forms of grief response are recognized by both systems, though homeopathy provides a more extensive list of physical sequelae following bereavement. Controlled trials of homeopathy in grief states are recommended.

Source: Davidson, J. R., & Gaylord, S. (1998). Homeopathic and psychiatric perspectives on grief. *Alternative Therapies in Health and Medicine, 4*(5), 30–35.

APPENDIX 2: INTEGRATIVE CARE CENTERS AND WELLNESS CENTERS

INTRODUCTION

This appendix gives examples of what an integrative care center or a wellness center might look like from the perspective of where they are and what services they offer.

UNIVERSITY OF ARIZONA PROGRAM IN INTEGRATIVE MEDICINE

The University of Arizona in Tucson established the first program in integrative medicine in the country in the 1980s. To advance research and education in this field, the Program in Integrative Medicine has the following components:

- Two-year fellowship
- Associate fellowship, distance learning
- Rotations for medical students and residents
- Continuing education
- Research
- Clinic

MARINO FOUNDATION FOR INTEGRATIVE MEDICINE

The Marino Foundation for Integrative Medicine in Cambridge, Massachusetts, is a not-for-profit organization integrating a variety of medical and alternative healing traditions to meet the needs of all the individuals it serves. The goal of this center is to synthesize conventional and alternative medicine into a collaborative partnership. This new paradigm for medicine offers patients safe and effective medical options while protecting them from unproven or unnecessary therapies. It houses a collaborative team of compassionate, innovative practitioners who provide acute, chronic, and preventative health care along with health education, training, and research.

The Marino Center is a full-service medical clinic offering such services as primary care, acupuncture, chiropractic and massage therapy, chelation therapy, nutrition, vitamin therapy, and more. They accept most major insurances.

Their mission statement includes:

- First doing no harm to patients, co-workers, and communities
- Respecting the natural forces of healing in the mind and body
- Evaluating its effectiveness through scientific research and self-scrutiny
- Affirming the importance of connection in people's lives
- Facilitating the evolution of integrative medicine in other organizations and communities
- Weekly meetings to share ideas, educate others, and discuss diagnostic and treatment options

MIND BODY WELLNESS CENTER

The Mind Body Wellness Center (MBWC) in Meadville, Pennsylvania, opened in 1997 under the direction of Barry Bittman, a neurologist with 16 years of experience. The center is a department of the Meadville Medical Center (MMC) and is located in a service area of 86,000 (per 1990 U.S. Census). The MBWC offers ongoing integrative disease-based programs for patients with diabetes, chronic obstructive pulmonary disease, cardiovascular disease, and cancer. All programs include nutrition, exercise, stress management/coping skills, and relaxation techniques tailored to the specific group's needs. Patients may perform aerobic exercises using equipment or mind-body exercises such as tai chi or yoga. Data collection is also an integral component of each program.

This freestanding center, owned and operated by the Meadville Medical Center, is innovative and provides a variety of whole-person integrative programs within a traditional health care setting. It offers programs incorporating modalities that have a documented scientific research base.

The MBWC operates on the basis of a tight-knit integration with traditional medicine plus an outcome-based research system that not only assures optimal care but also provides documentation for insurance providers of the validity of a whole-person approach. Under the direction of Barry Bittman and colleagues, psychoneuroimmunological based scientific research is also performed.

Facts about the MBWC

- Staffing data:
  Physicians: 1 + subspecialist program directors
  RNs: 2 (including one certified diabetes educator)
  LPNs: 1

■ Support staff:
Massage therapist
Acupuncturist
Licensed social workers (3)
Registered dietitian
Physical therapist (also a Feldenkrais practitioner)
Respiratory therapist
Research assistant
Marketing director
Independent contractors who perform yoga, tai chi, and Drumming
Clerical support staff

Client Visits

Patients are seen individually by clinicians, plus most practitioners also participate as members of interdisciplinary teams in disease-based programs. Many patients are seen by a team of practitioners in order to maximize the synergistic effect and healing potential.

Number of Programs Offered

The MBWC uses the word *program* to refer to any disease-based program and the word *class* to refer to wellness promotion opportunities. All programs are ongoing throughout the year. Classes (such as yoga, tai chi/qigong, Feldenkrais) are generally offered fall-spring and not during the summer months.

Special Events Associated with the Center

Annual conference: *Speaking from the Soul* (1–2-day conference/workshops)
Syndicated National Pubic Radio (NPR) show: Mind Body Matters
Weekly newspaper column: *Mind Over Matter*
Conferences associated with EcaP: The center operates Exceptional Cancer Patients (EcaP), a group started by Bernie Siegel that offers both professional and patient training programs and provides additional resources.

The MBWC's focus is on integration with traditional medicine. The center recently received a grant funded through the Pennsylvania Department of Health for cardiac risk reduction, a preventive and restorative approach. MBWC's mind-body approach is the basis for the Heart-to-Heart cardiac rehabilitation program at Meadville Medical Center for those patients who have a diagnosis of myocardial infarction, unstable angina, or bypass. Grant dollars are also used to offer a "lifestyle" change program.

Breathing Easy, the Pulmonary Rehabilitation program, and Diabetes Self-Management Skills, a diabetes education program, are covered by most insurers. Highmark Blue Cross/Blue Shield is the first major insurance company in the nation to cover Insights for Living Beyond Cancer, a whole-person approach for cancer patients developed with Bernie Siegel. Weigh to Be, a weight management program, is for the most part self-pay, as insurance companies customarily do not cover weight management modalities.

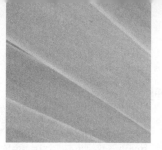

GLOSSARY

Many of the following terms are used in this book. Others, however, are not included in the book but are added here to supplement the knowledge base of complementary and alternative vocabulary.

A

Acupressure– Based on the principles of acupuncture, this ancient Chinese technique involves the use of finger pressure on specific points along the body to treat ailments such as tension, stress, aches, pains, cramps, or arthritis.

Acupuncture– Fine needles are inserted at specific points to stimulate, disperse, and regulate the flow of chi, or vital energy, and restore a healthy energy balance.

Adjustment– In chiropractic, a small controlled thrust that moves a joint slightly beyond its normal range of motion.

Alexander technique– F. Matthias Alexander created the method after concluding that bad posture was responsible for his own chronic voice loss. Practitioners use gentle hands-on guidance and verbal instruction to teach simple, efficient ways of moving as a means of improving balance, posture, and coordination and relieve tension and pain.

Allopathy– The treatment of disease by creating conditions that are opposite or hostile to the conditions resulting from the disease itself; from Greek roots meaning "other" and "disease." Drugs and surgery are allopathic treatments. The term is sometimes used to refer to conventional Western medicine to contrast it with alternative therapies, particularly homeopathy, which is based on like curing like.

AMMA therapy– System of bodywork therapy that uses traditional Oriental medicine to restore, promote, and maintain optimum health through the treatment of the physical body, bioenergy, and emotions. It is a form of acupressure used for a wide range of conditions.

Ancestor worship– Ritualized propitiation and invocation of dead kin, based on the belief that spirits influence the fate of the living. A widespread ancient practice.

Animism– Belief that a spirit or force resides in every animate and inanimate object, every dream and idea, giving individuality to each. The related Polynesian concept of mana holds that the spirit in all things is responsible for good and evil.

Applied kinesiology– A diagnostic technique and therapy developed in the 1960s by a chiropractor (George Goodheart). Applied kinesiology posits that organ or gland dysfunctions show up as weaknesses in certain muscles. Using gentle pressure, applied kinesiologists test muscle strength to identify health problems and nutritional deficiencies. After diagnosis, treatment may involve exercises to strengthen a muscle, hands-on manipulation of the muscles and bones and reflex points, and vitamin or mineral supplements.

Aquatherapy– Use of water in all its physical forms—hot water, cold water, tepid water, steam, vapor mist, and ice—to augment the healing process. In addition, the sensory, visual, and auditory sounds of water such as sitting by a waterfall, listening to raindrops, or relaxing by a stream or beach are all a part of aquatherapy.

Aromatherapy– Uses essential oils from flowers, trees, roots, herbs, berries, and fruits to treat emotional disorders such as stress and anxiety as well as a wide range of other ailments and to promote physical, mental, and emotional wellness. Oils are either massaged into the skin in diluted form, inhaled, placed in baths, or applied on and around the body. Aromatherapy is often used in conjunction with massage therapy, acupuncture, reflexology, herbology, chiropractic, and other wholistic healing.

Atomistic– Has to do with contemporary medicine's approach based on treatments using remedies producing effects opposite from those produced by the disease being treated.

Ayurvedic medicine– Practiced in India for over 5000 years. Ayurvedic tradition holds that illness is a state of imbalance among the body's systems and can be corrected through massage, natural medications, meditation, and other modalities used to address a spectrum of ailments, from allergies to AIDS.

B

Behavior therapy/modification– Aims at modifying behavior by reinforcing acceptable behavior and suppressing undesirable behavior. The therapist employs any of various techniques of reward and punishment, including aversion therapy, desensitization, and guided imagery. The learning theory of the psychologist B.F. Skinner and others is the basis for most behavior therapies. In Skinner's principle of extinction, a behavior pattern that is not reinforced, or rewarded, will be extinguished or rendered inoperative. For example, if smoking is made unpleasant for the smoker, then the smoking habit may be curbed or given up. Behavior therapy is used in private and institutional therapy and group and individual settings to treat such disorders as drug addiction, alcoholism, and phobias.

Bioenergetics– Holds that repressed emotions and desires affect the body and psyche by creating chronic muscular tension and diminished vitality and energy. Through physical exercises, breathing techniques, verbal psychotherapy, or other forms of emotional-release work, the therapist attempts to loosen this character armor and restore natural well-being.

Biofeedback– Technique used especially for stress-related conditions such as asthma, migraines, insomnia, and high blood pressure. Biofeedback is a way of monitoring minute metabolic changes in one's body with the aid of sensitive machines.

Biofield– An energy field that suffuses living bodies and extends several inches beyond the body. This concept is employed in therapies such as healing touch, medical qigong, therapeutic touch, and reiki. In these therapies, the biofield, from a practitioner's hands, is joined to the recipient's biofield in order to treat an illness or promote health. There is no consensus on what a biofield is; some say it is spiritual energy, others say it is an electromagnetic field.

Body-mind centering– A movement reeducation approach that explores how the body's systems contribute to movement and self-awareness. The approach also emphasizes movement patterns that develop during infancy and childhood. Incorporates guided movement, exercise, imagery, and hands-on work.

Body-oriented psychotherapy– Seeks to enhance the psychotherapeutic process by incorporating a range of massage, bodywork, and movement techniques. Acknowledging the mind-body link, practitioners may use light touch, soft or deep-tissue manipulation, breathing techniques, movement, exercise, or body awareness techniques to help address emotional issues.

Breathwork– General term for a variety of techniques that use patterned breathing to promote physical, mental, and/or spiritual well-being. Some techniques use the breath in a calm, peaceful way to induce relaxation or manage pain, while others use stronger breathing to stimulate emotions and emotional release.

C

Chakras– A term used in the Indian system of medicine that refers to the seven vital energy centers of the body. The chakras extend from the base of the spine to the crown of the head. Located in the perineal area, below the navel, at the solar plexus, at the heart, at the neck, between the eyebrows, and on the crown of the head. Each chakra corresponds to certain colors, emotions, organs, nerve networks, and energies.

Chelation therapy– Typically administered in an osteopathic or medical doctor's office, chelation therapy is a series of intravenous injections of the synthetic amino acid ethylenediaminetetraacetic acid (EDTA), designed to detoxify the body. Often used to treat arteriosclerosis, angina, and Alzheimer's disease. The Federal Drug Administration (FDA) approved chelation therapy removing lead and other heavy metals from the bloodstream. One theory holds that chelation removes the calcium in arterial plaque; another suggests that EDTA works as an antioxidant. Proponents say that chelation also reverses gangrene, relieves the pain associated with lupus and arthritis, and reverses memory loss.

Chiropractic– The chiropractic system is based on the premise that the spine is literally the backbone of human health. Misalignments of the vertebrae caused by poor posture or trauma result in pressure on the spinal nerve roots, which may lead to diminished function and illness. The chiropractor seeks to analyze and correct these misalignments through spinal manipulation or adjustments.

Colon hydrotherapy– Involves the cleansing of the large intestine with warm, purified water. A single colonic treatment is said to be equivalent to several enemas in removing toxic debris from the colon.

Craniosacral therapy– A manual procedure for remedying distortions in the structure and function of the craniosacral mechanism—the brain and spinal cord, the bones of the skull, the sacrum, and interconnected membranes. It is used to treat chronic pain, migraine headaches, temporomandibular joint (TMJ), and a range of other conditions.

D

Deep-tissue bodywork– General term for a range of therapies that seek to improve the function of the body's connective tissues and/or muscles. Among the conditions treated are whiplash, low back and neck pain, and degenerative diseases such as multiple sclerosis.

Dentistry, wholistic– Wholistic dentists are licensed dentists who bring an interdisciplinary approach to their practice, often incorporating such methods as homeopathy, nutrition, and acupuncture into their treatment plans. Most wholistic dentists emphasize wellness and preventive care and avoid silver-mercury fillings.

Diathermy– Deep-heat therapy that uses high-frequency electric currents to produce heat in body tissues. Physical therapists and sports physicians use diathermy to treat arthritis, bursitis, and fractures.

Dietary supplement– A product intended to supply nutrients and other healthful substances that may be lacking in a diet. Term used to apply only to vitamins, minerals, and proteins. Herbs are now classified as dietary supplements, and the definition also includes amino acids, glandulars (processed animal glands), enzymes, fish oils, and various extracts, such as flower essences. While their labels may not make any claims to cure, prevent, treat, or mitigate a disease, they can claim to help a structure or function of the body. Unlike food additives and prescription and over-the-counter drugs, dietary supplements do not require FDA approval to be sold on the market.

DMSO (dimethyl sulfoxide)– Solvent capable of passing through body tissues, approved by the FDA to treat one medical condition, interstitial cystitis (an uncommon bladder inflammation). Proponents and manufacturers claim that DMSO heals a wide range of problems (including bruises, pimples, and herpes) and relieves pain from conditions such as muscle strains. They credit DMSO with the ability to kill bacteria and fungi, improve circulation, and stimulate the immune system. DMSO produces strong garlic breath in users, even when used topically or intravenously.

Dream therapy– Mental activity associated with the rapid-eye-movement period of sleep. Generally consists of visual images and may reflect bodily disturbances or external stimuli. In primitive and ancient cultures, dreams played an extensive role in myth and religion. Freud emphasized dreams as keys to the makeup of the individual and distinguished between the experienced content of a dream and the actual meaning of the dream. Jung held that dreams are not limited to the personal unconscious but may also be shaped by archetypes that originate in the collective unconscious of the human species.

Drug therapy– Various drugs are used to alleviate symptoms of some mental illnesses. Lithium is used in alleviating symptoms of manic depression. Tranquilizers are used to reduce anxiety. All drugs have side effects, such as Ritalin, which is prescribed for hyperactive children and can retard physical growth.

E

Ear candling– Also called ear coning. Involves placing the narrow end of a specially designed hollow candle at the entry of the ear canal, while the opposite end is lit. Primarily used for relieving wax buildup and related hearing problems, ear candling is also used for ear infections and sinus infections.

Energy field work– Practitioners look for weaknesses in the energy field in and around the client's body and seek to restore its proper circulation and balance. Energy channeled through the practitioner is directed to strengthen the body's natural defenses and help the client's physical, mental, emotional, and/or spiritual state.

Enzyme therapy– A form of therapy that employs supplements of plant and animal enzymes to improve digestive function and other conditions. During digestion, the body's digestive enzymes are not the only ones at work; the enzymes present in raw fruits and vegetables also contribute to the breakdown of food in the stomach. Enzyme therapy advocates supplementation to reduce the work that the body has to do and because plant enzymes are destroyed in cooking. Since enzymes cannot be synthetically manufactured, supplements are derived from plants or from animal tissues. Some practitioners inject liquid enzymes to treat cancer and multiple sclerosis. Enzyme supplements are available over the counter, singly or in combination, in capsule, tablet, powder, and liquid form.

Essential– A nutritional term applied to vitamins, minerals, and amino acids; refers to anything that the body does not manufacture and that must be obtained through the diet.

Expressive therapies– Use the arts to promote physical and mental health and personal growth. Examples of expressive therapies include art therapy, dance therapy, drama therapy, music therapy, poetry, and psychodrama.

F

Feng shui– An ancient Chinese practice of configuring home or work environments to promote health, happiness, and prosperity. Feng shui literally means "wind water" and was used to help situate a house or garden to be in the ideal relationship to the natural environment. Modern feng shui practitioners more frequently focus on the interiors of the home. Feng shui consultants may advise clients to make adjustments in their surroundings, from color selection to furniture placement, to promote a healthy flow of chi, or vital energy.

Flower essences– Intended to alleviate negative emotional states that may contribute to illness or hinder personal growth. Drops of a solution infused with the captured essence of a flower are placed under the tongue or in a beverage. The appropriate essences are chosen, focusing on the client's emotional state rather than on a particular physical condition.

G

Glandulars– Animal glands, processed into pill form and taken internally. Typically made from cow, sheep, or pig glands, glandulars on the market include adrenal, testicular, ovary, pancreas, pituitary, prostate, and thymus products. Critics point out that these supplements are unlikely to boost gland function because digestion breaks down and inactivates the DNA in a glandular. In addition, using glandulars may encourage the client's glands to reduce hormone production. Other risks include bacterial contamination of the product and the antibiotics and pesticides present in the glands of the livestock from which they are taken.

The FDA generally prohibits glandulars containing hormones because they are classified as drugs. Armour Thyroid is straight bovine thyroid gland. Many "natural" oriented medical doctors prescribe it in place of synthroid on the presumption that cofactors in the whole gland may have other synergistic effects. Nutritionists, chiropractors, and naturopaths use these products to nourish and help repair the target gland.

Glucosamine sulfate– A natural amino sugar found in joint spaces. As a dietary supplement, it is said to stimulate the repair of arthritic joints by building up the protective cartilage that arthritis destroys.

H

Healing touch– Practiced by registered nurses and others to accelerate wound healing, relieve pain, promote relaxation, prevent illness, and ease the dying process. The practitioner uses light touch or works with his or her hands near the client's body in an effort to restore balance to the client's energy system.

Hellerwork– A system of somatic education and structural bodywork that is based on the inseparability of body, mind, and spirit, making the connection between movement, body alignment, and personal awareness. During sessions, the structural balance of the body is realized through the systematic release of muscle and connective tissue to restore the body's optimal natural balance, posture, and flexibility. Myofascial release, movement awareness, and dialogue are the essence of the sessions enabling one to move more fluidly and have increased stamina, strength, and energy.

Herbalism– Uses natural plants or plant-based substances to treat a range of illnesses and to enhance the functioning of the body's systems. Though herbalism is not a licensed professional modality in the United States, herbs are prescribed by a range of practitioners, from holistic medical doctors to acupuncturists to naturopaths.

HIV therapies– Practitioners offer a range of therapies that aim to treat the human immunodeficiency virus AIDS or its symptoms. Due to the life-threatening nature of this disease, these therapies are often used as complements to conventional approaches to HIV.

Holistic/wholistic– An adjective meaning "targeted to the whole person"—mind, body, and spirit. Wholistic medicine considers not only physical health but also the emotional, spiritual, social, and mental well-being of the person.

Homeopathy– A medical system that uses infinitesimal doses of natural substances to stimulate a person's immune and defense system. Homeopathic remedies are named for the plant or animal ingredient from which they are made.

Hydrosol– The water that is obtained along with essential oil after plant materials are distilled. In distillation, plant materials are heated in water to release plant oils. The steam and vapor are channeled through a tube to a condensing coil, where they cool and return to liquid form. The essential oils float on top of the water. The hydrosol contains water-soluble plant constituents and trace amounts of essential oil. Hydrosols are sometimes used in aromatherapy together with the essential oils and may be spritzed in the air and on the face and body.

Hypnosis– Although the condition resembles normal sleep, scientists have found that the brain wave patterns of hypnotized subjects are much closer to the patterns of deep relaxation. Hypnosis is now generally viewed as a form of attentive, receptive, highly focused concentration in which external events are omitted or disregarded. Widely used by surgeons, dentists, and psychotherapists to relieve anxiety or as an anesthetic. Used to relax a patient, reduce resistance to therapy, facilitate memory, and address stopping smoking, eating less, or fighting fears.

I

Iridology– Diagnostic system based on the premise that every organ has a corresponding location within the iris of the eye, which can serve as an indicator of the organ's health or disease. Used by naturopaths and other practitioners, particularly when diagnosis achieved through standard methods is unclear.

J

Jin shin do– Developed by a psychotherapist, it combines acupressure, Taoist yogic breathing, and Reichian segmental theory (addresses how emotional tension affects the physical body) with the goal of releasing physical and emotional tension and armoring. Aims to promote a state in which the patient can address the emotional factors that underlie various physical conditions.

Kinesiology– The study of muscles and their movement. Applied kinesiology is a system that uses muscle testing procedures, in conjunction with standard methods of diagnosis, to gain information about a patient's overall state of health.

L

Light box– A set of bright, full-spectrum light bulbs inside a box with a reflective background and diffusing screen; produces light that is 10–20 times stronger than ordinary indoor light. Used to treat winter depression, or SAD (seasonal affective disorder). Treatment typically involves spending 15 minutes to 3 hours in front of a light box every day in the fall, winter, and early spring. Research suggests that bright lights help regulate the body's internal clock, which controls hormone secretion and sleep patterns.

Light-emitting diodes (LEDs)– Tiny light sources (frequently used in digital watches and electronic equipment) that have been used in the field of phototherapy. Their power output is low enough to be safe for human exposure but strong enough to stimulate the biological responses involved in healing. Research indicates that LEDs may accelerate the healing of skin wounds and certain other conditions.

M

Magnetic therapy– Magnetic field therapy or biomagnetic therapy involves the use of magnets, magnetic devices, or magnetic fields to treat a variety of physical and emotional conditions, including circulatory problems, certain forms of arthritis, chronic pain, sleep disorders, and stress.

Manipulation– Application of manual force for healing. Term describes the techniques used in osteopathy, chiropractic, massage, and other bodywork therapies. Manipulation may involve various forms of massage, muscle pressure, and joint realignment or adjustment.

Mantra– In Hinduism and Buddhism, mystic word used in ritual and meditation. It is believed to have power to bring into being the reality it represents. Use of such mantras usually requires initiation by a guru, or spiritual teacher.

Massage therapy– A general term for a range of therapeutic approaches with roots in both Eastern and Western cultures. Involves the practice of kneading, stroking, compression, tapping, pinching, plucking, scraping, or otherwise manipulating a person's muscles and soft tissue.

Medicine, holistic/wholistic– A broadly descriptive term for a healing philosophy that views a patient as a whole person, not as just a disease or a collection of symptoms. In the course of treatment, wholistic medical practitioners may address emotional and spiritual dimensions as well as the nutritional, environmental, and lifestyle factors that may contribute to an illness. Many wholistic practitioners combine conventional forms of treatment with natural or alternative treatments.

Meditation– Discipline in which the mind is focused on a single point of reference. Employed since ancient times in various forms by all religions, the practice gained greater notice in postwar United States as interest in Zen Buddhism rose. Meditation is now used by many nonreligious adherents as a method of stress reduction; known to lower levels of cortisol, a hormone released in response to stress. Enhances recuperation and improves the body's resistance to disease.

Megavitamin therapy– *See* Orthomolecular medicine.

Melatonin– Hormone produced by the pineal gland in the brain and released mainly at night in the absence of light on the retina. Regulates the onset and timing of sleep and seasonal changes in the body, such as winter weight gain. Levels of melatonin decline with age. Melatonin is being investigated as a sleep promoter and to prevent or reduce jet lag. Synthetic melatonin and melatonin derived from bovine pineal glands are available as over-the-counter dietary supplements. Melatonin occurs naturally in some foods but in fairly small amounts. Reported side effects include reduced fertility, inhibition of male sexual drive, hypothermia, and damage to the retina. Some physicians and scientists advise against taking melatonin as a long-term supplement.

Meridians– Within traditional Oriental medicine theory, meridians are the pathways of a set of unseen but present energy lines that run longitudinally throughout the body and are carriers of chi. The meridian system includes the 12 main meridians, the "8 extras," which serve as reservoirs of chi, the divergent meridians, and the tending muscular meridians.

Midwifery– Midwives provide education and support during pregnancy, assist the mother during labor and delivery, and provide follow-up care. Practitioners of childbirth support include childbirth educators, childbirth assistants, and women labor coaches who also provide postpartum home care.

Myofascial release– Trauma, posture, or inflammation can create a binding down of fascia resulting in excessive pressure on nerves, muscles, blood vessels, osseous structures, and/or organs. This hands-on technique seeks to free the body from the grip of tight fascia, or connective tissue, thus restoring normal alignment and function and reducing pain. Therapists apply mild, sustained hand pressure in order to gently stretch and soften fascia. Treatment is used to treat neck and back pain, headaches, recurring sports injuries, scoliosis, and other conditions.

N

Network chiropractic– Uses network spinal analysis, a method characterized by the sequential application of a number of gentle, specific chiropractic adjusting techniques. Care progresses through a series of levels that parallel spinal and quality-of-life changes.

Neural therapy– A form of therapy based on the idea that illness is the result of disruptions in biological energy and that the disruptions are caused by changes in the electric activity of the autonomic nervous system (which controls involuntary functions like breathing).

Neurotopic injection– Treatment involves dozens of injections of small amounts (0.5 cc or less) of sterile saline solution (0.9% salt) into the muscles at both sides of the spine near the places where the nerves enter into the back muscles. According to this theory, salt injection helps the nerves function better, leading to improved circulation, control of pain, and healing of numerous disorders. Statistics on successful treatment of back and neck pain, sciatica, disk problems, headaches, arthritis, prostate and thyroid problems, asthma, and allergies have been presented at more than 15 international medical congresses. Technique is being evaluated in double-blind studies at the National College of Naturopathic Medicine in Oregon.

Nosode– A homeopathic remedy made from diseased tissue or bodily secretions rather than from a plant or animal. Taken like a homeopathic immunization to build up an immune response against a specific disease. Nosodes are often named for the disease present in the material from which they were made—for example, the flu nosode and the infectious mononucleosis nosode.

O

Orthomolecular medicine– A form of nutrient therapy that uses combinations of vitamins, minerals, and amino acids normally found in the body to maintain good health and treat specific conditions, such as asthma, heart disease, depression, and schizophrenia. "Orthomolecular" means an approach based on a correct ("ortho") balance of substances present in the body.

P

Pet therapy– A therapeutic approach based on the idea that expressing affection for a pet helps people feel happier, maintain a positive outlook, and therefore improve their health. According to several studies, having a pet can reduce stress, lower blood pressure, and ward off loneliness and depression. Many nursing homes and some prisons have developed pet therapy programs, with excellent results.

Polarity therapy– Based on a theory of energy flow in the body developed by Randolph Stone, a doctor of naturopathy, osteopathy, and chiropractic. Asserts that balancing the flow of energy in the body is the foundation of health. Specific points along the currents are said to hold positive or negative energies. Practitioners use gentle touch and guidance in diet, exercise, and self-awareness to help clients balance their energy flow, thus supporting a return to health.

Prana– The yogic concept of a cosmic energy or life force, similar to the Chinese idea of chi, that enters the body with the breath. Prana is thought to flow through the body, bringing health and vitality. It is considered the vital link between the spiritual self and the material self.

Pranayama– A term from Yoga and Ayurveda meaning breath control.

Probiotics– Substances such as *Acidophilus* and *Bifidus* that restore the beneficial bacteria normally present in the intestines. Stress, poor diet, antibiotics, and oral contraceptives can throw off the normal balance of bacteria and fungi. This imbalance may be manifested as a yeast infection or as symptoms such as diarrhea or gastrointestinal disturbances.

R

Rebirthing– Also known as conscious-connected breathing or vivation. A technique in which the therapist guides clients through breathing exercises to help them reexperience past memories—including birth—and let go of emotional tensions stored in the body.

Reflexology– Based on the idea that specific points on the feet and hands correspond with organs and tissues throughout the body. With fingers and thumbs, the practitioner applies pressure to these points to treat a wide range of stress-related illnesses and ailments.

Regression– Psychological defense mechanism, viewed as a return to an earlier mode of behavior, thought, or feeling. The unconscious process that helps the mind resolve conflicts or lessen anxiety by returning to forms of gratification previously abandoned.

Reiki– Practitioners of this ancient Tibetan healing system use light hand placements to transmit healing energies to the recipient. While the practitioners may vary widely in technique and philosophy, Reiki is commonly used to treat emotional and mental distress as well as chronic and acute physical problems as well as to assist the recipient in achieving spiritual focus and clarity.

Rolfing– Uses deep manipulation of the fascia to restore the body's natural alignment, which may have become rigid through injury, emotional trauma, and inefficient movement habits. The process, developed by biochemist Ida P. Rolf, involves 10 sessions, each focusing on a different part of the body.

Rubenfeld synergy method– Gentle touch, movement, verbal exchange, and imagination used to access memories and emotions locked in the body. Integrates elements of the Alexander technique, Feldenkrais method, gestalt, and hypnotherapy. Combines bodywork and psychotherapy. May be used for physical or emotional problems or for personal growth.

S

Self-actualization– Fully realizing one's individual human potential.

Self-awareness– Self-conscious state of focusing attention on oneself.

Shaman– Among tribal peoples, a magician, medium, or healer who owes his powers to mystical communion with the spirit world. Characteristically, a shaman goes into autohypnotic trances, during which he contacts spirits. Shamans are found among the Siberians, Eskimos, and Native American tribes and in southeast Asia and Oceania. There is currently also a development of shamanic healers and practitioners in North America. (*See* Spiritual/shamanic healing.)

Shark cartilage– A supplement touted as a cancer treatment. Sharks, whose frames are composed of cartilage, not bone, get cancer infrequently. Proponents of this treatment claim sharks get cancer infrequently because something in their cartilage inhibits the ability of tumors to create the blood supply needed to continue growing. Shark cartilage is also promoted as an immune system stimulant and remedy for joint pain, swelling, and stiffness.

Shiatsu– A form of acupressure used in Japan for over 1000 years to treat pain and illness and for general health maintenance. Practitioners apply finger pressure at specific points on the body in order to stimulate chi, or vital energy. Used to treat stress, circulatory problems, depression, asthma, headaches, diarrhea, and bronchitis.

Sounding the body– A diagnostic and therapeutic technique used in sound healing. Sound healers read a patient's body by singing a series of tones and listening for imbalances in the natural frequencies of the body or its energy fields. Imbalances are said to be indicated by changes in the tone of the healer's voice. To correct a problem, the sound healer applies sound to the patient's body by singing certain tones near the affected organ or by applying tuning forks or electronic vibratory instruments to the body.

Spiritual/shamanic healing– Practitioners who regard themselves as conductors of healing energy or sources from the spiritual realm. Both may call upon spiritual helpers such as power animals, angels, inner teachers, the client's higher self, or other spiritual forces. Both forms of healing can be used for a range of emotional and physical illnesses.

Structural examination/diagnosis– An osteopathic diagnostic technique, it involves a visual, hands-on assessment by an osteopathic physician of the skeleton, joints, muscles, ligaments, and tendons.

Subluxation– In chiropractic, a misalignment of bones within joints said to interfere with the flow of nervous impulses and diminish the body's ability to stay healthy.

T

Teleology– The philosophical belief that natural processes are not determined by mechanism but rather by their utility in an overall natural design.

TENS (transcutaneous electrical nerve stimulation)– Delivery of an electric current through the skin to the nerves. Used in physical therapy and to relieve painful conditions such as neuralgia, sciatica, and arthritis. The low-voltage electric current blocks the nerves' reception of pain signals and possibly stimulates the production of endorphins, the body's pain-killing chemicals.

Therapeutic touch– Practiced by registered nurses and others to relieve pain and stress. Practitioner assesses where a person's energy field is weak and congested, then uses his or her hands to direct energy into the field to balance it.

Therapy– Treatment and care of someone to combat disease, injury, or mental disorder.

Tonic– Herbal remedy made from herbs taken to maintain health or ward off illness, rather than to treat an illness. Also known as a normalizer.

Toning– In sound healing, projection of a nonverbal sound to balance the body's energy fields.

Trager bodywork– Movement education approach that gently rocks, cradles, and moves the client's body. Meant to promote relaxation and increase mobility and mental clarity. Used by athletes for performance enhancement and by people with musculoskeletal and back problems.

V

Vibrational healing/medicine– Promotes healing by balancing the body's energy field. Can include acupuncture, homeopathy, flower essences, sound and color healing, crystals, gems, aromatherapy, and energy-based bodywork. *See* Reiki, Therapeutic touch, and Polarity therapy.

Y

Yin and yang– Positive (sometimes termed female) and negative (sometimes termed male) energies described in Oriental medicine with many attributes accorded to each. They function as interdependent, complementary opposites.

Yoga therapy– Emerging field of practices that use Yoga to address mental and physical problems while integrating body and mind. Practitioners work one-on-one or in a group setting.

Z

Zero balancing– Method for aligning body structure and body energy. Through touch akin to acupressure, practitioner seeks to overcome imbalances in the body's structure/energetic interface, which is said to exist beneath the level of conscious awareness. Often used for stress reduction.

Zone therapy– Another name for reflexology. (*See* Reflexology.)

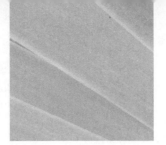

INDEX

A

AAAOM. *See* American Association of Acupuncture and Oriental Medicine (AAAOM)

AANP. *See* American Association of Naturopathic Physicians (AANP)

AATA. *See* American Art Therapy Association, Inc. (AATA)

ABMP, Associated Bodywork and Massage Professionals (ABMP)

Academy for Guided Imagery, 172, 446

ACAOM. *See* Commission for Acupuncture and Oriental Medicine (ACAOM)

Acetylcholine (ACh) biosynthesis, 412

ACh biosynthesis. *See* acetylcholine (ACh) biosynthesis

ACHS. *See* Australasian College of Herbal Studies (ACHS)

ACTH. *See* Adrenocorticotropic hormone (ACTH)

Acupressure, 211, 224–29
  advice to patients, 229
  integrative, 226
  Jin Shin Do bodymind, 226–27
  jin shin jyutsu, 227
  overview of, 224
  practitioners, 224–25
  reflexology, 227–28
  resources, 281–82, 440–44
  shiatsu, 228
  treatment, 225–29
  trigger point/myotherapy, 229

Acupressure Institute, 440

Acupuncture, 71, 269–78
  advice to patients, 275–76
  certification, 272–73
    conditions addressed, 275
    frequently asked questions about, 276
    history of, 271–72
    opioid system and, 475
    overview of, 269–72
    practitioners, 272–73
    research, 276–78, 472–75
    resources, 438–39
    in Taiwan, 474–75
    theories of, 270–71
    treatment, 273–75

Acute viral myocarditis, 478

AD. *See* Alzheimer's disease (AD)

ADA. *See* American Dietetic Association (ADA)

Adrenocorticotropic hormone (ACTH), 385, 389

ADTA. *See* American Dance Therapy Association (ADTA)

Aerobic fitness, 418–20
  intensity of workout, 420
  length of workout, 418–19
  sample programs, 420

AHCPR. *See* U. S. Agency for Health Care Policy and Research (AHCPR)

AK. *See* applied kinesiology (AK)

Alexander, F. Matthius, 191

Alexander technique (AT), 191–92, 208

Alexander Technique International, 441

All-Natural Healthcare Association (ANHA), 154

Allopathic (Western) medicine, 5–6
  history of, 5
  holistic health, 5–6

Alternative medical systems, 71–72
  acupuncture, 71
  naturopathy, 72

Alternative medical systems (*cont.*)
  oriental medicine, 71
  traditional indigenous systems, 72
  unconventional western systems, 72
Alternative Medicine, Expanding Medical Horizons, 65
Alternative therapy. *See* complementary and alternative medicine (CAM)
Altruism, 313
Alzheimer's disease (AD), 269, 468
AMA. *See* American Medical Association (AMA)
American Academy of Environmental Medicine, 446
American Alliance of Aromatherapy, 439
American Art Therapy Association, Inc. (AATA), 164, 166, 187
American Association of Acupuncture and Oriental Medicine (AAAOM), 272
American Association of Homeopathic Pharmacists, 450
American Association of Naturopathic Physicians (AANP), 11, 151, 455
American Association of Oriental Medicine, 438
American Board of Homeotherapeutics, 134–35
American Board of Hypnotherapy, 452
American Board of Pain Medicine (ABPM), 273
American Botanical Council, 447
American Cancer Society, 112
American Chiropractic Association, 444
American College for Advancement in Medicine, 456
American College of Acupuncture and Chinese Medicine, 438
American Dance Therapy Association (ADTA), 193, 203
American Dietetic Association (ADA), 112, 115, 127, 456
American Foundation for Homeopathy, 132
American Foundation of Traditional Chinese Medicine, 438
American Health and Herbs, 53
American Herbalist Guild, 447

American Holistic Health Association, 448
American Holistic Medical Association, 448
American Holistic Nurses Association, 279, 449
American Holistic Veterinary Medical Association, 448
American Institute of Homeopathy, 450–51
American Massage Therapy Association (AMTA), 210, 214, 231, 352, 441
American Medical Association (AMA), 139, 176, 237
American Music Therapy Association (AMTA), 169–70, 188, 455
American Naturopathic Medical Association, 455
American Oriental Bodywork Therapy Association (AOBTA), 224–25, 231, 441
American Polarity Therapy Association, 441
American Preventive Medical Association, 448
American School of Osteopathy, 13
American Society for Clinical Hypnosis, 452
American Society for Clinical Nutrition (ASCN), 127
American Society for the Alexander Technique, 441
American Vegan Society, 459
American Yoga Association, 204–5
AMMA therapy, 278–80
  advice to patients, 280
  nurses certificate program in, 450
  overview of, 278–79
  practitioners, 279
  resources, 282
  training requirements, 279
  treatment, 279–80
AMTA. *See* American Massage Therapy Association (AMTA); American Music Therapy Association (AMTA)
Ancient Greece, healing in, 28
Anger, 386
ANHA. *See* All-Natural Healthcare Association (ANHA)

Animism, 25
Antiaging regimens, 118–19
Antigen-presenting cells (APCs), 410
Antiobiotics, 5, 17–18
Antioxidants, 121–22
AOBTA. *See* American Oriental Bodywork Therapy Association (AOBTA)
APCs. *See* antigen-presenting cells (APCs)
Applied kinesiology (AK), 7, 283
   history, 292
   practitioners, 292
   treatment, 292–93
The Aquarian Conspiracy (Ferguson), 32
Aquatherapy, 283, 284–85
Archetypes, 162
Arnot, Bob, 118
Aromatherapy, 283, 285, 286, 300, 439
Aromatherapy for Health Professionals, 439
Art therapy, 164–68
   expressive therapies, 166
   journaling, 166–67
   modalities, 165
   practitioners, 165–66
   research, 168
   training requirements, 166
   treatment, 166–67
Art Therapy Credentials Board, 166
Asanas, 203–4
Asclepions, 28, 38
Asclepius, 28
ASCN. *See* American Society for Clinical Nutrition (ASCN)
Aspartame, 428
Associated Bodywork and Massage Professionals (ABMP), 214, 231, 442
Association for Applied Psychophysiology and Biofeedback, 440
Association for Transpersonal Psychology, 453, 457
Association of Humanistic Psychology, 453
Association of Vegetarian Dietitians & Nutrition Educators, 459
Asthma, 179, 469
Aston, Judith, 192
Aston Patterning, 192
Astragalus, 428

Astrology, 283, 285
AT. *See* Alexander technique (AT)
Atkins, Robert, 109, 113, 116
Atkins Diet, 113
ATM. *See* awareness through movement (ATM)
Atomistic approach, 29
Attention to detail, healing through, 335–37
Aura fields, 16
Aura-soma color therapy, 287
Auriculotherapy, 274
Australasian College of Herbal Studies (ACHS), 150
Authenticity, 306
Awareness
   barriers to, 371
   creativity and, 372
   in healing, 368–74
   theories of, 369–71
   types of, 369
Awareness through movement (ATM), 194
Ayurvedic Institute, 439
Ayurvedic medicine, 6, 26–27, 76, 439–40

B
Baby boomers, 34–35
Bach, Edward, 10
Back pain, chronic
   hydrotherapy and, 479
   magnets and, 262
   tai chi and, 203
Bailey, Covert, 116
Barbara Brennan healing science, 249
Bastyr University, 11, 149, 150, 151, 455
B cells, 409
Behavioral medicine, 70
Behavioral psychology, stress management and, 400
Bioelectromagnetics, 75
Bio-Electro-Magnetics Institute, 444
Bioenergetics, 249–50
Biofeedback, 250, 440
Biofeedback Certification Institute of America, 440
Biofield medicine, 74–75

Biologically based therapies, 73–74
Biological terrain assessment (BTA 1000), 250
Biotechnology, 52
Birthing pools, 479
Bittman, Barry, 486
Black cohosh, 101
Bland, Jeffrey, 114
Bloodletting, 130
Blood pressure, tai chi and, 200–201
Body-mind centering, 192
Body-mind therapy. *See* mind-body medicine
Body-oriented psychotherapy, 161
Bodywork, 210, 217–22
    Bonnie Prudden myotherapy, 218
    Breema, 218
    craniosacral therapy, 218
    deep-tissue, 218–19
    Hellerwork, 219
    kripalu, 220
    myofascial release, 220
    naprapathy, 220
    neuromuscular therapy, 220–21
    ohashiatsu, 221
    ortho-bionomy, 221
    resources, 440–44
    Rolfing, 219
    Rubenfeld synergy method, 221
    soma neuromuscular integration, 221
    structural integration, 222
    Trager, 222
Bone marrow, 408
Bonnie Prudden myotherapy, 218
Botanical medicine, 100
Breast cancer, 118, 415–17
The Breast Cancer Prevention Diet (Arnot), 118
Breathwork, 283, 287, 291
Breema bodywork, 218
Brennan, Barbara, 249, 250
Bressler, David, 172
British Institute of Homeopathy, 451
Brown, Joy, 52–53
BTA 1000. *See* biological terrain assessment (BTA 1000)
Burn patients, massage and, 470

C

CAM. *See* complementary and/or alternative medicine (CAM)
Canadian Academy of Homeopathy, 134
Canadian College of Naturopathic Medicine (CCNM), 11, 12, 149, 151
Canyon Ranch Health Resort, 86
Caring, 321–22
Carpal tunnel syndrome (CTS), 122, 206–7
Carson, Rachel, 354
Catholic Church, healing and, 28
CBT. *See* cognitive-behavioral therapy (CBT)
CCE. *See* Council on Chiropractic Education (CCE)
CCNH. *See* Clayton College of Natural Health (CCNH)
CCNM. *See* Canadian College of Naturopathic Medicine (CCNM)
Celebration (hospital), 52
Center for Mind/Body Medicine, 453
Center for Natural Medicine and Prevention, 68
Center for the Improvement of Human Functioning, 453
Central nervous system (CNS), 412
Chakras, 27, 204
Chanting, 283, 287–88
Charaka, 295
CHD. *See* coronary heart disease (CHD)
Chelation therapy, 283, 288
Chi, 25, 198, 199, 271–72
Childbirth
    acupuncture for pain relief during, 472
    assistants, 11
    educators, 11
Children
    good eating habits for, 346–47
    obesity in, 346
    reducing television viewing to prevent obesity, 348
China, 25–26, 48
Chinese medicine. *See* traditional Chinese (Oriental) medicine (TCM)
ChiroNet, 48

Chiropractic, 6–7, 234–46
  adjustments, 239–40
  basis of, 235
  cautions, 241–42
  history of, 235
  licensure, 237
  overview of, 234–35
  practitioners, 236–37
  research, 242–44
  resources, 246, 444
  training requirements, 236–37
  treatment, 238–40
Chopra Center for Well-Being, 454
Christianity, healing and, 28–29
Christian Science, 16
Chronic diseases, increase in, 46
Circadian rhythm, 295–96
Circle of human potential, 339
Clayton College of Natural Health
  (CCNH), 150
Client-centered therapy, 370
CNME. *See* Council on Natruropathic
  Medicine Education (CNME);
  Council on Naturopathic Medical
  Education (CNME)
CNS. *See* central nervous system
Cognitive-behavioral therapy (CBT),
  163–64
Colds, stress and, 394
College of Maharishi Ayur-Veda Health
  Center, 440
Colon therapy, 283, 288–91
  hazards, 290
  history of, 289–90
  research, 288–89
Colorado Center for Healing Touch, 444
Commission E, 101–2
Commission for Acupuncture and Orien-
  tal Medicine (ACAOM), 275
Community visits, 58
Compassion, 313–16
Complementary/alternative practice
  (CAP), 87–89
Complementary and alternative medicine
  (CAM)
  classification of practices, 69–76
  costs, 79
  defined, 64
  discussion with clients about, 79–80
  education changes and, 49–50
  effectiveness of, 76–77
  financial factors and, 43–45
  fundamental premises of, 41
  increase in chronic diseases and, 46
  managed care and, 50–51
  medical school courses involving, 49, 50
  nature of, 63–64
  organizations and, 50–51
  overreliance on prescription drugs
    and, 46
  physician referrals and, 47
  practitioner's expertise, 77–78
  projections for future, 57–58
  relationship of healing to, 4
  resources, 437–65
  safety of, 76–77
  service delivery, 78–79
  societal change and, 51–52
  state and regional differences in, 47–49
  strategies for use and practice, 76–80
  surge in, 41–47
  use by individuals with physical disabili-
    ties, 45
  use of, 41–43
*Complementary and Alternative Therapies in
  Nursing* (Snyder and Lindquist), 50
Computers, 53–54
Conditioning, 412–13
Conferences, 465
Consciousness
  awakening, 366–68
  healing and, 365–79
Controlled breathing, 376–77
Coping statements, 399–400
Core energetics, 161–62
Coronary heart disease (CHD), 33,
  117–18, 164
Corporal works of mercy, 28, 29
Council for Responsible Nutrition,
  456–57
Council on Chiropractic Education
  (CCE), 236
Council on Naturopathic Medicine Educa-
  tion (CNME), 11, 149, 151

Counselors, 160
Craniosacral therapy, 218
CTS. *See* carpal tunnel syndrome (CTS)
Culture, characteristics of, 36
Cupping, 275
Curing, healing versus, 21–22
Cystic fribrosis, 469–70

D

Daily ritual, 367–68
Dance/movement therapies, 192–93, 208
Deep-tissue bodywork, 218–19
Dehydroepian drosterone (DHEA), 103,
   429–30
Dendritic cells, 410
Dentistry
   acupuncture in, 473–74
   holistic, 8
Depression, 163
Deqi, 273
DHA. *See* docosahexaenoic acid (DHA)
DHEA. *See* dehydroepian drosterone
   (DHEA)
DHHS. *See* U. S. Department of Health
   and Human Services (DHHS)
Diabetic neuropathy, acupuncture for, 473
Diabetic peripheral neuropathy (DPN),
   262–63
Diamond, Harvey, 116
Diamond, Marilyn, 116
Diet, healthy, 348–50
Dietary Goals for the United States (U. S.
   Senate Select Committee on
   Nutrition and Human Needs), 32
Dietary Supplement Health and Education
   Act, 102
Dietician, 109
Diet therapy. *See* nutrition and special diet
   therapy
Dioscorea, 122
Disease prevention, 72–73, 85
Diseases of adaptation, 387
Docosahexaenoic acid (DHA), 426
The Doctor Dean Edell Show, 53
Doctors Online Radio Network, 53
Dossey, Barbara, 30
Dossey, Larry, 37

Doulas, 11
DPN. *See* diabetic peripheral neuropathy
   (DPN)
Dunbar, Flanders, 31
Dunn, Halpert, 31
Dynamic Learning Center, 456

E

Eastern cultures, healing in, 25–26
Echinacea, 427
Edell, Dean, 53
EDTA. *See* ethylenediaminetetraacetic acid
   (EDTA)
Education, 49–50
   medical schools, 50
   nursing programs, 50
   telemedicine in, 55
Educational kinesiology (Edu-K), 283, 293
Edu-K. *See* educational kinesiology (Edu-
   K)
Effleurage, 215, 216
Electro-acupuncture, 274
ELHILL, 356
Empathy, healing through, 331–35
Encyclopedia of Alternative Medicine classifi-
   cation system, 75
Energy therapies, 16, 247–66
   advice to patients, 261
   history of, 248
   modalities, 249–61
   overview of, 247–48
   practitioners, 248–49
   research, 261–62, 471
   resources, 265–66, 444- 45
Environment
   healing, 354–58
   joint work space, 357–58
   overview of problems, 355–56
   personal space, 357
Environmental Health & Light Research
   Institute, 452
Environmental medicine, 7, 446
EPA. *See* U. S. Environmental Protection
   Agency (EPA)
Eras of medicine, 37–38
Esalen Institute, 458
Essential oils, 285, 286

Ethnic groups, predominant in United States, 35
Ethylenediaminetetraacetic acid (EDTA), 288
Eupsychia Institute, 458
Evening primrose oil *(oenothera biennis),* 108
Exercise, 350, 415–23
  aerobic fitness, 418–20
  beginning a program of, 417–18
  breast cancer and, 415–17
  enjoyment of, 423
  healing through, 419
  immune suppression and, 420, 421, 423
  recovery phase, 420, 421, 423
  swimming, 421
  twenty-minute running plan, 421

F

Faith healing, 15
Family practitioner, 51
FDA. *See* U. S. Food and Drug Administration (FDA)
Feldenkrais, Moshe, 193
Feldenkrais Guild, 442
Feldenkrais method, 193–94
Feng shui, 283, 291
FI. *See* functional integration (FI)
Fiber, 114
Fight-or-flight response, 384–89
Finsen, Niels, 295
Fit for Life (Diamond and Diamond), 116
Fit or Fat? (Bailey), 116
Five C's of Caring, 322
Flax, 425–26
Flower essences, 10, 266, 446
Flower Essence Society, 446
Food
  harmful, 428
  herbs as immune boosting, 425–26
Food guide pyramid, 110, 346
Food Quality Protection Act (FQPA), 356
Forgiveness, 306–9
FQPA. *See* Food Quality Protection Act (FQPA)
Framework Convention on Climate Change, 354

France, 101
Freud, Sigmund, 158, 370
Fruitarians, 111
Functional integration (FI), 194
Functional medicine, 114

G

GAS. *See* general adaptation syndrome (GAS)
General adaptation syndrome (GAS), 31, 387–88, 392
Germany, 48, 101–2
Germ theory, 5
Gestalt therapy, 162, 370
Ginko biloba, 105, 109
Ginseng, 102
Glucosamine sulfate, 154–55
Goodheart, George J., Jr., 292
Government initiatives, 36–37
Granulocytes, 409–10
Gratitude journal, 167
Green tea, 426
Grief, homeopathy and, 484
Group Health Cooperative of South Central Wisconsin, 48
Group visits, 58
Guided imagery, 172–74, 446
Gyrokinetics, 194
Gyrotonics, 194

H

Hahnemann, Samuel, 130–31
Hahnemann College of Homeopathy, 134
Hakomi Institute, 442
Harman, Willis, 365
Healers
  altruism and, 313
  compassion and, 313–16
  forgiveness and, 306–9
  guiding principles, 304–5
  living from place of authenticity, 306
  love and, 309–12
  process of becoming, 303–17
Healing
  ancient Greek and Roman period, 28–29
  in antiquity, 24–29
  in the arts, 52–53

Healing (*cont.*)
  awareness in, 368–74
  baby boomers and, 34–35
  beliefs about, 15–17
  for caregivers, 338–54
  centers, 38–39
  changing demographics and, 34
  computer influence on, 53–54
  in contemporary times, 34–36
  versus curing, 21–22
  defined, 3
  Eastern cultures and, 25–26
  faith, 15
  government initiatives and, 36–37
  Indian cultures and, 26–27
  joining of Eastern and Western philoso-
    phies of, 19–20
  mental, 16
  multicultural impact on, 35–36
  natural, 17–19
  in new millennium, 37–39
  new world view and, 29–33
  philosophies of, 4–15, 467
  primitive cultures and, 24–25
  projections for future, 57–58
  relationship to alternative and comple-
    mentary care, 4
  spirituality and, 378–79
  touch, 250–52, 444–45
Healing attitudes, 318–25
  caring for others as extension of self,
    321–22, 323–25
  humor, 320
  joy and empowerment through service,
    318–21
  joyful disposition, 320–21
  sense of purpose, 322, 325
Healing behaviors, 325–37
  attention to detail, 335–37
  being fully present, 325–28
  empathy, 331–35
  listening, 328–31
Healing room, for in-house staff, 358
Healing Touch International, 445
Health care practitioners
  abbreviations used for state licenses,
    98–99

  broadest national training standards for,
    96–98
  in new millennium, 39
  selecting, 77–78
  in wellness centers, 85–86
Health kinesiology, 283, 293
Health maintenance organizations
  (HMOs), 43
  coverage of alternative care by, 50–51
  reasons for adding alternative care, 44
  types of alternative care offered by, 44
HealthNet, 55
Health promotion, 73, 84–85
Health Science Centers, 55
HealthStyles Radio, 53
Healthwise, 53
Health World Online, 461
Healthy People
  2000, 37
  2010, 36, 37
  background, 36–37
  focus areas and objectives, 37
Heart disease, stress and, 395–96
HeartNet International, 458
Heller, Joseph, 219
Hellerwork, 219
Hellerwork International, 442
Herbalists, 104, 107
Herbal medicine, 7–8, 73, 100–109
  advice to patients, 107
  overview of, 100–103
  practitioners, 103–4
  research, 107–9
  resources, 127–29, 447
  training requirements, 104
  treatment, 104–7
  Web sites, 128–29
Herb Research Foundation, 447
Herbs
  classification of, 8
  healing, 429
  as immune boosting foods, 425–26
  as medicine, 427–28
  quality control, 103
  regulation of, 102–3
  risks and interactions, 106
  standardization of, 102

Heyer, Lucy, 195
High fiber diet, 114
High-level wellness, 31
Hippocrates, 5, 28
HIV. *See* human immunodeficiency virus (HIV)
HMOs. *See* health maintenance organizations (HMOs)
Holism, model of journey to, 305
Holistic Alliance of Professional Practitioners, Entrepreneurs, and Networks, 449
Holistic dentistry, 8
Holistic Dentists Association, 449
Holistic health care, 5–6
  modern movement, 33
  new world view and, 29–33
  nursing, 305–6
  reawakening of, 31
  resources, 448–50
Holistic Nursing Certification Corporation, 449
Holotrophic breathwork, 283, 291
Homeopathic Academy of Naturopathic Physicians, 451
Homeopathic Educational Services, 451
Homeopathic Pharmacopoeia of the United States, 135
Homeopathy, 8–10
  advice to patients, 138–39
  certification, 134
  clinical effects of, 9
  flower essences, 10
  history of, 132
  overview of, 130–32
  versus placebo, 139–40, 141
  practitioners, 133–35
  principles of, 130–31
  regulation of, 132–33
  research, 139–43, 481–84
  resources, 145–46, 450–52
  training requirements, 134–35
  treatment, 135–38
  types of therapy, 136–38
  Web site, 146
Hope, immune system and, 414
Hormones, 122

Horvath, Juliu, 194
Hospitals
  alternative therapy programs in, 48, 87–89
  Internet and, 54
Huang Di Nei Jing (Yellow Emperor's Classic of Internal Medicine), 268, 271
Human Ecology Action League, 446
Human immunodeficiency virus (HIV), 407
Humours, 28
Huxley, Laura, 306
Hydrotherapy, 283, 285, 479–81
Hypertension, tai chi for, 19–20
Hypnosis, 17, 176–80
  characteristics of, 176
  overview of, 176
  past-life regression therapies, 177
  patients' questions about, 178
  practitioners, 176–77
  research, 179–80
  resources, 452
  routine endoscopy and, 180
  smoking cessation and, 179–80
  therapeutic, 370–71
  treatment, 177

I

Illness care, 85
Illness dialogue journal, 167
IMA. *See* International Massage Association (IMA)
Imagery, 171–75
  guided, 172–74, 446
  history of, 172
  mindful eating, 174
  neurolinguistic programming, 174–75
  nurses certificate program in, 450
  overview of, 171–72
  practitioners, 172
  rebirthing, 175
  research, 175
  senses and, 414
  treatment, 173–75
Immune system, 406–31
  cells of, 408–10
  conditioned response, 412–13

Immune system (*cont.*)
exercise and, 415–23
fuel for, 428–30
hope and, 414
imbalance in, 430
immune response, 410
as internal army, 407
joy and, 414
learning and, 412–14
malnutrition and, 430–31
memory and, 412–14
neuropeptides, 411–12
nutrition and, 423–31
optimism and, 414–15
organs of, 408
psychedelic drugs and, 413–14
stress and, 411–12, 431
therapeutic touch and, 471
vigorous exercise and suppression of,
420, 421, 423
Indian cultures, healing in, 26–27
Integrative medicine, 82–90
budgetary considerations, 90
business aspects of, 89–90
continuing education in, 86–87
existing hospital practice implications,
87–89
factors influencing development of,
82–83
focus of care, 84–85
model centers of, 83–84
projections for future, 90
International and American Associations of
Clinical Nutritionists, 459
International Association of Yoga
Therapists, 461
International Chiropractors Association,
444
International Foundation for Homeopathy,
134
International Institute of Reflexology, 443
International Massage Association (IMA),
214, 443
International Medical and Dental
Hypnotherapy Association, 452
International Society for Orthomolecular
Medicine, 457

Internet
cautions, 464–65
commercial health Web sites, 463–65
herbal medicine resources, 128–29
hospitals and, 54
libraries, 461
online health services, 56
Internet Public Library, 461
Ipriflavone, 123
Iridology, 283, 291
Iridology: The Diagnosis (Lahn), 291
Isoflavones, 112, 113, 121

J
Jaundice, 297–98
Jensen, Bernard, 291
Jin Shin Do bodymind acupressure, 226
Jin shin jyutsu, 227
Johns Hopkins Gazette, 53
Journaling, 166–67
Joy
as healing attitude, 318–21
immune system and, 414
Jukebox Radio, 53
Jung, Carl, 158, 162

K
Kava, 101
Kinesiology, 283, 292–95
advice to patients, 293
applied, 7, 283, 292–93
educational, 283, 293
health, 283, 293
research, 293–95
Koop, C. Everett, 54
Krieger, Delores, 248
Kripalu bodywork, 220
Kripalu yoga, 205–6
Kunz, Dora, 248

L
Lactovegetarians, 111
Lahn, Henry, 291
Legumes, 121
Library of Congress, 461
Life Sciences Institute of Mind/Body
Health, 454

Lifestyle, 72–73
Lifestyle Heart Trial study, 117–18
Light therapy, 283, 295–98
  at home, 297
  jaundice in newborns, 297–98
  resources, 452
  seasonal affective disorder, 295–96
Ling, Per Henrik, 212, 213
Listening
  healing through, 328–31
  skills checklist, 332
Love, 309–12
Lower urinary tract infection (UTI), 472
Lucid dreaming, 14
Lymph nodes, 408

M

Macrobiotics, 110, 111
Macrophages, 410, 428
Magnet therapy, 43, 252–56
  criticism of, 255
  precautions, 254
  rationales for, 253–56
  recommendations for, 253
  treatment, 253
Maharishi AyurVed, 6
Maharishi Mahesh Yogi, 6
Managed-care organizations (MCOs),
  47–48
Manipulative and body-based systems, 74
Mantra, 204
Marino Foundation for Integrative Medicine, 485–86
Massage therapy, 211, 212–23
  advice to patients, 222, 353–54
  bodywork, 217–22
  classification of movements, 216
  growth of, 213
  history of, 212–13
  infant, 217
  medical conditions helped by, 352
  neonates and, 223
  overview of, 212–13
  phlebitis and, 353
  physiological benefits of, 217
  practitioners, 214
  regulation, 214

  research, 223, 353, 469–70
  resources, 440–44
  as self-care, 352–54
  sleep and, 223
  sports, 352
  Swedish, 212, 215, 352
  therapeutic backrubs, 213
  treatment, 214–17
MBWC. *See* Mind Body Wellness Center
  (MBWC)
MCOs. *See* managed-care organizations
  (MCOs)
M.D. Anderson Cancer Center, 55
Medical schools, 50
Meditation, 180–85
  behavioral aspects of, 375
  behavioral modification and, 376
  eight-step program for, 377
  elements of, 375
  focusing, 182
  forms of, 180–81
  history of, 181
  menopausal symptoms and, 184
  mindfulness, 182
  modern medicine and, 374–75
  practice of, 181
  practitioners, 181
  process of, 374
  relaxation response, 182–83
  research, 183–85
  transcendental, 68, 183
MEDLINE
  alternative medicine journals in,
    462–63
  searching, 462
Melatonin, 122, 296
Mental therapies, 15, 453, 467
Mentgen, Janet, 250
Meridians, 25, 26, 198, 272, 273
Mesmer, Franz Anton, 252
Mesmerism, 16, 252
Metaphysical/mental healing, 16
Microfee-for-service, 58
Micronutrients, 120
Midwifery, 10–11
Mind/Body Health Sciences, 460
Mind/Body Medical Institute, 449, 454

Mind-body medicine, 70–71
  art therapy, 164–68
  hypnosis, 176–80
  imagery, 171–75
  meditation, 180–85
  methods, 70
  modalities, 70
  music therapy, 168–71
  psychotherapy, 158–64
  religion and spirituality, 70, 71
  resources, 187–88, 453–55
  social and contextual areas, 70
  subcategories of, 70
  systems, 70
Mind Body Wellness Center (MBWC),
      486–88
  client visits, 487
  facts about, 486–87
  number of programs offered, 487
  special events associated with,
      487–88
Mind cures, 15
Mindful living, 366–67
Mobility. *See* posture and mobility
      modalities
Mother Teresa, 320
Movement therapies, 190–96
  advice to patients, 196
  Alexander technique, 191–92
  Aston Patterning, 192
  body-mind centering, 192
  dance/movement therapies, 192–93
  Feldenkrais method, 193–94
  Gyrotonics, 194
  Pilates method, 194–95
  practitioners, 191
  research, 196
  resources, 208–9
  Rosen method, 195
Moxibustion, 274–75
MRFIT. *See* Multiple Risk Factor Inter-
      vention Trial (MRFIT)
MT. *See* music therapy (MT)
Mucor, 155
Multiple Risk Factor Intervention Trial
      (MRFIT), 33
Muscle testing, 107

Music therapy (MT), 168–71
  history of, 169–70
  overview of, 168–70
  practice location and music's effect, 171
  practitioners, 170
  research, 170–71, 468
  resources, 455
  treatment, 170
Myofascial release, 220

N

NAAMT. *See* North America Academy for
      Magnetic Therapy (NAAMT)
NAHA. *See* National Association for
      Holistic Aromatherapy (NAHA)
Naprapathy, 220
National Acupuncture and Oriental
      Medicine Alliance, 438
National Association for Holistic
      Aromatherapy (NAHA), 300, 439
National Board of Chiropractic Examiners
      (NBCE), 237
National Center for Complementary and
      Alternative Medicine (NCCAM),
      65–66, 68. *See also* Office of Com-
      plementary and Alternative Medicine
      (OAM)
  budget of, 66
  classification system, 69–75
  history of, 65
  mission of, 66
  purpose of, 66
  Web site, 461
National Center for Homeopathy, 132,
      134, 451
National Center for Nutrition and Diet-
      etics (NCND), 115, 127
National Certification Board for Thera-
      peutic Massage and Bodywork
      (NCBTMB), 214, 232
National College of Naturopathic
      Medicine (NCNM), 11, 150, 151
National Commission for the Certifi-
      cation of Acupuncturists (NCCA),
      272
National Council Against Health Fraud
      (NCAHF), 289

National Council of Acupuncture Schools and Colleges (NCASC), 272
National Guild of Hypnotists (NGH), 177, 178, 452
National Institutes of Health (NIH), 64, 65
National Music Therapy Registry (NMTR), 170
National Public Radio (NPR), 53
Natural healing, 17
    for headache, 18
    resurgence of, 17–19
Natural killer (NK) cells, 381, 409, 428
Natural Woman Institute, 461
Naturopathic medicine, 11–12, 72, 76
    accredited institutions, 11
    advice to patients, 153–54
    history of, 147–48
    licensure requirements, 151
    overview of, 147–48
    practitioners, 12, 149–51
    principles of, 148
    regulation, 151
    research, 154–55
    resources, 156–57, 455–56
    schools of, 149–50
    training requirements, 149–50
    treatment, 151–53
    typical clinical practice modalities, 152–53
    Web site, 157
Naturopaths, 104, 107, 114
NBCE. See National Board of Chiropractic Examiners (NBCE)
NCAHF. See National Council Against Health Fraud (NCAHF)
NCBTMB. See National Certification Board for Therapeutic Massage and Bodywork (NCBTMB)
NCCA. See National Commission for the Certification of Acupuncturists (NCCA)
NCCAM. See National Center for Complementary and Alternative Medicine (NCCAM)
NCND. See National Center for Nutrition and Dietetics (NCND)

NCNM. See National College of Naturopathic Medicine (NCNM)
NDE. See near-death experience (NDE)
Near-death experience (NDE), 14
Neurofeedback, 256
Neurolinguistic programming, 174–75, 456
Neuromuscular therapy, 220–21
New England Female Medical College, 132
A New Perspective on the Health of Canadians (LaLonde), 32
NGH. See National Guild of Hypnotists (NGH)
NHPA. See Nurse Healers Professional Associates (NHPA)
Nightingale, Florence, 5, 30
Nightingale Institute for Health and the Environment, 450
NK cells. See natural killer (NK) cells
NLM. See U. S. National Library of Medicine (NLM)
NLP Comprehensive, 456
NMTR. See National Music Therapy Registry (NMTR)
Noise, 355–56
North America Academy for Magnetic Therapy (NAAMT), 256
North American Society of Acupuncture and Alternative Medicine, 273
North American Society of Teachers of the Alexander Technique, 443
North American Vegetarian Society, 460
Northrup, Christiane, 105
Notes on Nursing (Nightingale), 30
NPR. See National Public Radio (NPR)
Nurse Healers Professional Associates, 445
Nurse Healers Professional Associates (NHPA), 259
Nurse practitioner, 51
Nurses
    herbal medicine and, 103–4
    holistic, 305–6, 449–50
    modern holistic health movement and, 33
Nurses' Health Study, 118
Nursing programs, 50

Nutritional supplements, 119–23
  advice to patients, 121
  overview, 119–21
  practitioners, 121
  research, 121–23
Nutrition and special diet therapy, 73,
    109–19
  advice to patients, 115–17
  basic plan, 424–25
  cautions, 430
  optimum diet, 116–17
  overview, 110–14
  practitioners, 114–15
  research, 117–19
  resources, 127, 456–57
  treatment, 115
Nutritionists, 114

O

OAM. *See* Office of Complementary and
    Alternative Medicine (OAM)
Obesity, 344–46
  childhood, 346
  underlying causes of, 346
Office of Complementary and Alternative
    Medicine (OAM), 64–69, 237, 462.
    See also National Center for Comple-
    mentary and Alternative Medicine
    (NCCAM)
  budget of, 66
  Evaluation Program, 69
  functional areas, 67
  history of, 65
  mission of, 66
  programs, 66–67
  purpose of, 66
  research centers, 68
  Research Database Program, 68–69
  sponsored research, 67–68
Ohashiatsu, 221
Olive oil, 349
Omega Institute for Holistic Studies,
    458–59
OOBE. *See* out-of-body experience
    (OOBE)
Opioid system, acupuncture and, 475

Optimism, immune system and, 414–15
Optimum diet, 116–17
Orbisiconography, 26
Oriental medicine. *See* Traditional Chinese
    medicine (TCM)
Ornish, Dean, 109, 113, 116
Ornish Diet, 113
Ortho-bionomy, 221
Osteoarthritis, 261
Osteopathic medicine, 13
Osteoporosis, 123
Out-of-body experience (OOBE), 14
Ovolactovegetarians, 111

P

Pain management, 164, 179
Palmer, David Daniel, 6, 235
Parkinson's disease, 468
Pathwork, 162
Pavek, Richard, 158
Penicillin, 17–18
Perls, Frederick S., 370
Personal health coach, 58
Personal space, 357
Pesticides, 356
Pet therapy, 283, 298
Pharmacists, 84
Phillips Publishing, 460
Phlebitis, 353
Phoenix rising yoga therapy, 205
Physicians
  herbal medicine and, 103–4
  referrals by, 47
Phytoestrogens, 120–21
Phytomedicine, 100
Phytotherapy, 73, 100
Pilates, Joseph H., 194
Polarity therapy, 256–57
Polymorphonuclear (PMN) leukocytes,
    409–10
Population demographics, 83
Posture and mobility modalities, 189–209
  movement therapies, 190–96
  resources, 208–9
  tai chi, 196–203
  yoga, 27, 203–7

PPO. *See* preferred provider organization (PPO)
Preferred provider organization (PPO), 48, 51
Prescription drugs
  abuse of, 46
  overreliance on, 46
Presence, healing through, 326–28
President's Initiative on Race, 36
Pressure point therapy, 352
Pressure ulcers, hydrotherapy and, 480
Primitive cultures, healing in, 24–25
Pritikin, Nathan, 109
Pritikin Diet, 113
Psychedelic drugs, immune system and, 413–14
Psychodynamic theory, 370
Psychosynthesis, 370
Psychosynthesis International, 459
Psychotherapists
  degrees held by, 159, 160
  licensed, 159–60
Psychotherapy, 158–64
  advice to patients, 162–63
  body-oriented, 161
  core energetics, 161–62
  gestalt, 162
  group, 161
  one-to-one, 161
  pathwork, 162
  practitioners, 159–60
  training requirements, 159–60
  treatment, 160–61

Q

Qi. *See* chi
Qigong, 198, 199–200, 457
Qigong Institute, 457

R

Radio, 52–53
Ramey, David, 255
Rapid eye technology (RET), 283, 298
Rebirthing, 175
Reflexology, 227–28
Reiki, 257–58, 445

Reiki Alliance, 445
Relaxation response, 182–83
Relaxation techniques, 350–51
  deep breathing, 350
  eye breaks, 351
  music, 351
  naps, 351
  stretch breaks, 351
  water, 351
Religion, 70, 71
Religious groups, predominant in United States, 35
Rheumatoid arthritis, 284, 478
Ritual, daily, 367–68
RMPA. *See* Rosen Method Professional Association (RMPA)
Robert Jaffe advanced healing energy, 258
Rogers, Carl, 370
Rolf, Ida, 192, 219
Rolfing, 192, 219
Rolf Institute, 443
Rosen, Marion, 195
Rosen method, 195
Rosen Method Professional Association (RMPA), 195, 209, 443
Rossmean, Martin, 172
Rubenfeld, Ilana, 221
Rubenfeld Synergy Center, 445
Rubenfeld synergy method, 221
Running, twenty-minute plan for, 421

S

Safety, of alternative therapies, 76–77
Saw palmetto *(serenoa repens)*, 108
Schaub, Bonney, 172
Schaub, Richard, 172
Schlesinger, Laura, 52–53
The Science and Practice of Iridology (Jensen), 291
Scientific Revolution, 29
SCNM. *See* Southwest College of Naturopathic Medicine (SCNM)
Scott, Jimmy, 293
Sears, Barry, 109, 113, 116
Seasonal affective disorder (SAD), 295–96
Seeds and Bridges, 450

Selective serotonin reuptake inhibitor (SSRI), 105
Self-care, 338–54
  assessment, 339–42
  basic approaches for, 343–54
  children's eating habits, 346–47
  chronic disease and, 343
  components of healthy diet, 348–50
  exercise, 350
  healthy digestion, 348
  obesity, 344–46
  personal options to stay fit, 342–43
  relaxation techniques, 350–51
Self-medication, 103
Selye, Hans, 31, 387–88
SEN. *See* Spiritual Emergence Network (SEN)
Sense of purpose, as healing attitude, 322, 325
Shamanism, 13–14
Shen Nung, 271
SHEN therapy, 258
Shiatsu, 228
Siegel, Bernie, 488
Sinarteriology, 26
Skin disease, stress and, 394–95
Smith, Timothy, 118
Smoking cessation, 179–80
Smuts, Jan, 30
Social workers, 160
Society for Light Treatment & Biological Rhythms, 452
Society of Teachers of the Alexander Technique (STAT), 192
Sohn, Tina, 278
Soma neuromuscular integration, 221
Sound therapy. *See* music therapy (MT)
Southwest College of Naturopathic Medicine (SCNM), 11, 150, 151
Soy foods, 112–13
Sperry, Roger, 365
Spiritual Emergence Network (SEN), 459
Spiritualism, 16
Spirituality, healing and, 71, 258, 378–79, 457–59
Spleen, 408

Sports massage, 352
SSRI. *See* selective serotonin reuptake inhibitor (SSRI)
St. John's wort, 105
STAT. *See* Society of Teachers of the Alexander Technique (STAT)
Sterile technique, 5
Still, Andrew Taylor, 13
Stream-of-consciousness morning journal, 167
Stress, 381–403
  behavioral psychology and, 400
  capacity, 399
  changes in body under, 390–91
  changing anxiety to concern, 398
  colds and, 394
  coping statements, 399–400
  coping with, 402–3
  defined, 382–83
  determining levels of, 384
  effect of negative, 389
  exercise and, 401–2
  factors contributing to, 383–84
  fight-or-flight response, 384–89
  heart disease and, 395–96
  illness and, 385–87, 392–96
  immunity and, 393–94, 411–12, 431
  management, 396–400
  meditation and, 395, 396
  skin disease and, 394–95
  spiral, 391
  tolerance to, 398–99
  types of stressors, 390
  weak links and, 387
Stress Reduction and Relaxation Program, 454–55
Structural integration, 222
Sugar, 428
Sulfa, 148
Support groups, 465
Swedish massage, 212, 215, 352
Swimming, 421

T

TAC-TIC therapy. *See* touching and caressing, tender in caring (TAC-TIC) therapy

Tai chi, 196–203
  advice to patients, 200–201
  effects on blood pressure, 200
  history of, 197
  for hypertension, 19–20
  practice of, 198
  practitioners, 198
  research, 200–203, 478
  for stress reduction, 401–2
Taiwan, acupuncture utilization in,
    474–75
Taoism, 198
T cells, 408–9
TCM. *See* traditional Chinese medicine
    (TCM)
Technology, 52
Telematics, 52
Telemedicine, 55–57
  cautions, 57
  consumer use, 56–57
  in education, 55
  for providers, 55–56
  Web sites, 56
Television, association with obesity, 348
Teologic approach, 33
Therapeutic hypnosis, 370–71
Therapeutic touch, 259–61
  practitioners, 259
  recommendations for, 260
  research, 471
  treatment, 259–61
Thich Nhat Hanh, 366
Thymus, 408
TM. *See* transcendental meditation
    (TM)
Tornatis, Alfred, 287
Touching and caressing, tender in caring
    (TAC-TIC) therapy, 217
Touch therapies, 210–33, 469
  acupressure, 211, 224–29
  bodywork, 210, 217–22
  effects, 210
  massage therapy, 211, 212–23
  modalities, 211
  resources, 230–33
Tough love, 310–12
Tower Handle Unit, 194

Toxicology Data Network (TOXNET),
    356
TOXNET. *See* Toxicology Data Network
    (TOXNET)
Traditional Chinese medicine (TCM),
    14–15, 25–26, 71, 76
  Alzheimer's disease and, 269
  history of, 267–68
  research, 476–78
  resources, 281–82, 438–39
Trager, Milton, 222
Trager bodywork, 222
Trager Institute, 443
Transcendental meditation (TM), 68, 183
Trigger point/myotherapy, 229

U
U. S. Agency for Health Care Policy and
    Research (AHCPR), 242–43
U. S. Department of Agriculture (USDA),
    346
U. S. Department of Health and Human
    Services (DHHS), 65
U. S. Environmental Protection Agency
    (EPA), 356
U. S. Food and Drug Administration
    (FDA), 66–67, 132–33
U. S. National Library of Medicine
    (NLM), 77, 461, 462–63
UHDs. *See* ultrahigh dilutions (UHDs)
Ultrahigh dilutions (UHDs), 141–42,
    482–83
Unconventional therapy. *See* comple-
    mentary and alternative medicine
    (CAM)
UNEP. *See* United Nations Environment
    Program (UNEP)
United Nations Environment Program
    (UNEP), 354
University of Arizona Program in Integra-
    tive Medicine, 485
University of Texas Medical Branch
    (UTMB), 55
Upledger Institute, 444
Urology, 477
USDA. *See* U. S. Department of Agricul-
    ture (USDA)

UTI. *See* lower urinary tract infection (UTI)
UTMB. *See* University of Texas Medical Branch

V
Vedic system. *See* Ayurvedic medicine
Vegan Action, 460
Vegans, 111
Vegetarian Education Network, 460
Vegetarianism, 111–12
    categories of, 111
    resources, 459–60
Vegetarian Resource Group, 460
Vermillion, Ryan, 255
VidiMedix, 55–56
Virtual clinics, 56
Vitamins, 121–22
Vitex agnus-castus (chasteberry), 101, 108–9

W
Wall, Vicki, 287
Walt Disney Company, 52
Warts, 140
Washington State, as model for alternative therapy insurance coverage, 47
Weil, Andrew, 109, 114, 116
Wellness
    centers, 84, 85–86
    paradigm, 31–33

Westbrook University, 150
Western medicine. *See* allopathic (Western) medicine
Western States Training Associates, 456
Whirlpool therapy, 480–81
WHO. *See* World Health Organization (WHO)
Whole foods, 349–50
Women's health, 460–61
World Health Organization (WHO), 226

Y
Yin and yang, 14–15, 25, 198, 269–70
Yoga, 27, 203–7
    advice to patients, 206
    common forms of, 204
    kripalu, 205–6
    lipid profiles and, 207
    phoenix rising, 205
    practitioners, 204–5
    research, 206–7
    resources, 209, 461
    techniques, 205

Z
Zone diet, 113–14
The Zone (Sears), 116